Basic, Advanced, and Robotic Laparoscopic Surgery

FEMALE PELVIC SURGERY VIDEO ATLAS SERIES

Series Editor:

Mickey Karram, MD
Director of Urogynecology
The Christ Hospital
Clinical Professor of Obstetrics and Gynecology
University of Cincinnati
Cincinnati, Ohio

Other Volumes in the Female Pelvic Surgery Video Atlas Series

Hysterectomy for Benign Disease
Mark D. Walters & Matthew D. Barber, Editors

Management of Acute Obstetric Emergencies
Baha M. Sibai, Editor

Pelvic Organ Prolapse
Mickey Karram & Christopher Maher, Editors

Posterior Pelvic Floor Abnormalities
Tracy Hull, Editor

Urinary Incontinence
Roger Dmochowski & Mickey Karram, Editors

Urologic Surgery for the Gynecologist and Urogynecologist
John B. Gebhart, Editor

Vaginal Surgery for the Urologist
Victor Nitti, Editor

FEMALE PELVIC SURGERY VIDEO ATLAS SERIES
Mickey Karram, Series Editor

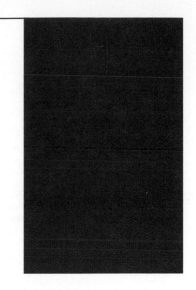

Basic, Advanced, and Robotic Laparoscopic Surgery

Tommaso Falcone, MD, FRCSC, FACOG
Professor and Chair
Obstetrics and Gynecology & Women's Health Institute
Vice Chair, Office of Professional Staff Affairs
Cleveland Clinic
Cleveland, Ohio

Jeffrey M. Goldberg, MD
Professor and Section Head
Reproductive Endocrinology and Infertility
Department of Obstetrics and Gynecology
Cleveland Clinic
Cleveland, Ohio

Illustrated by **Joe Chovan, Milford, Ohio**

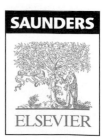

SAUNDERS

ELSEVIER

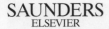

SAUNDERS
ELSEVIER

1600 John F. Kennedy Blvd.
Ste 1800
Philadelphia, PA 19103-2899

BASIC, ADVANCED, AND ROBOTIC LAPAROSCOPIC SURGERY   ISBN: 978-1-4160-6264-6

Library of Congress Cataloging-in-Publication Data (in PHL)

Basic, advanced, and robotic laparoscopic surgery / [edited by] Tommaso Falcone, Jeffrey M. Goldberg ; illustrated by Joe Chovan. – 1st ed.
    p. ; cm.
  Includes bibliographical references.
  ISBN 978-1-4160-6264-6
  1. Laparoscopic surgery.   I. Falcone, Tommaso.   II. Goldberg, Jeffrey M.
  [DNLM: 1. Genital Diseases, Female–surgery.   2. Gynecologic Surgical Procedures–methods.   3. Laparoscopy–methods.   4. Robotics–methods.   5. Surgery, Computer-Assisted–methods.   WP 660 B3105 2010]
  RD33.53.B37 2010
  618.1′059–dc22

2010007298

Acquisitions Editor: Rebecca S. Gaertner
Development Editor: Arlene Chappelle
Publishing Services Manager: Anitha Raj
Project Manager: Mahalakshmi Nithyanand
Design Direction: Louis Forgione

Printed in Canada
Last digit is the print number: 9 8 7 6 5 4 3 2

Contributors

Marjan Attaran, MD
Department of Obstetrics and Gynecology, Cleveland Clinic, Cleveland, Ohio
Laparoscopic Surgery for Mullerian Anomalies, Incompetent Cervix, and Ovarian Transposition

Mohamed A. Bedaiwy, MD, PhD
Associate Professor, Department of Obstetrics and Gynecology, Assiut School of Medicine, Assiut, Egypt, Clinical Fellow, Department of Obstetrics and Gynecology, University Hospitals Case Medical Center, Case Western Reserve University Cleveland, Ohio
Laparoscopic Surgery for Mullerian Anomalies, Incompetent Cervix, and Ovarian Transposition

Andrew Brill, MD
Director, Minimally Invasive gynecology, Reparative Pelvic Surgery, and Surgical Education, California Pacific Medical Center, San Francisco, California
Instrumentation and Energy Sources Utilized During Laparoscopic Procedures

Chi Chiung Grace Chen, MD
Assistant Professor, Department of Gynecology and Obstetrics, Johns Hopkins Bayview Medical Center, Baltimore, Maryland
Complications of Laparoscopic Surgery

Gouri B. Diwadkar, MD
Fellow, Female Pelvic Medicine and Reconstructive Surgery, Department of Obstetrics and Gynecology, Obstetrics, Gynecology, and Women's Health Institute, Cleveland Clinic, Cleveland, Ohio
RoboticSurgery

Richard D. Drake, MD
Department of Obstetrics and Gynecology, Cleveland Clinic, Cleveland, Ohio
Laparoscopic Management of Adnexal Masses

Richard L. Drake, PhD
College of Medicine, Cleveland Clinic Main Campus, Cleveland, Ohio
Abdominal Wall and Pelvic Anatomy for Laparoscopists

Pedro Escobar, MD
Department of Obstetrics and Gynecology, Cleveland Clinic, Cleveland, Ohio
Laparoscopic and Robotic Advances in Gynecologic Malignancies

Tommaso Falcone, MD
Profressor and Chair, Obstetrics and Gynecology & Women's Health Institute, Vice Chair, Office of Professional Staff Affairs, and Department of Obstetrics and Gynecology, Cleveland Clinic, Cleveland, Ohio
Abdominal Wall and Pelvic Anatomy for Laparoscopists; Laparoscopic Management of Adnexal Masses; Indications and Techniques for Laparoscopic Myomectomy; Indications and Techniques for Total and Subtotal Laparoscopic Hysterectomy; Laparoscopic Surgery for Mullerian Anomalies, Incompetent Cervix, and Ovarian Transposition; Indications and Techniques for Laparoscopic Management of Pelvic Endometriosis; Robotic Surgery; Complications of Laparoscopic Surgery

Amanda Nickles Fader, MD
Director of GYN Robotic Surgery, Greater Baltimore Medical Center (GBMC); Assistant Professor, Gynecologic Oncology, Johns Hopkins Medical Institutions, Baltimore, Maryland
Laparoscopic and Robotic Advances in Gynecologic Malignancies

Jeffrey M. Fowler, MD
Division of Gynecologic Oncology, Department of Obstetrics and Gynecology, Ohio State University College of Medicine, Columbus, Ohio
Laparoscopic and Robotic Advances in Gynecologic Malignancies

Jeffrey M. Goldberg, MD
Professor and Section Head, Reproductive Endocrinology and Infertility, Department of Obstetrics and Gynecology, Cleveland Clinic, Cleveland, Ohio
Indications and Contraindications for Laparoscopy; Instrumentation and Energy Sources Utilized During Laparoscopic Procedures; Indications and Techniques for Laparoscopic Myomectomy; Laparoscopic Tubal Surgery; Indications and Techniques for Laparoscopic Management of Pelvic Endometriosis; Laparoscopic Treatment of Pelvic Pain; Complications of Laparoscopic Surgery

William W. Hurd, MD
Division Chief, Reproductive Endocrinology and Infertility, Department of Obstetrics and Gynecology, University Hospitals Case Medical Center, Cleveland, Ohio
Abdominal Wall and Pelvic Anatomy for Laparoscopists

Sarah Kane, MD
Department of Obstetrics and Gynecology, MetroHealth Medical Center, Cleveland, Ohio
Techniques for Laparoscopic Suturing

Amy J. Park, MD
Director of Benign Gynecology, Section of Female Pelvic Medicine and Reconstructive Surgery, Washington Hospital Center; Assistant Professor, Departments of Obstetrics/Gynecology and Urology, Georgetown University School of Medicine, Washington, DC
Indications and Techniques for Laparoscopic Management of Pelvic Endometriosis

Minita S. Patel, MD
Division of Urogynecology, Hartford Hospital, Hartford, Connecticut
Trocar Insertion—Choosing the Appropriate Position and Techniques for Placement

We would like to acknowledge our residents and fellows who assist with the care of our patients. It is gratifying to know that they will use what we have taught them to benefit their own patients as well as the patients of the trainees that they will in turn teach. We want to thank our very understanding and supportive families for allowing us to spend the many hours on evenings and weekends away from them in order to complete this project and other time consuming professional endeavors.

Beri M. Ridgeway, MD
Female Pelvic Medicine and Reconstructive Surgery, Department of Obstetrics and Gynecology, Obstetrics, Gynecology, and Women's Health Institute, Cleveland Clinic, Cleveland, Ohio
Indications and Techniques for Total and Subtotal Laparoscopic Hysterectomy

Leigh G. Seamon, DO
Assistant Professor, Gynecologic Oncology, Markey Cancer Center, University of Kentucky College of Medicine, 331 E Whitney-Hendrickson Building, 800 Rose Street, Lexington, Kentucky
Laparoscopic and Robotic Advances in Gynecologic Malignancies

Kevin J. Stepp, MD
Assistant Professor, Case Western Reserve University, Cleveland, Ohio; Section Head, Urogynecology and Pelvic Reconstructive Surgery, Carolinas Medical Center, Charlotte, North Carolina
Techniques for Laparoscopic Suturing

Paul K. Tulikangas, MD, FACOG, FACS
Assistant Professor, Division of Urogynecology, Hartford Hospital/University of Connecticut, Hartford, Connecticut
Trocar Insertion—Choosing the Appropriate Position and Techniques for Placement

Devorah R. Wieder, MD, MPH
Associate Staff, Center for Specialized Womens Health, Obstetrics, Gynecology, and Women's Health Institute, Cleveland Clinic, Cleveland, Ohio
Indications and Techniques for Laparoscopic Myomectomy

Video Contributors

Floor J. Backes, MD
Clinical Instructor, Department of Obstetrics and Gynecology, Ohio State University College of Medicine, Columbus, Ohio
Video: *Robotic Radical Hysterectomy for Cervical and Endometrial Carcinomas*

Stephanie L. Cogan, MD
St. Louis Urological Surgeons, Chesterfield, Missouri
Video: *Laparoscopic Myomectomy for a Pedunculated Fibroid; Laparoscopic Supracervical Hysterectomy*

David E. Cohn, MD
Associate Professor, Department of Obstetrics and Gynecology, Ohio State University College of Medicine, Columbus, Ohio
Video: *Appropriate Steps for Setting Up the Robot; Robotic Hysterectomy and Lymphadenectomy for Endometrial Carcinoma*

Anna Frick, MD
Obstetrics, Gynecology and Women's Health Institute, Cleveland Clinic, Cleveland, Ohio
Video: *Diagnostic Laparoscopy; Laparoscopic Trocar Placement*

A. Marcus Gustilo-Ashby, MD
Department of Obstetrics and Gynecology, Cleveland Clinic, Cleveland, Ohio
Video: *Principles and Techniques of Laparoscopic Suturing; Laparoscopic Lateral Ovarian Transposition*

Jason D. Hurt, MD
Division of Gynecologic Oncology, Department of Obstetrics and Gynecology, Ohio State University College of Medicine, Columbus, Ohio
Video: *Robotic Hysterectomy and Lymphadenectomy for Endometrial Carcinoma*

Lynda Jayjohn, RN
Nurse Manager, Ohio State University Medical Center, Columbus, Ohio
Video: *Appropriate Steps for Setting Up the Robot*

Cathy Jenson
Video: *Appropriate Steps for Setting Up the Robot*

Justin Juliano, MD
Department of Radiation Oncology, Cleveland Clinic, Cleveland, Ohio
Video: *Laparoscopic Lateral Ovarian Transposition*

Keri Lee
Surgical Technologist, Ohio State University Medical Center, Columbus, Ohio
Video: *Appropriate Steps for Setting Up the Robot*

Harout Margossian, MD
NY Urogynecology, Brooklyn, New York
Video: *Pelvic Anatomy by Laparoscopy; Laparoscopic Management of Endometriosis Overlying the Ureter; Laparoscopic Management of Endometriosis Involving the Internal Iliac Artery; Laparoscopic Management of Cul-de-Sac Prior to Hysterectomy in a Patient with Stage 4 Endometriosis; Laparoscopic Management of Deep Rectosigmoid Endometriosis*

Tristi W. Muir, MD
Director, Division of Female Pelvic Medicine and Reconstructive Surgery, University of Texas Medical Branch, Galveston, Texas
Video: *Laparoscopic Transabdominal Cerclage in a Patient with a Bicornuate Uterus*

Edward Nickerson
Support Analyst, Robotic Surgery Program, Ohio State University Medical Center, Columbus, Ohio
Video: *Appropriate Steps for Setting Up the Robot; Robotic Hysterectomy and Lymphadenectomy for Endometrial Carcinoma*

Marie Fidela R. Paraiso, MD
Section Head, Center of Urogynecology and Reconstructive Pelvic Surgery; Co-Director, Female Pelvic Medicine and Reconstructive SSurgery; Director of Pelvic Floor Disorders Center, Lakewood Hospital; Assistant Professor of Surgery, Department of Obstetrics and Gynecology, Obstetrics, Gynecology, and Women's Health Institute, Cleveland Clinic, Cleveland, Ohio
Video: *Principles and Techniques of Laparoscopic Suturing; Laparoscopic Management of Adnexal Masses; Laparoscopic Transabdominal Cerclage in a Patient with a Bicornuate Uterus*

Debra L. Richardson, MD
Department of Obstetrics and Gynecology, Southwestern Medical Center, Dallas, Texas
Video: *Appropriate Steps for Setting Up the Robot; Robotic Hysterectomy and Lymphadenectomy for Endometrial Carcinoma*

Anthony J. Senagore, MD
Spectrum Health System, Grand Rapids, Michigan
Video: *Laparoscopic Management of Deep Rectosigmoid Endometriosis*

Andrew I. Sokol, MD
Associate Director of Minimally Invasive Surgery, Washington Hospital Center, Washington, DC
Video: *Laparoscopic Management of an Ovarian Remnant; Laparoscopic Myomectomy of Large Intramural Fibroids; Criteria for Planning Optimal Myometrial Incision During Laparoscopic Myomectomy*

Susan Valmadre, MB,BS
Division of Obstetrics and Gynaecology, The Mater Hospital, Sydney, NSW, Australia
Video: *Appropriate Steps for Setting Up the Robot*

Mark D. Walters, MD
Professor and Vice Chair of Gynecology, Department of Obstetrics and Gynecology, Obstetrics, Gynecology, and Women's Health Institute, Cleveland Clinic, Cleveland, Ohio
Video: *Pelvic Anatomy by Laparoscopy*

James L. Whiteside, MD
Assistant Professor, Dartmouth-Hitchcock Medical Center, Dartmouth Medical School, Lebanon, New Hampshire
Video: *Laparoscopic Management of Adnexal Masses; Laparoscopic Management of an Ovarian Remnant*

Preface

"See one, do one, teach one" is the old adage for learning clinical procedures. As many surgeons tend to be visual learners, seeing better should improve the acquisition of new skills. This book further enhances the visual experience by including videos of the procedures in addition to static color images. The book has chapters that demonstrate the most important basic concepts of laparoscopy such as anatomy, instrumentation, and principles of laparoscopic suturing. Most chapters have an organ- or disease-based approach. The only instrument-based approach is the chapter on robotics. In the future, robotics may simply be incorporated as an option for any surgical procedure. It is our hope that this book and accompanying videos will facilitate the attainment of the knowledge and skills required to perform these procedures because the patients will ultimately reap the rewards of a minimally invasive surgical approach.

Tommaso Falcone, MD, FRCSC, FACOG
Jeffrey M. Goldberg, MD

Contents

Abdominal Wall and Pelvic Anatomy for Laparoscopists

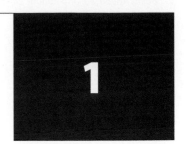

1

Tommaso Falcone M.D.
Richard L. Drake Ph.D.
William W. Hurd M.D.

Video Clips on DVD

1-1 Pelvic Anatomy by Laparoscopy
(13 minutes/23 seconds)

Introduction

The objective of reproductive surgery is to treat gynecologic conditions using the procedures and techniques least likely to compromise fertility. The primary goal is to restore normal anatomy whenever possible. In order to optimize outcomes and minimize complications, every reproductive surgeon requires a thorough knowledge of abdominal wall and pelvic anatomy. This chapter will review practical surgical anatomy of the anterior abdominal wall and pelvis important to gynecologists, with special emphasis on the laparoscopic approach.

Anterior Abdominal Wall

The abdominal wall is made up of four structural layers beneath the skin: (1) subcutaneous tissue (superficial fascia), (2) muscles and transversalis fascia, (3) deep fascia of the rectus sheath and the extraperitoneal fascia, and (4) parietal peritoneum (Figure 1-1). Interspersed among these layers are several important nerves and blood vessels.

Subcutaneous Tissue

The layer collectively referred to by most surgeons as "subcutaneous" tissue (superficial fascia) is actually made up of a superficial fatty layer (Camper's fascia) and a deep membranous layer (Scarpa's fascia). These connective tissue layers contain the superficial abdominal wall vessels, and are the most common site of postoperative wound infections.

Muscles and Transversalis Fascia

The abdominal wall is made up of five pairs of muscles. In the midline, the **rectus abdominis** muscles extend along the whole length of the front of the abdomen from the xiphoid process and costal cartilages of the fifth through seventh ribs to the pubic crest and symphysis. This broad strap muscle is divided into four segments by three

Figure 1-1. Muscle groups of the anterior abdominal wall; the superficial inguinal ring with the critical structures.

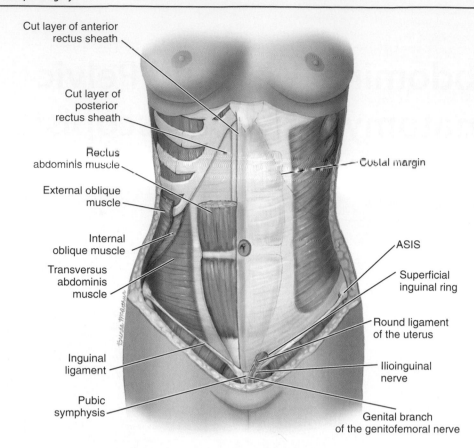

fibrous intersections attached to the anterior, but not the posterior rectus sheath (Figure 1-2). This allows the inferior (deep) epigastric vessels to pass along the posterior surface of the muscle without encountering a barrier.

The **pyramidalis** muscle is a small triangular muscle that lies in front of the rectus abdominis muscle at the lower part of the abdomen and is contained within its fascial sheath. It arises from the front of the pubis and the anterior pubic ligament bilaterally and inserts into the linea alba, between the umbilicus and pubis. This muscle is commonly absent on one or both sides.

There are three sets of lateral muscles. The **external oblique** muscle is the most external and arises from the lower eight ribs. The fibers run anteriorly and inferiorly ending in an aponeurosis that extends anteriorly to the midline. An **aponeurosis** is a fibrous membrane resembling a flattened tendon that binds muscles to each other or to bone. Beneath the external oblique, the **internal oblique** muscle arises from the lumbar fascia, the iliac crest, and the lateral two thirds of the inguinal ligament, and runs anteriorly and superiorly ending in an aponeurosis. The most internal of the lateral muscles is the **transversus abdominis.** It arises from the lateral third of the inguinal ligament, from the anterior three fourths of the iliac crest, from the costal cartilages of the sixth through eighth ribs (interdigitating with the diaphragm), and from the lumbodorsal fascia, and ends anteriorly as an aponeurosis. Deep to the transversus abdominis muscle is the transversalis fascia, a continuous layer of specialized investing fascia that lines the abdominal cavity and continues into the pelvic cavity.

Deep Fascia of the Rectus Sheath and Extraperitoneal Fascia

The rectus abdominis muscle is enclosed anteriorly and posteriorly by fascia known as the **rectus sheath**. This sheath is formed from fusion of the aponeuroses of all three lateral abdominal muscles. These aponeuroses fuse lateral to the rectus abdominis muscles as the **linea semilunares**, and again in the midline as the **linea alba**, which

Figure 1-2. The external oblique aponeurosis has been cut on the left side exposing the two nerve bundles.

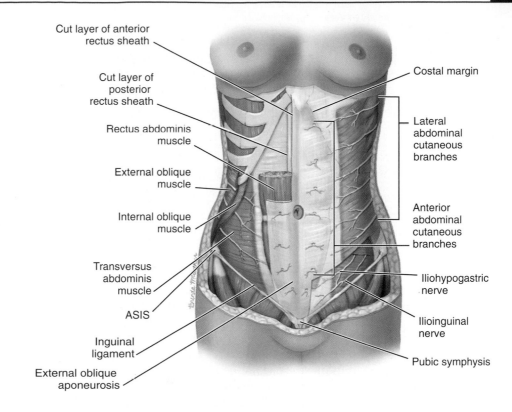

Cut layer of anterior rectus sheath

Cut layer of posterior rectus sheath

Rectus abdominis muscle

External oblique muscle

Internal oblique muscle

Transversus abdominis muscle

ASIS

Inguinal ligament

External oblique aponeurosis

Costal margin

Lateral abdominal cutaneous branches

Anterior abdominal cutaneous branches

Iliohypogastric nerve

Ilioinguinal nerve

Pubic symphysis

extends from the xiphoid process to the pubic symphysis. The **arcuate line** is a transverse line midway between the umbilicus and pubic symphysis. Above this line, the aponeuroses of the lateral muscles split to enclose the rectus abdominis muscles both anteriorly and posteriorly; below this line, these aponeuroses all pass anterior to the rectus abdominis muscles. Inferiorly, the aponeurosis of the external oblique attaches to the anterior superior iliac spine (ASIS) and the pubic tubercle, forming the **inguinal ligament**.

The inguinal canal is about 4 cm long and runs parallel to the inguinal ligament. The inguinal canal has an anterior wall formed by the aponeurosis of the external oblique, an inferior wall (floor) formed by the inguinal ligament, a superior wall (roof) formed by arching fibers of the internal oblique and transversus abdominis muscles, and a posterior wall formed by the transversalis fascia. A defect, or more precisely a tubular evagination, of the transversalis fascia forms the deep (internal) inguinal ring through which the round ligament enters the inguinal canal. This ring lies midway between the ASIS and the pubic symphysis. Medial to the deep (internal) inguinal ring are the inferior epigastric vessels. The opening of the aponeurosis of the external oblique superior to the pubic tubercle is the superficial (external) inguinal ring. Through it the round ligament, the terminal part of the ilioinguinal nerve, and the genital branch of the genitofemoral nerve exit the inguinal canal (see Figure 1-1).

Deep to the transversalis fascia and the rectus sheath is the extraperitoneal fascia, a layer of connective tissue that separates the transversalis fascia from the parietal peritoneum. This layer contains a varying amount of fat, lines the abdominal cavity, and is continuous with a similar layer lining the pelvic cavity. Viscera in the extraperitoneal fascia are referred to as being retroperitoneal.

Parietal Peritoneum

The parietal peritoneum is a one-cell-thick membrane that lines the abdominal cavity and in certain places reflects inward to form a double layer of peritoneum called mesentery.

Nerves

There are four categories of nerves that supply the anterior abdominal wall, each of which contains both motor and sensory fibers. The **thoracoabdominal nerves** originate from T7 through T11, travel anteroinferiorly between the internal oblique and transversus abdominis muscles, and have the following distribution:

- T7-T9 – superior to the umbilicus
- T10 – at level of umbilicus
- T11 – inferior to umbilicus

The **subcostal nerves** originate from T12 and travel anteroinferiorly between the internal oblique and transversus abdominis muscles to innervate the abdominal wall inferior to the umbilicus.

The iliohypogastric nerve and ilioinguinal nerve both originate from L1. Like the thoracoabdominal and subcostal nerves, these nerves begin their course anteroinferiorly between the internal oblique and transversus abdominis muscles. However, at the anterior superior iliac spine (ASIS), they both pierce the internal oblique muscle to travel between the internal and external oblique muscles (see Figure 1-2). The iliohypogastric nerve innervates the abdominal wall lateral and inferior to the umbilicus. The ilioinguinal nerve enters the inguinal canal and emerges from the superficial (external) inguinal ring and is sensory to the labia majora, inner thigh, and groin.

These nerves are particularly at risk in lower abdominal incisions, which are the commonest causes of abdominal wall pain as a result of nerve entrapment by suture or scar tissue. For this reason, knowledge of the course of the ilioinguinal and iliohypogastric nerves in the anterior abdominal wall can help avoid their injury during laparotomy and laparoscopic surgery. Data from cadaveric studies suggest that injury to these nerves can be minimized during laparoscopy by making transverse skin incisions and by placing laparoscopic trocars at or above the level of the ASIS. In cases of chronic abdominal pain caused by these nerves, an injection of local anesthetic at a site approximately 3 cm medial to the ASIS will often provide relief.

Blood Vessels

The major vessels in the anterior abdominal wall can be divided into deep and superficial vessels. The superficial vessels include the **superficial epigastric** and the **superficial circumflex iliac** vessels (Figure 1-3). These vessels are branches of the femoral artery and vein. They course bilaterally through the subcutaneous tissue (superficial fascia) of the abdominal wall, branching as they proceed toward the head of the patient.

To avoid vessel injuries, these superficial vessels can often be seen prior to secondary laparoscopic port placement by transillumination of the abdominal wall using the intra-abdominal laparoscopic light source. Injury to these vessels during trocar placement can result in a palpable hematoma that will be found to be located anterior to the fascia on CT scan. In unusual cases, the hematoma can dissect down into the labia majora.

The deep vessels consist of the **inferior epigastric** artery and vein, which are also bilateral. These vessels originate from the external iliac artery and vein and course along the peritoneum until they dive deeply into the rectus abdominis muscles midway between the pubic symphysis and the umbilicus (Figure 1-4). The inferior epigastric vessels are the lateral border of an inguinal triangle known as Hesselbach triangle. This triangle is bound medially by the rectus abdominis muscle and inferiorly by the inguinal ligament.

The course of the inferior epigastric vessels can often be visualized at laparoscopy as the lateral umbilical fold because of the absence of the posterior rectus sheath below the arcuate line. Injury to these vessels can result in life-threatening hemorrhage that must be quickly controlled by occluding the lacerated vessels with electrosurgery or precisely-placed sutures.

If these vessels cannot be visualized (usually because of excess tissue), trocars should be placed approximately 8 cm lateral to the midline and 8 cm above the sym-

Figure 1-3. The superficial vessels are branches of the femoral artery.

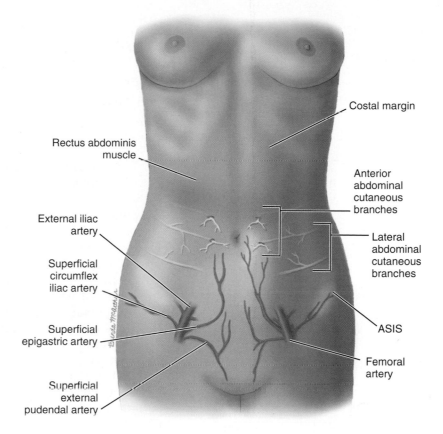

Costal margin

Rectus abdominis muscle

Anterior abdominal cutaneous branches

External iliac artery

Lateral abdominal cutaneous branches

Superficial circumflex iliac artery

Superficial epigastric artery

ASIS

Femoral artery

Superficial external pudendal artery

Figure 1-4. The inferior epigastric artery courses medially towards the rectus muscle. The round ligament courses from the uterus to the deep inguinal ring lateral to the inferior epigastric vessels.

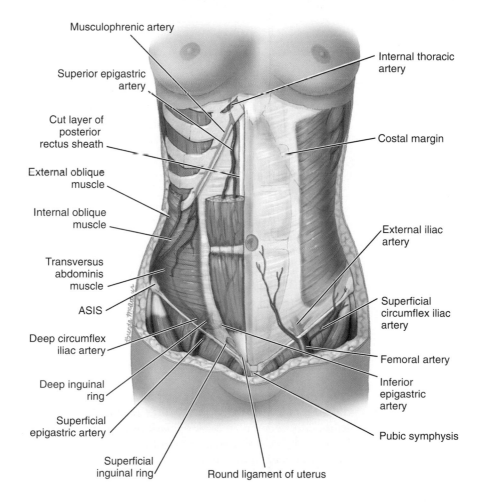

Musculophrenic artery

Superior epigastric artery

Internal thoracic artery

Cut layer of posterior rectus sheath

Costal margin

External oblique muscle

Internal oblique muscle

External iliac artery

Transversus abdominis muscle

ASIS

Superficial circumflex iliac artery

Deep circumflex iliac artery

Femoral artery

Deep inguinal ring

Inferior epigastric artery

Superficial epigastric artery

Pubic symphysis

Superficial inguinal ring

Round ligament of uterus

Figure 1-5. The relative anatomy of the abdominal wall vessels and nerves relative to the trocar sites (marked with *circles*). The trocars at the level of the umbilicus are placed with advanced laparoscopic surgery.

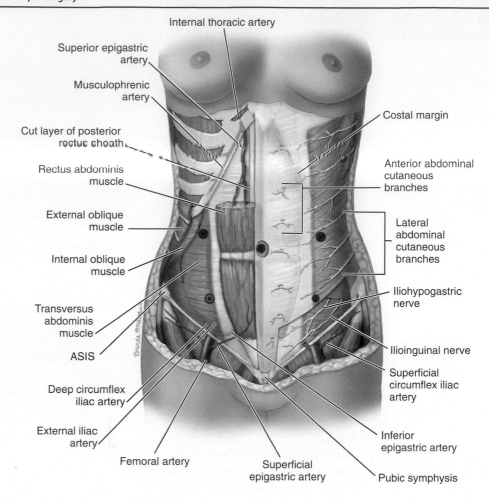

physis. On the right side of the abdomen, this point approximates "McBurney point," located at one third the distance from the ASIS to the umbilicus. The corresponding point on the left is sometimes referred to as "Hurd point" (Figure 1-5).

Peritoneal Landmarks

Several useful landmarks can often guide the laparoscopic surgeon so as to avoid injury to important retroperitoneal structures. Two midline and two bilateral pairs of **peritoneal folds** can usually be seen on the anterior abdominal wall at laparoscopy. The **falciform ligament**, which is the remnant of the ventral mesentery and contains the obliterated umbilical vein in its free edge, can be seen in the midline above the umbilicus extending to the liver. The **median umbilical fold**, which contains the urachus, can usually be seen in the midline below the umbilicus extending to the bladder. Although the urachus normally closes before birth, it should be avoided during secondary trocar placement both because it can be difficult to penetrate, and because in rare cases, it can remain patent to the bladder.

On each side of the urachus lie the **medial umbilical folds**. These landmarks contain the obliterated umbilical arteries, and extend from the umbilicus to the anterior division of the internal iliac artery (Figure 1-6). Lateral to these, the **lateral umbilical folds** can be seen in 82% of patients. These are the most important structures to the laparoscopists, because they contain the inferior epigastric vessels; knowing their location can avoid injury to these large vessels during placement of secondary laparoscopic ports.

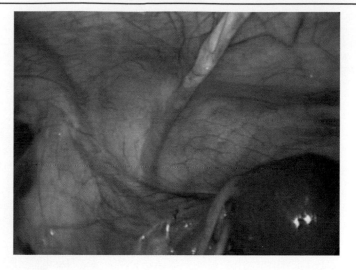

Figure 1-6. This figure demonstrates the left round ligament entering the deep inguinal ring. Medial to this is the lateral umbilical fold, which contains the inferior epigastric vessels, and the medial umbilical fold, which contains the obliterated umbilical artery.

Peritoneal pouches normally exist between the pelvic organs. The **vesicouterine pouch** is located anteriorly between the uterus and bladder. The ventral margin of the bladder can be visualized in approximately half of the patients behind the anterior abdominal wall peritoneum, and is important for secondary trocar placement especially after previous abdominal surgery. The dorsal bladder margin can often be visualized on the anterior uterus and is used as a landmark for dissections during hysterectomy.

The **rectouterine pouch (pouch of Douglas)** is located between the anterior surface of the rectum and the posterior surface of the vagina, cervix, and uterus. Endometriosis often involves the rectouterine pouch, and in severe cases, completely obliterates it. Inferiorly, an extraperitoneal fascial plane called the **rectovaginal septum** extends from the rectouterine pouch to the perineal body. It lies between the posterior wall of the vagina and the anterior wall of the rectum, and when involved with endometriosis, can be felt on pelvic exam as nodularity.

Upper Abdomen

In the past, the reproductive surgeon had little need to understand the anatomy of the upper abdomen. However, for laparoscopists who utilize the "left upper quadrant" primary trocar placement for laparoscopy, an understanding of the anatomy of this area becomes important.

For the left upper quadrant technique, the Veress needle and primary trocar are placed into the abdomen 2 cm below the subcostal arch, at the midclavicular line. It is important to know what anatomic structures lie close to this area to avoid injury during insertion of the primary cannula. The anatomic structures at risk of injury in this area include (from closest to furthest to the entry point) the stomach, the left lobe of the liver, the pancreas, the aorta, the spleen, the inferior vena cava, and the left kidney. The splenic flexure of the colon has a variable distance from the entry point. Although relatively few injuries using the left upper quadrant approach have been reported, it appears that the colon may be the organ at greatest risk of injury when using this technique (Figure 1-7).

Posterior Abdominal Wall and Pelvic Sidewalls

Structures of the posterior abdominal wall anterior to the vertebral column and the pelvic sidewalls are of interest to the reproductive surgeon for several reasons. First, retroperitoneal dissection can be required in these areas during some gynecologic procedures such as treatment of deep endometriosis and removal of pelvic masses

Figure 1-7. This figure shows the branches of the external iliac artery. The relationship of the left upper quadrant trocar at the left costal margin with the regional anatomy is shown.

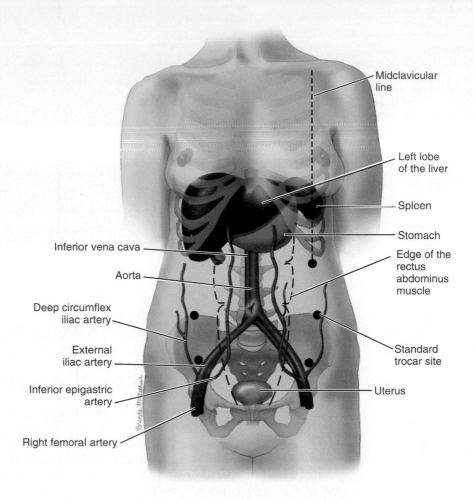

Midclavicular line

Left lobe of the liver

Spleen

Stomach

Edge of the rectus abdominus muscle

Inferior vena cava

Aorta

Deep circumflex iliac artery

External iliac artery

Inferior epigastric artery

Right femoral artery

Standard trocar site

Uterus

adherent to the peritoneum. Second, an understanding of the course of retroperitoneal nerves is a useful reminder to the surgeon to be aware of the position of self-retaining retractor blades during laparotomy, because permanent nerve injury can result from prolonged pressure on these structures. Finally, with the use of closed techniques for primary laparoscopic trocar placement, injury to the retroperitoneal structures can occur and knowledge of this anatomy is essential for effective and expedient management.

Like the anterior abdominal wall, the posterior abdominal wall and pelvic sidewalls contain multiple, well-defined muscles. Other important structures include several large nerves and blood vessels and the ureters.

Muscles

There are several muscles of importance in the posterior abdominal wall lateral to the vertebral column that can be seen lateral to the pelvic inlet. The **diaphragm** forms the roof of the abdomen and extends down to form the most superior aspect of the posterior abdominal wall. The **psoas major** muscle runs longitudinally from the transverse processes of the upper lumbar vertebrae to the lesser trochanter of the femur, and makes up a large part of the posterior and medial wall. The tendon of the **psoas minor** muscle can be seen anterior to the psoas major during dissection near the external iliac vessels. The **quadratus lumborum** muscle runs lateral and posterior to the psoas major from the transverse process of lumbar vertebrae and ribs to the iliac crest. The **iliacus** muscle spans the iliac fossa. Finally, the **piriformis** muscle begins on the anterior surface of the sacrum and passes through the greater sciatic foramen to attach to the greater trochanter of the femur. It lies immediately beneath the internal iliac vessels.

Nerves

Multiple nerves enter or trasverse the pelvic sidewalls. Deep nerves of the pelvis, such as the **superior and inferior gluteal** nerves, supply several of the pelvic muscles but are not visible during reproductive surgery. Likewise, the **obturator** nerve traverses the pelvis. The obturator nerve originates at spinal cord levels L2 through L4 and descends in the psoas major muscle until the pelvic brim where it emerges medially to lie on the obturator internus muscle lateral to the internal iliac artery and its branches (Figure 1-8). It descends on the obturator internus muscle to enter the obturator canal and exits in the thigh. It is sensory to the medial side of the thigh and motor to the muscles in the medial compartment of the thigh (the adductor muscles). It can easily be seen during pelvic sidewall dissections for endometriosis or lymph node dissection.

The genitofemoral nerve (from spinal cord levels L1 and 2) lies on the anterior surface of the psoas major muscle (Figure 1-9). It has two branches, the femoral and genital nerves. The femoral branch enters the thigh under the inguinal ligament and the genital branch enters the inguinal canal. The genitofemoral nerve is sensory to the skin over the anterior surface of the thigh. Injury to this nerve is seen after appendectomy or when the fold of peritoneum from the sigmoid colon to the psoas major muscle is incised.

The **femoral** nerve (spinal cord levels L2 through L4) is not usually seen during pelvic surgery, but may be injured by compression at laparotomy. It is a branch of the lumbar plexus and descends within the substance of psoas major muscle, emerging at its lower lateral border. The nerve continues between the psoas and iliacus muscles and then passes posterior to the inguinal ligament to supply the skin of the anterior thigh region as well as the muscles in the anterior compartment of the thigh (Figure 1-10). Pressure on the psoas major muscle for prolonged periods may cause temporary or permanent damage to the femoral nerve. For this reason, caution must be taken when using self-retaining retractors to make certain that the lateral blades do not put pressure on the pelvic sidewalls.

Figure 1-8. The course of the obturator nerve on the obturator internus muscle into the obturator foramen is demonstrated.

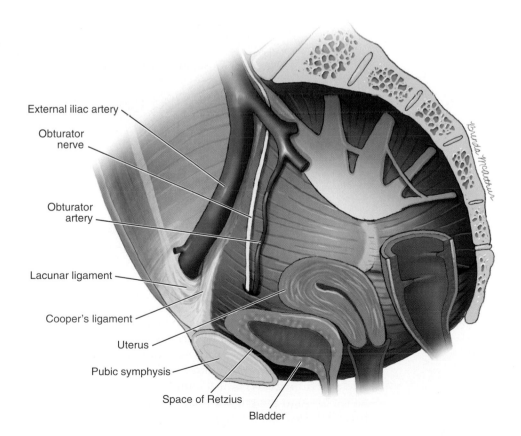

External iliac artery

Obturator nerve

Obturator artery

Lacunar ligament

Cooper's ligament

Uterus

Pubic symphysis

Space of Retzius

Bladder

Figure 1-9. This figure shows the genitofemoral nerve as it branches on the psoas muscle. The genital branch enters the inguinal canal and exits the superficial inguinal ring.

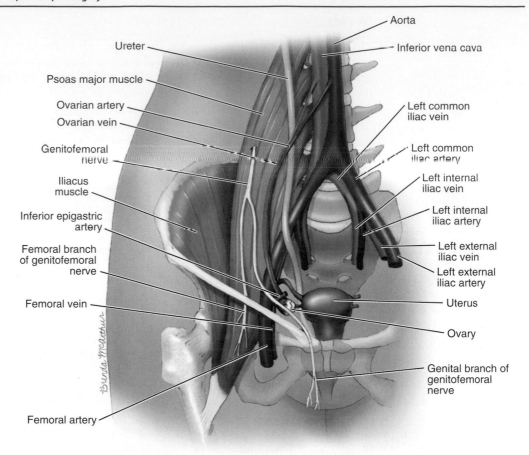

Figure 1-10. The contents of the inguinal canal are demonstrated. Note the course of the femoral nerve under the inguinal ligament.

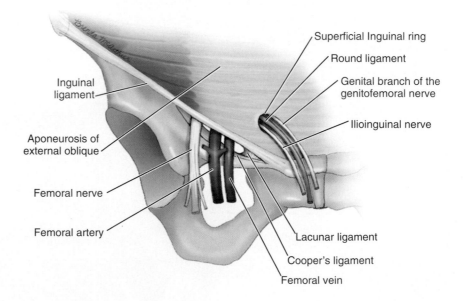

The **sacral and coccygeal nerve plexuses** are located anterior to the piriformis muscle beneath the branches of the internal iliac artery. The most important nerves in this area are the sciatic and pudendal nerves. The **sciatic** nerve (from spinal cord levels L4 through S3) lies anterior to the piriformis muscle and exits the pelvic cavity through the greater sciatic foramen, inferior to the muscle. Anterior to the sciatic nerve are many branches of the internal iliac artery. The **pudendal** nerve (from spinal cord levels S2 through S4) is also found anterior to the piriformis muscle and exits the pelvic cavity through the greater sciatic foramen, inferior to the piriformis muscle. It courses around the sacrospinous ligament and ischial spine, re-enters the lesser sciatic foramen, and continues into the perineum. Endometriosis may involve the sciatic nerve at this level and cause a pain syndrome related to the course of this nerve.

Blood Vessels

The major blood vessels are perhaps the most important structures of the pelvis. Successful pelvic surgery requires a thorough understanding of their anatomy. The **aorta** bifurcates at the level of L4 into the left and right common iliac arteries (Figure 1-11). The **common iliac artery** passes laterally, anterior to the common iliac vein to the pelvic brim. At the lower border of L5, the common iliac artery divides into internal and external iliac branches. The **external iliac artery** gives off only two branches, the inferior epigastric artery and the deep circumflex iliac artery, and then becomes the femoral artery, after passing under the inguinal ligament, which is the primary blood supply to the lower limb. (Figure 1-12)

The **internal iliac artery** supplies all of the organs within the pelvis and sends branches out through the greater sciatic foramen to supply the gluteal muscles. A branch also exits through the greater sciatic foramen and re-enters the lesser sciatic foramen to supply the perineum. After passing over the pelvic brim, the internal iliac arteries divide into anterior and posterior trunks. The **posterior trunk** consists of three branches: the iliolumbar, lateral sacral, and superior gluteal arteries. These vessels are closely related to the nerve plexus on the piriformis muscle (Figure 1-13A). The superior gluteal artery is the largest branch of the internal iliac artery and supplies the muscles and skin of the gluteal region. Accidental occlusion of this artery during uterine fibroid embolization can result in necrosis of the gluteal region.

The **anterior trunk** of the internal iliac artery has several branches that are routinely seen during laparoscopic surgery. The **obliterated umbilical artery** is a fibrous band seen on the anterior abdominal wall as the medial umbilical fold, and can be traced back to its junction with the internal iliac artery (see Figure 1-13a). At this point, the **uterine artery** can be identified as it arises from the medial surface of the internal

Figure 1-11. In thin women, the bifurcation of the aorta is approximately at the level of the umbilicus.

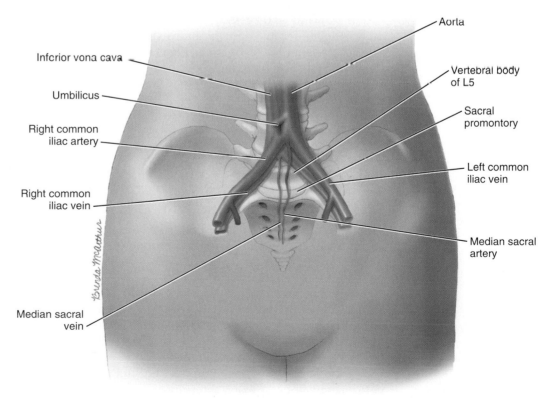

Aorta

Inferior vena cava

Vertebral body of L5

Umbilicus

Sacral promontory

Right common iliac artery

Left common iliac vein

Right common iliac vein

Median sacral artery

Median sacral vein

Figure 1-12. The round
ligament courses around the
inferior epigastric vessels to
enter the deep inguinal ring.

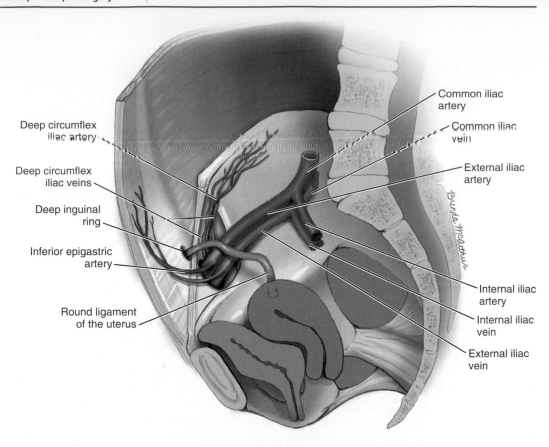

iliac. The **superior vesical artery** also arises near this point and courses medially and inferiorly to supply the superior aspect of the bladder and the distal ureter.

The **uterine artery** is of particular importance to the reproductive surgeon. After the umbilical artery emerges from the anterior trunk of the internal iliac arteries, the uterine artery runs parallel to the ureter and then crosses over it, at the level of the uterine cervix, in the base of the broad ligament (Figure 1-13B).

The **vaginal artery** most commonly originates from the uterine artery, but may arise independently from the internal iliac artery. The uterine, vaginal, and ovarian arteries anastomose with each other, with branches of the internal pudendal artery, and with the corresponding contralateral arteries.

The other important branches of the anterior trunk of the internal iliac artery are the **obturator artery**, which courses laterally and anteriorly towards the obturator canal, and the **middle rectal, internal pudendal,** and **inferior gluteal arteries**. The inferior gluteal artery is the largest branch of the anterior trunk.

Ureters

The ureters measure approximately 25 to 30 cm from kidney to bladder, and are occasionally duplicated on one or both sides for all or part of this course. Their abdominal segment lies behind the parietal peritoneum on the medial part of the psoas major muscle and crosses the common iliac vessels at the level of their bifurcation at the pelvic brim (Figure 1-14).

The pelvic segment of the ureter runs down the lateral wall of the pelvic cavity, along the anterior border of the greater sciatic notch, immediately beneath the parietal peritoneum. Here the ureters form the posterior boundary of the ovarian fossae. They then run medial and forward between the two layers of the broad ligaments. It is here that the ureters run parallel to the uterine arteries for about 2.5 cm before crossing under the arteries and ascending on the lateral aspects of the uterine cervix and upper part of the vagina to reach the bladder (see Figure 1-13A).

Figure 1-13. A, The pelvic side wall arteries and nerves are demonstrated. Note that the umbilical artery and the uterine artery invariably emerge from the anterior trunk of the internal iliac artery as a common artery and then branch off. The uterine artery courses laterally to the ureter until the level of the uterus where it crosses over the ureter to ascend the uterus. **B,** This is the left pelvic side wall with the peritoneum removed. The most lateral structure is the obturator nerve. The left ureter is the most medial structure. In between is a common trunk that bifurcates into the umbilical artery and the uterine artery. The umbilical artery courses toward the anterior abdominal wall. The uterine artery courses laterally to the ureter until the level of the uterus where it crosses over the ureter to ascend the uterus.

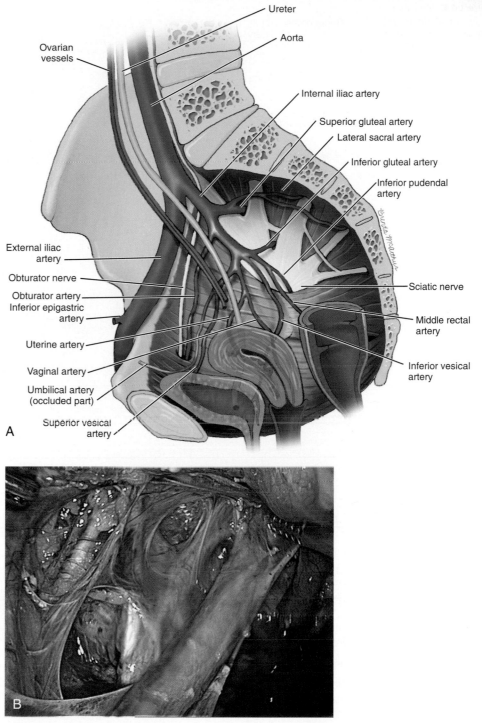

The average distance between the ureters and cervix is more than 2 cm. However, the reproductive surgeon should remember that this distance can be less than 0.5 cm in approximately 10% of women, which partially explains the relatively common occurrence of ureteral injury during hysterectomy.

Upon reaching the base of the bladder, the ureters run obliquely through the wall for about 2 cm and open by slit-like orifices at the angles of the trigone. When the bladder is distended during cystoscopy, these orifices are about 5 cm apart. When the bladder is emptied, this distance decreases by 50%.

Figure 1-14. The course of the ureter from the kidney to the bladder. Note the left ovarian vein enters the renal vein.

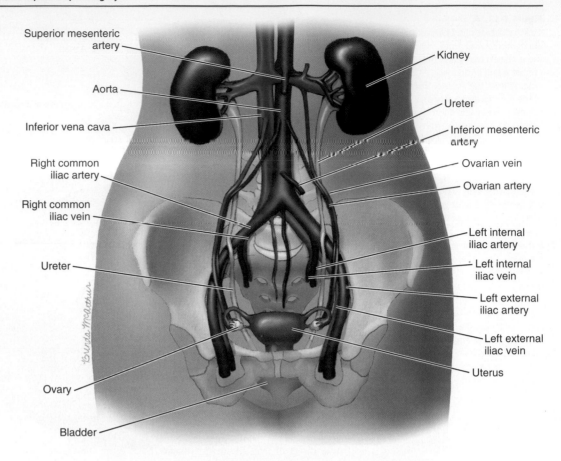

Superior mesenteric artery

Aorta

Inferior vena cava

Right common iliac artery

Right common iliac vein

Ureter

Ovary

Bladder

Kidney

Ureter

Inferior mesenteric artery

Ovarian vein

Ovarian artery

Left internal iliac artery

Left internal iliac vein

Left external iliac artery

Left external iliac vein

Uterus

Muscles of the Pelvic Floor

The pelvic floor consists of two closely related muscle layers: the **pelvic diaphragm** and the **deep perineal pouch.** Damage to these muscles or their innervation is common during vaginal delivery. A thorough understanding of this anatomy is imperative for anyone doing vaginal surgery for prolapse or urinary incontinence.

Pelvic Diaphragm

The **pelvic diaphragm** forms the muscular floor of the pelvis, and is made up of the **levator ani** and **coccygeus** muscles, all of whose components are attached to the inner surface of the minor pelvis (Figure 1-15). The levator ani is composed of three muscles. The innermost **puborectalis** muscle is attached to the pubic symphysis and encircles the rectum. The thicker, more medial **pubococcygeus** muscle runs from the pubis to the coccyx. This muscle is attached laterally to the obturator internus muscle by a thickened band of dense connective tissue called the arcus tendineus. The fusion of these bilateral muscles in the midline is called the levator plate and forms a shelf on which the pelvic organs rest. When the body is in a standing position, the levator plate is horizontal and supports the rectum and upper two thirds of vagina above it. The thinner, more lateral **iliococcygeus** muscle runs from the arcus tendineus and ischial spine to the coccyx. The posteriolateral margin of the pelvic diaphragm is the **coccygeus** muscle, which extends from the ischial spine to the coccyx and lower sacrum (see Figure 1-15).

Weakness or damage to parts of the pelvic diaphragm may loosen the sling behind the anorectum and cause the levator plate to sag. Women with prolapse have been shown to have an enlarged urogenital hiatus on clinical examination.

Figure 1-15. The components of the pelvic diaphragm.

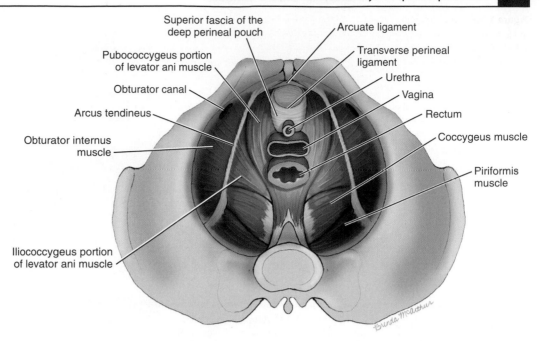

Superior fascia of the deep perineal pouch

Pubococcygeus portion of levator ani muscle

Obturator canal

Arcus tendineus

Obturator internus muscle

Iliococcygeus portion of levator ani muscle

Arcuate ligament

Transverse perineal ligament

Urethra

Vagina

Rectum

Coccygeus muscle

Piriformis muscle

Perineal Membrane, Deep and Superficial Perineal Pouches

The deep perineal pouch bridges the gap between the inferior pubic rami and the perineal body. It closes the urogenital hiatus and has a sphincter-like effect at the distal vagina. It provides structural support for the distal urethra and also contributes to continence because of its attachment to periurethral striated muscles. Knowledge of the anatomy of this area is necessary for surgical procedures that involve creation of a neo-vagina in patients with androgen insensitivity syndrome or correction of ambiguous genitalia.

The perineal membrane and the deep perineal pouch are musculofascial structures located over the anterior pelvic outlet below the pelvic diaphragm. The perineal membrane is a fascial layer attached to the ischiopubic rami. There are openings in this fascia for the urethra and vagina. The deep perineal pouch is located superior to this membrane and has several contiguous striated muscles: the **compressor urethrae** and sphincter **urethrovaginalis**, the **external urethral sphincter**, and the **deep transverse perineal muscles**.

The superficial perineal pouch contains the **ischiocavernosus, bulbospongiosus, and superficial transverse perineal muscles;** it also contains the greater vestibular glands (Bartholin glands).

Presacral Space

Reproductive surgeons are sometimes required to operate in the presacral space when performing a presacral neurectomy to control chronic pelvic pain. In this space lies the **superior hypogastric plexus**, which contains both sympathetic and parasympathetic nerve fibers. In reality this plexus is more prelumbar rather than presacral. The superior hypogastric plexus divides into two branches at about the level of the bifurcation of the aorta near L4 (Figure 1-16). In addition to visceral afferent fibers from the uterus, these nerve trunks also carry parasympathetic fibers that stimulate bladder contraction and modulate the activity of the distal colon. It is for this reason that presacral neurectomy can result in both bladder and bowel dysfunction.

Another risk of presacral neurectomy is blood vessel injury. The **left common iliac vein** makes up the left superior margin of the presacral area as it lies inferior to the bifurcation of the aorta and anterior to the vertebra, and it can be injured during this dissection. The **median sacral vessels** originate from the aortic bifurcation and

Figure 1-16. The bifurcation of the superior hypogastric plexus at the level of the bifurcation of the aorta.

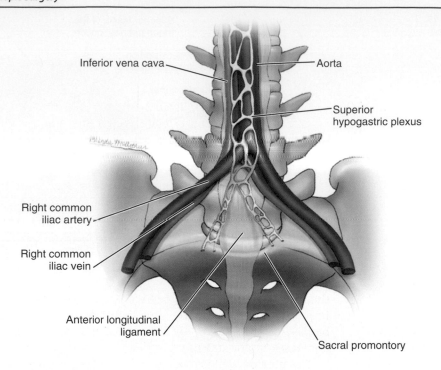

descend in the midline into the presacral area. Bleeding from these vessels and the **presacral venous plexus** can be potentially life-threatening.

Pelvic Viscera

The pelvic viscera include the rectum, urinary organs, and the internal genitalia, including vagina, uterus, uterine tubes, and ovaries.

The Rectum

The rectum of the adult is approximately 12 to 15 cm in length. It begins at the rectosigmoid junction in front of S3 and ends at the anorectal junction at the level of the tip of the coccyx. Unlike the colon, it lacks taeniae coli, haustra, and omental appendices.

The upper third of the rectum projects into the peritoneal cavity anteriorly and laterally. At its midpoint, the anterior peritoneum of the rectum extends onto the fornix of the vagina to form the rectouterine pouch. The distal one third is completely retroperitoneal.

The blood supply to the rectum includes the **superior rectal artery**, a branch from the inferior mesenteric artery; the **middle rectal artery**, a branch from the internal iliac artery; and the **inferior rectal artery**, a branch from the internal pudendal artery. The rectum is innervated by sympathetic fibers from the **inferior hypogastric plexus**, parasympathetic fibers that leave the sacral spinal cord (S2 through S4) as pelvic splanchnic nerves and enter the inferior hypogastric plexus before passing to the rectum, and sensory fibers from the rectum that join the inferior hypogastric plexus.

Vagina

The vagina is a musculomembranous sheath 7 to 9 cm in length that extends anteroinferiorly from the uterine cervix to the vestibule. Because the cervix enters the vagina along the anterior wall, the posterior wall is about 1 cm longer than the anterior wall.

Anterior and posterior to the cervix are vaginal fornices. Intraperitoneally, the vagina is separated from the rectum by the rectouterine pouch, and from the bladder by the vesicouterine pouch

The vagina receives its blood supply from the **uterine, vaginal, and middle rectal arteries,** which form an extensive anastomotic network. Innervation of the vagina is from the inferior hypogastric plexus and pelvic splanchnic nerves.

Uterus

The uterus is a fibromuscular organ that varies in size and weight according to life stage and parity. The uterus is divided into a body (corpus) and cervix. The part of the body of the uterus above the uterine tube is called the fundus. In a nulliparous woman the uterus is about 8 cm in length from the external os to the fundus, 5 cm in width at the fundus, and 2 to 3 cm anteroposteriorly. It weighs between 40 and 100 g.

The uterine cavity is triangular in shape, and the anterior and posterior walls approximate each other. Since the uterine cavity is a virtual space, ultrasound assessment of the uterus will only show a cavity when it is distended with fluid.

The length of the uterine cavity changes according to life stage, in part because of the profound effect of hormones on uterine size. In premenarchal girls the uterine length from the external os to the fundus is 1 to 3 cm. The cervix occupies two thirds of the uterine length in prepubertal girls and only one third after menarche. During the reproductive years, the expected length of the cavity is about 6 to 7 cm, which is important to remember when instrumenting the uterine cavity during endometrial biopsy, hysteroscopy, or embryo transfer. In postmenopausal women the uterus decreases to about 3 to 5 cm long.

The uterine wall is made up of three layers: endometrium, myometrium, and serosa. The endometrium is hormonally responsive and varies in thickness from 5 to 15 mm within a single menstrual cycle during the reproductive years. After menopause, it should be greater than 5 mm in thickness as measured by ultrasound.

The myometrium consists of three to four indistinct layers of smooth muscle approximately 1 to 1.25 cm thick during the reproductive years. It is thickest in the mid-portion of the uterine corpus and thinnest near the opening of the uterine tube. The outermost layer consists of mostly longitudinal fibers. The middle layer consists of circular and oblique fibers, and includes most of the blood vessels and loose connective tissue. The innermost layer is composed of mostly longitudinal fibers that are continuous with the uterine tubes and ligaments that surround the uterus.

The uterine blood supply is from the **uterine artery**, a branch of the internal iliac artery. The uterine artery courses along the lateral border of the uterus and forms extensive anastomoses with the ovarian and vaginal arteries. Approximately 6 to 10 blood vessels penetrate the uterus from the uterine artery and run circumferentially as the anterior and posterior arcuate arteries. Vessels from the sides anastomose in the midline, but no large blood vessels are found in the midline. Doppler studies have shown that the arcuate arteries are at the periphery of the uterus. The arcuate arteries supply the radial branches that deeply penetrate the myometrium to reach the endometrium. These radial arteries give rise to the spiral arteries of the endometrium.

Incisions on the uterus made during myomectomy should take into consideration the anatomy of the uterus. An incision made vertically in the midline is less likely to divide the large uterine vessels on the lateral border of the uterus. However, vertical uterine incisions may transect several arcuate arteries.

Uterine Tubes

The uterine tubes are contained within the uppermost margin of the broad ligament and measure about 10 to 12 cm (Figure 1-17). The tube is divided into several distinct anatomic segments: intramural (or interstitial), isthmic, ampullary, and infundibulum. The internal diameter of the tube ranges from less than 1 mm at the intramural portion to up to 10 mm at the infundibulum.

The intramural portion of the tube is usually 1.5 cm long, and may be tortuous. The tubal ostium where it opens into the uterine cavity can be seen at hysteroscopy at each angle of the fundus.

The isthmic portion is often the site of tubal ligation and therefore the site of tubal anastomosis. The lumen is approximately 0.5 mm. Although magnification is required

Figure 1-17. The ampullary portion of the right uterine tube and ovary. The fimbriae are normal. The ovaries are suspended by the mesovarium.

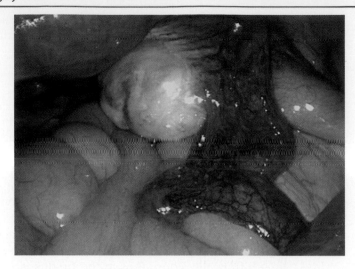

for anastomosis, the subsequent pregnancy rates are highest for procedures done in this area.

The ampulla comprises two thirds of the length of the tube and has 4 or 5 longitudinal ridges. It is the site of fertilization, and is thus the most common site of ectopic pregnancy. Tubal ligations are often performed at this more distal site. Although the lumen is much greater here, the pregnancy rates after anastomosis are lower.

The infundibulum is the distal section of the tube. It is not attached by peritoneum, and is open to the peritoneal cavity. Its delicate finger-like projections are called fimbriae.

The tubal wall consists of three layers: mucosa, muscularis, and serosa. The muscular layer has a somewhat indistinct external longitudinal layer and an inner circular layer of smooth muscle. The intramural portion has no anatomic sphincter but closure is sometimes seen during hysteroscopy. The blood supply to the tube runs in the mesosalpinx and consists of branches from the uterine and ovarian artries.

Ovaries

The ovaries are ovoid structures suspended from the posterior aspect of the broad ligament by the mesovarium (see Figure 1-17). This fold of peritoneum contains an extensive complex of blood vessels. The infundibulopelvic ligament enters the ovary along its superior pole and carries the ovarian vessels, lymphatics, and nerves. These vessels are in close proximity to the ureter at the pelvic brim. The ovarian ligament is located on the inferior pole of the ovary. The ovary is attached to the broad ligament by the mesovarium. It has a rich vascular supply. An arcade of vessels is formed from the anastomoses of the uterine and ovarian vessels. These vessels, called helicine because of their highly coiled structure, course through the mesovarium into the medulla. Veins then drain the medulla to form a plexus seen in the mesovarium. Dissection around this area during a lysis of tubal adhesion or cystectomy should be performed with great care to avoid bleeding.

The ovarian volume is dependent on both the life stage and the germ cell population. During the reproductive years, ovaries without functional cysts weigh approximately 20 to 35 g and measure approximately $4 \times 2 \times 1$ cm. Before menarche and after menopause the ovaries will be smaller.

Pelvic Fasciae and Ligaments

The pelvic viscera are attached to the pelvic sidewalls by (1) peritoneal folds, (2) condensations of pelvic fascia, and (3) remnants of embryonic structures. In the past, it was believed that these structures supported the uterus and prevented genital prolapse. Thus many of these structures were designated as "ligaments." However, it has become clear that none of these structures provide significant support for the pelvic viscera in the presence of pelvic floor defects.

Peritoneal Folds

The **broad ligament** is a double-layered transverse fold of peritoneum that encloses the uterus and uterine tubes and extends to the lateral walls and pelvic floor. It is made up of the **mesometrium** lateral to the uterus that encloses the uterine vessels and the ureters, the **mesovarium** that attaches the ovary to the broad ligament posteriorly (see Figure 1-17), and the **mesosalpinx** that connects the uterine tube near the base of the mesovarium.

The **suspensory ligament of the ovary**, often referred to as the "**infundibulopelvic ligament**," is a lateral continuation of the broad ligament beyond the uterine tube that connects the ovary to the pelvic brim and contains the ovarian artery and vein. The ureter crosses beneath these vessels near the point where this ligament joins the pelvic sidewall.

Fascial Ligaments

The **cardinal (transverse cervical) ligament** is a connective tissue condensation lateral to the cervix that is bordered anteriorly and posteriorly by the leaves of the broad ligament and inferiorly by the pelvic floor. It is continuous with the paracervix, a dense fibrous sheath around the lower cervix and the upper vagina, and is attached to the pelvic walls laterally. It usually contains major branches of the uterine vessels.

The **uterosacral ligament** is a connective tissue band arising from the posterior paracervix that fans out to attach to the sacrum and rectum. It contains some smooth muscle fibers.

Gubernacular Ligaments

The **ovarian ligament** runs in the broad ligament and attaches the medial pole of the ovary to the posterior lateral uterine surface beneath the uterine tube. The **round ligament** is the forward continuation of the uterine attachment of the ovarian ligament. This fibromuscular structure traverses the deep (external) inguinal ring and terminates as fibrous strands in the connective tissue of the labium majora. (See Video 1-1 🎞️)

Suggested Reading

Delancey JO, Hurd WW: Size of the urogenital hiatus in the levator ani muscles in normal women and women with pelvic organ prolapse, *Obstet Gynecol* 91(3):364-368, 1998.

Drake RL, Vogl W, Mitchell AWM: *Gray's Anatomy for Students*, 2nd ed. Philadelphia: Churchill Livingstone, Elsevier, 2010.

Herschorn S: Female pelvic floor anatomy: the pelvic floor, supporting structures, and pelvic organs, *Rev Urol* 6 (suppl 5):S2-S10, 2004.

Hurd WW, Amesse LS, Gruber JS, Horowitz GM, Cha GM, Hurteau JA: Visualization of the epigastric vessels and bladder before laparoscopic trocar placement, *Fertil Steril* 80(1):209-212, 2003.

Hurd WW, Bude RO, DeLancey JOL, Newman JS: The location of abdominal wall blood vessels in relationship to abdominal landmarks apparent at laparoscopy, *Am J Obstet Gynecol* 171:642-646, 1994.

Hurd WW, Chee SS, Gallagher KL, Ohl DA, Hurteau JA: Location of the ureters in relation to the uterine cervix by computed tomography, *Am J Obstet Gynecol* 184(3):336-339, 2001.

Patsner B: Laparoscopy using the left upper quadrant approach, *J Am Assoc Gynecol Laparosc* 6(3):323-325, 1999.

Stultz P: Peripheral nerve injuries resulting from common surgical procedures in the lower abdomen, *Arch Surg* 117:324-327, 1982.

Tulikangas PK, Nicklas A, Falcone T, Price LL: Anatomy of the left upper quadrant for cannula insertion, *J Am Assoc Gynecol Laparosc* 7:211-214, 2000.

Whiteside J., Barber M, Walters M, Falcone T: Anatomy of ilioinguinal and iliohypogastric nerves in relation to trocar placement and low transverse incisions, *Am J Obstet Gynecol* 189:1574-1578, 2003.

Indications and Contraindications for Laparoscopy

Jeffrey M. Goldberg M.D.

Jeffrey M. Goldberg M.D.

2

Introduction: History of Laparoscopy

The indications and contraindications for laparoscopic surgery have evolved as technologic advances reduce the limitations to performing increasingly more complex procedures. The following is a brief timeline of the most significant events in the development of operative laparoscopy.

1901 – Georg Kelling, a gastroenterologist from Dresden, Germany, performs "coelioscopy" on a dog. This visionary procedure uses a trocar and insufflation device (Politzer air pump) to create a pneumoperitoneum, and a Nitze cystoscope.

1910 – Hans Christian Jacobaeus in Stockholm, Sweden, uses a cystoscope to inspect the abdominal cavity in humans and calls the procedure laparoscopy. Concurrently, Bctram Bernheim at Johns Hopkins performs the first laparoscopy in the US and calls his procedure organoscopy. Neither uses pneumoperitoneum.

1912 – Severin Nordentoft utilizes the Trendelenburg position to improve visualization.

Over the next half century, laparoscopy is almost exclusively the domain of gastroenterologists who use it to inspect the liver.

1920 – Benjamin Orndoff develops a sharp pyramidal trocar to facilitate entry into the abdomen.

1921 – Otto Goetze develops an insufflator and Korbsch develops the first needle for creating a pneumoperitoneum.

1924 – Richard Zollikofer recommends using carbon dioxide for the pneumoperitoneum.

1929 – Heinz Kalk increases the viewing angle of the laparoscope (as well as developing angled scopes) and describes the use of a second port to enable operative procedures.

1938 – Janos Veress, a Hungarian chest physician, publishes an article on the use of a special insufflation needle for creating a pneumothorax in patients with tuberculosis. The needle is then used to establish the pneumoperitoneum. (The needle still bears his name.)

1938 – P.F. Boesch in Germany performs the first laparoscopic tubal ligation.

1941 – F.H. Power and A.C. Barnes utilize the Bovie high-output generator to perform tubal ligation. This replaces the low-output generators used to deliver monopolar electrocautery in the 1930s.

1944 – Raoul Palmer, a French gynecologist, promotes the use of laparoscopy in gynecology, especially for tubal ligation. He advises monitoring intra-abdominal pressure. In patients with previous laparotomy, he recommends inserting the initial trocar in the left upper quadrant below the costal margin, "Palmer's point."

1952 – N. Fourestier introduces the use of a quartz light rod lens and H.H. Hopkins, the glass rod lens, to replace the series of glass lenses and distal incandescent lamp in earlier generation endoscopes. This provides a brighter and clearer image with reduced heat.

1957 – Basil Hirschowitz introduces fiberoptic technology to endoscopy which further improves light delivery.

1960s-1970s – Kurt Semm of Kiel, Germany, a gynecologist and engineer, develops a complete set of laparoscopic instruments and describes their use for performing all of the basic gynecologic laparoscopic procedures. He also develops a pressure-controlled insufflator, the endocoagulator, a suction/irrigator, a morcellator, and methods for suturing with intracorporeal and extracorporeal knot-tying. He is responsible for establishing advanced operative laparoscopic surgery.

1971 – Richard Fikentscher and Kurt Semm introduce bipolar electrocautery for laparoscopic surgery, initially for tubal ligation.

Late 1970s – Camran Nezhat popularizes the use of a video camera and monitor to perform operative laparoscopy.

1985 – Erich Muhe of Germany performs the first laparoscopic cholecystectomy. This procedure is responsible for the wide acceptance of operative laparoscopy and leads to the virtual explosion of new laparoscopic devices and procedures.

1990 – Harry Reich performs the first laparoscopic hysterectomy, introducing the modern era of advanced laparoscopic surgery.

1999 – T. Falcone and J.M. Goldberg perform the first fully robotic surgery, a tubal anastomosis.

Indications

Current laparoscopic instrumentation enables any gynecologic procedure done by laparotomy to be performed laparoscopically. The only difference is the route of access. The main advantage of laparoscopy is that it is usually performed as an outpatient procedure. Numerous high-quality clinical trials have demonstrated that most gynecologic procedures can be safely accomplished by laparoscopy (Table 2-1). Although laparoscopic procedures frequently take longer to perform and require additional disposable items, the increased operative costs are offset by averting the need for hospitalization.

Because patients are ambulatory within a few hours, the risk of thromboembolism is much less. Wound infections are also greatly reduced with the small laparoscopy puncture sites. Also, avoiding hospitalization eliminates nosocomial urinary and pulmonary infections. Postoperative ileus, common with laparotomy, is much less frequent with laparoscopy.

Comparative studies between laparotomy and laparoscopy for various procedures such as hysterectomy, linear salpingostomy for ectopic pregnancy, and myomectomy

Table 2-1 Laparoscopic Procedures

- Diagnostic laparoscopy
- Laparoscopic sterilization
- Tubal surgery

  Ectopic pregnancy
  Reconstructive surgery – anastomosis, neosalpingostomy/fibrioplasty
  Salpingectomy

- Lysis of adhesions
- Treatment of endometriosis – all stages
- Ovarian cystectomy and oophorectomy
- Myomectomy
- Hysterectomy – total laparoscopic, laparoscopic supracervical, laparoscopic-assisted vaginal hysterectomy
- Surgery for pelvic support

have demonstrated numerous advantages with the laparoscopic approach. These include less postoperative discomfort and analgesia use, and more rapid return to activity. While second-look laparoscopy has demonstrated a significant reduction in de novo adhesions, it is unknown whether that translates into improved pregnancy rates or reduced chronic pelvic pain. Finally, the small laparoscopic punctures are usually considered to be more cosmetic than the large laparotomy incision. However, a survey of 100 women found that about two thirds preferred the cosmetic appearance of a low Pfannenstiel incision to the multiple punctures required to perform laparoscopic hysterectomy.

While not a specific indication, laparoscopy may be a better approach for patients with morbid obesity. Laparotomy is an ordeal in the morbidly obese due to compromised visualization and surgical access. It is associated with increased intraoperative blood loss as well as higher rates of postoperative complications such as wound infections, respiratory problems, and thromboembolic disease.

Morbid obesity also significantly increases the risks and difficulty of laparoscopic surgery. The thick abdominal wall makes it difficult to establish a pneumoperitoneum, impedes access to the pelvic structures, and hinders the excursions of the trocars. Closing the fascia on larger incisions is also more of a challenge, predisposing the patient to incisional hernias. The increased intra-abdominal fat in the omentum and bowel mesentery compromises exposure. Visibility is further limited by the inability of the patient to tolerate steep Trendelenburg and the higher intra-abdominal pressures needed to elevate the heavy abdominal wall. Proper preoperative counseling and postoperative management are important to optimize the surgical outcome.

Absolute Contraindications

Perhaps the patients that laparoscopy benefits the most are the poorest candidates for surgery in general, i.e., those with compromised cardiopulmonary status, renal failure, or morbid obesity, as well as the oldest and youngest patients. It is imperative to optimize such patients' medical status prior to surgery. While there are many relative contraindications to laparoscopic surgery, the few absolute contraindications include shock, markedly increased intracranial pressure, retinal detachment, and inadequate surgical equipment or anesthesia monitoring.

Relative Contraindications

Compromised Cardiopulmonary Status

Cardiopulmonary disease and hypovolemia require careful monitoring by the anesthesiologist, including central monitoring and arterial blood gas analysis to reduce the risk of respiratory failure and cardiac arrest. Less Trendelenburg and lower intra-abdominal pressures may be necessary to maintain adequate ventilation and cardiac output.

Ventriculoperitoneal or Peritoneojugular Shunts

Though no longer considered an absolute contraindication, patients with ventriculoperitoneal or peritoneojugular shunts are at risk for shunt malfunction and increased intracranial pressure with neurologic compromise or brain herniation. At present there is no standard management of these patients, but some have advocated minimizing intra-abdominal pressure and Trendelenburg, clamping the distal end of the shunt, and monitoring intracranial pressure.

Pregnancy

In terms of fetal safety and technical ease, the ideal time for surgery during pregnancy is early in the second trimester. There is a concern that transperitoneal absorption of the CO_2 pneumoperitoneum can lead to hypercarbia and fetal acidosis. However, this can be avoided if the anesthesiologist increases minute ventilation to compensate for the increased P_{CO_2} to a higher degree than with the nonpregnant patient. The end-tidal P_{CO_2} in pregnant patients should be kept lower than in nonpregnant patients, to reflect the physiologic compensated respiratory alkalosis of pregnancy. Transperitoneal absorption of CO_2 may also be avoided by the use of gasless laparoscopy. The other concern is injury to the uterus, which may be reduced by using the open technique or the left upper quadrant technique for the initial trocar insertion. Finally, the large third-trimester uterus reduces exposure and working space which may be somewhat overcome with higher trocar placement and the use of a 30° laparoscope.

Large Pelvic Masses

Similar to the third-trimester uterus, large pelvic masses present difficulty with exposure and access, necessitating higher, more lateral placement of the trocars. Very large cysts such as in mucinous cystadenomas may be better approached with a minilaparotomy incision for technical ease and reduced risk of rupture while still being minimally invasive.

Ovarian Cancer

In general, ovarian cancer is managed by laparotomy by a gynecologic surgeon with special expertise. Laparoscopic staging of ovarian cancer has been described. Laparoscopic management of stage IA, grade 1 or 2 invasive cancer or tumors of low malignant potential has been reported. The risk of rupture of an early-stage invasive cancer has significant management consequences.

Small Bowel Obstruction

While there are reports of successful laparoscopic treatment of small bowel obstruction, the dilated loops of bowel restrict exposure and increase the risk for bowel injury.

Suggested Reading

Al-Mufarrej F, Nolan C, Sookhai S, Broe P: Laparoscopic procedures in adults with ventriculoperitoneal shunts, *Surg Laparosc Endosc Percutan Tech* 15:28-29, 2005.

Currie I, Onwude JL, Jarvis GJ: A comparative study of the cosmetic appeal of abdominal incisions used for hysterectomy, *Br J Obstet Gynaecol* 103:252, 1996.

Chi DS, Abu-Rustum NR, Sonoda Y, Ivy J, Rhee E, Moore K et al: The safety and efficacy of laparoscopic surgical staging of apparent stage I ovarian and fallopian tube cancers, *Am J Obstet Gynecol* 192:1614-1619, 2005.

Dubuisson JB, Fauconnier A, Chapron C, Kreiker G, Norgaard C: Second look after laparoscopic myomectomy, *Hum Reprod* 13:2102-2106,1998.

Falcone T, Goldberg J, Garcia-Ruiz A, Margossian H, Stevens L: Full robotic assistance for laparoscopic tubal anastomosis: first case report, *J Laparoendosc Adv Surg Tech A* 9(1): 107-113, 1999.

Gerges FJ, Kanazi GE, Jabbour-Khoury SI: Anesthesia for laparoscopy: a review, *J Clin Anesth* 18:67-78, 2006.

Goldberg JM, Maurer WG. A randomized comparison of gasless laparoscopy and CO2 pneumoperitoneum, *Obstet Gynecol* 90:416-420,1997.

Lau WY, Leow CK, Li AKC: History of endoscopic and laparoscopic surgery, *World J Surg* 21:444-453, 1997.

Lundorff P, Hahlin M, Kallfelt B, Thorburn J, Lindblom B: Adhesion formation after laparoscopic surgery in tubal pregnancy: a randomized trial versus laparotomy, *Fertil Steril* 55:911-915, 1991.

Mais V, Aossa S, Guerriero S, Mascia M, Solla E, Melis GB: Laparoscopic versus abdominal myomectomy: a prospective randomized trial to evaluate benefits in early outcome, *Am J Obstet Gynecol* 174:654-658, 1996.

Modlin IM, Kidd M, Lye KD: From the lumen to the laparoscope, *Arch Surg* 139:1110-1126, 2004.

Operative Laparoscopy Study Group. Postoperative adhesion development after operative laparoscopy: evaluation at early second-look procedures, *Fertil Steril* 55:700-704,1991.

Seracchioli R, Rossi S, Govoni F, Rossi E, Venturoli S, Bulletti C, Flamigni C: Fertility and obstetric outcome after laparoscopic myomectomy of large myomata: a randomized comparison with abdominal myomectomy, *Hum Reprod* 15:2663-2668, 2000.

Trocar Insertion
Choosing the Appropriate Position and Techniques for Placement

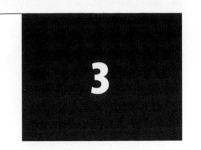

Minita S. Patel M.D.
Paul Tulikangas M.D.

 Video Clips on DVD

3-1 Laparoscopic Trocar Placement 4:49
3-2 Diagnostic Laparoscopy 1:04
3-3 Technique of Left Upper Quadrant Trocar Insertion with Case Demonstrations of Takedown of Midline Adhesions,

Removal of Large Ovarian Cysts and Laparoscopic Cystectomy in a Pregnant Patient (6 minutes/54 seconds)

Introduction

Establishing access to the abdomen is the first step in any laparoscopic procedure. Attention must be paid to this part of the operation because it is a common time for complications. Thoughtful placement of primary and secondary laparoscopic trocars allows for excellent surgical exposure and angles that expedite the operative procedure.

Studies evaluating laparoscopic trocar insertion are limited by the relatively rare occurrence of the major complications associated with different techniques. As with most surgical complications, they are also probably underreported. In this chapter we present the recommended techniques that should be utilized to facilitate safe and effective trocar placement, as well as clinical caveats we have developed through experience.

Trocar Insertion and Relevant Anatomy

Prior to a discussion on trocar insertion, a thorough understanding of the anatomy of the anterior abdominal wall is necessary. The abdominal wall extends from the xiphoid process of the sternum cephalad, to the pubic bone caudad. The layers of the abdominal wall from outside in are: skin; subcutaneous tissue; the external oblique, internal oblique, and transversus abdominis muscles with their aponeuroses; transversalis fascia; preperitoneal fat; and peritoneum. There are also nerves, blood vessels, and lymphatics. The location of the relevant intraperitoneal structures, specifically the aorta, the vena cava and its bifurcation into the common iliacs, the epigastric vessels, bowel, and bladder varies depending on body habitus and surgical history.

The umbilicus is the location on the abdominal wall which has the shortest distance from skin to peritoneum. For this reason, it is commonly selected as a site for the first trocar insertion. Depending on body mass index (BMI), the bifurcation of the aorta can vary anywhere from directly underneath (for those with a normal BMI) to 3 to 4 cm caudad (in the obese) (Figure 3-1).

The superficial and inferior epigastric and superficial circumflex iliac arteries are important vascular structures of which to be mindful when inserting accessory trocars.

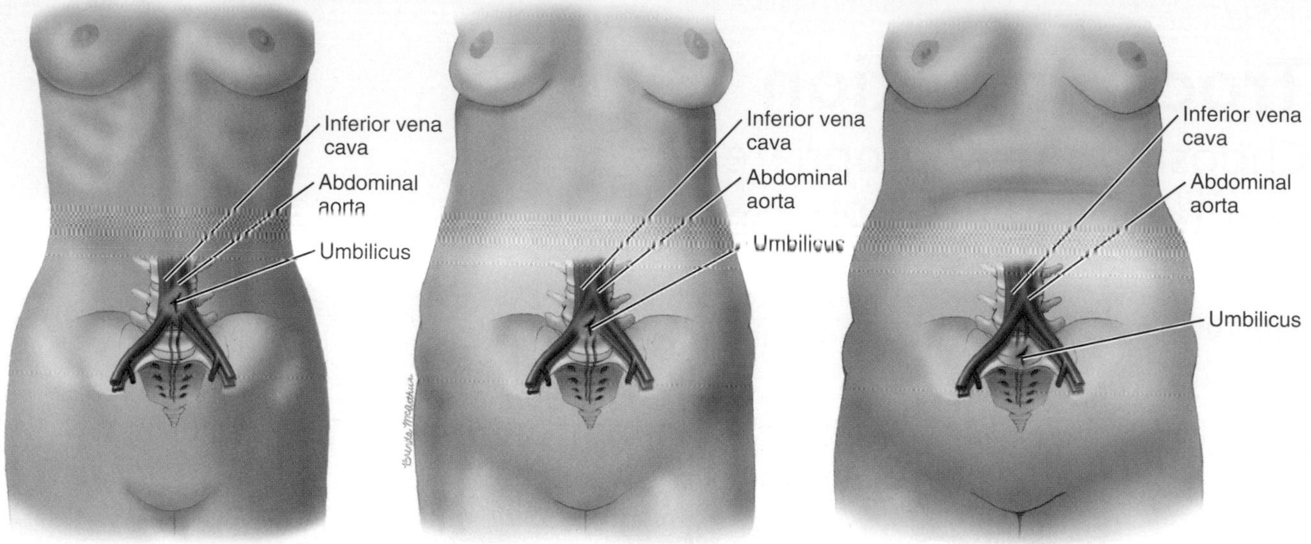

Figure 3-1. Location of the major retroperitoneal blood vessels in relationship to the umbilicus. This relationship varies with BMI.

To avoid injury, the inferior epigastric vessels should be visualized directly before insertion of additional trocars. They are identified by following the round ligament to the deep (internal) inguinal ring. There, the inferior epigastric vessels are seen passing cranially on the anterior abdominal wall. The superficial epigastric vessels may be visualized by illuminating the anterior abdominal wall with a laparoscopic light source.

The lateral trocars are usually placed 3 to 5 cm superior to the pubic symphysis and 4 to 8 cm lateral to the midline. The inferior epigastric and superficial epigastric arteries are 5 to 6 cm lateral from the midline. The superficial circumflex iliac arteries course lateral to the epigastric arteries, approximately 9.5 cm (SD: 1.6 cm) lateral from the midline. In patients with portal hypertension, these vessels are often engorged and easily injured.

In cases where intra-abdominal adhesions are suspected or difficulty with establishing intraperitoneal access through the umbilicus is encountered, the left upper quadrant can be used for the primary trocar insertion site (Figure 3-2). This site is also helpful in pregnant women and in patients with large pelvic masses.

For the left upper quadrant trocar insertion, the primary trocar is inserted 3 cm below the left subcostal margin in the midclavicular line. At this location, there is less subcutaneous fat and, usually, no adhesions. However, the liver, spleen, stomach, and lungs are at risk for injury, and this technique should not be used in those with hepatosplenomegaly, prior gastric or splenic surgery, or masses of the stomach or pancreas. A gastric drainage tube should always be placed prior to left upper quadrant trocar insertion. A study of the distance between these organs and the left upper quadrant insertion site found that as BMI increased, so did the distance to these organs.

The iliohypogastric and ilioinguinal nerves (Figure 3-3) provide sensory innervation to the gluteal and hypogastric regions, the groin, the inner thigh, and the labia majora. These are vulnerable to injury during insertion and fascial closure of the lateral trocar ports used in laparoscopy. An anatomic study has demonstrated that the ilioinguinal nerve starts 3.1 cm (SD: 1.5 cm) medial and 3.7 cm (SD: 1.5 cm) inferior to the anterior superior iliac spine (ASIS) and ends 2.7 cm (SD: 0.9 cm) lateral to the midline and 1.7 cm (SD: 0.9 cm) superior to the pubic symphysis. The iliohypogastric nerve starts 2.1 cm (SD: 1.8 cm) medial and 0.9 cm (SD: 2.8 cm) inferior to the ASIS and ends 3.7 cm (SD: 2.7 cm) lateral to the midline and 5.2 cm (SD: 2.6 cm) superior to the pubic symphysis. Fascial closure of ports greater than 5 mm in diameter is recommended due to the risk for hernia formation. Given the proximity of the iliohypogastric and ilioinguinal nerves to these lateral ports, care should be taken during fascial closure.

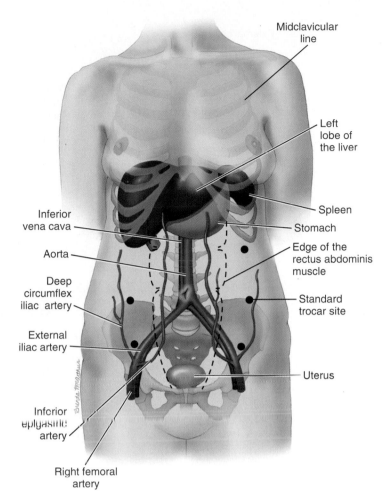

Preoperative considerations prior to trocar insertion include a history of anterior abdominal wall surgery (TRAM flaps or abdominoplasty) where there may no longer be an umbilicus to use for trocar insertion. These patients may be good candidates for left upper quadrant trocar insertion for easier identification of critical landmarks (sternal border, midclavicular line). The left upper quadrant site also provides a panoramic view of the abdomen for placement of secondary trocars. A history of prior ventral hernia repair should not be a contraindication to laparoscopy because trocars can be inserted through the mesh. However, trocars should not be inserted blindly or directly at the site of the hernia repair. The bowel can be adherent to the repair site, so again, left upper quadrant insertion may be warranted in order to perform lysis of adhesions at the umbilical and lower quadrant sites as well as to place these additional trocars under direct visualization to minimize the risk of bowel injury. If a trocar is passed through a permanent mesh, we typically close the mesh with a permanent suture.

Positioning during Laparoscopy

Positioning during laparoscopy is also important in order to ensure ease of operation and reduce strain on the patient and surgeon. Most patients are placed in the lithotomy position with Allen or "Yellofin" type stirrups supporting the legs (Figure 3-4). Care should be taken not to hyperflex or extend the hips. In short patients, check the popliteal fossa to be sure there is no compression of the peroneal nerve. If the surgeon anticipates perineal exposure will be needed (for example, LAVH), then extending the leg at the knee in the Yellofin stirrup will improve exposure.

In general, tucking the arms of the patient after intubation will increase the surgeons' mobility during laparoscopy (Figure 3-5), especially because after insertion of

Figure 3-3. Location of the ilioinguinal and iliohypogastric nerves in the lower anterior abdominal wall.

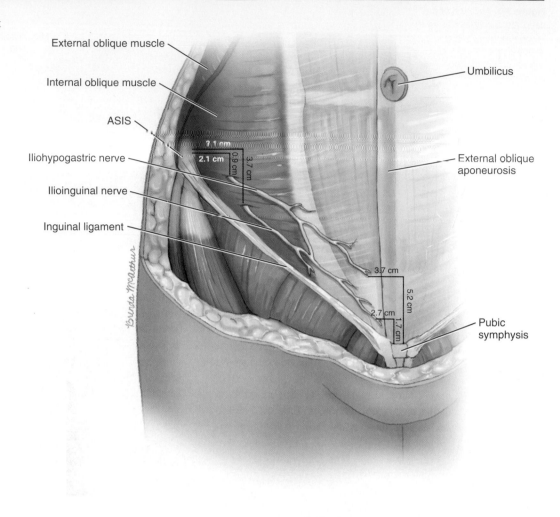

External oblique muscle

Internal oblique muscle

ASIS

Iliohypogastric nerve

Ilioinguinal nerve

Inguinal ligament

Umbilicus

External oblique aponeurosis

Pubic symphysis

2.1 cm
0.9 cm
3.7 cm
3.7 cm
5.2 cm
2.7 cm
1.7 cm

Figure 3-4. Proper support of lower extremities in Yellofin stirrups.

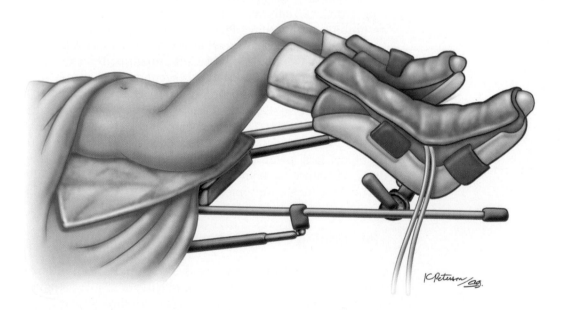

trocars, the surgeons turn their bodies to operate facing screens rather than standing facing the patient. Additionally, with upper abdominal and lateral ports, surgeons tend to stand further cephalad relative to the patient than for laparotomy.

If significant Trendelenburg may be needed, some pelvic surgeons secure the patient's upper abdomen to the table with padded straps to keep her in position.

Figure 3-5. Recommended position of the patient's arms, tucked by her side and supported.

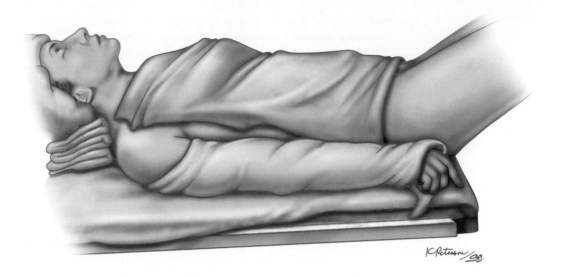

Selection of Site and Technique for Primary Trocar Insertion

View DVD: Videos 3-1 and 3-2

Insertion of the primary trocar carries the highest risk for injuries sustained during laparoscopy, because the trocar is often placed blindly. The primary trocar is inserted, followed by insufflation of the peritoneal cavity and insertion of a camera for visualization of subsequent trocar placement and surgery. Locations for primary trocar placement and insufflation are the umbilicus, left upper quadrant, above the umbilicus, cul-de-sac, and the fundus of the uterus.

The umbilicus is most commonly used, because the distance from the skin to the peritoneal cavity is the shortest on the abdominal wall. However, those with prior abdominal surgery or a history of peritonitis or radiation may have bowel adherent to the umbilicus; in these cases, blind insertion of a Veress needle for insufflation of the peritoneal cavity may increase the risk of injury to the bowel. In obese patients, entry through the umbilicus may be technically challenging and there is higher risk for preperitoneal insufflation due to an increased distance between skin and peritoneal cavity from increased preperitoneal fat.

In those with a history of umbilical hernia repair or suspected bowel adhesions, entry above the umbilicus may allow for easier visualization of the sacrum and structures above the pelvis. Insufflation through the cul-de-sac or fundus of the uterus has been reported. For insufflation through the fundus of the uterus, the patient is placed in steep Trendelenburg position. A long Veress needle is inserted through the fundus of the uterus. It has been reported to be effective in women with BMI over 25 kg/m^2. A similar technique can be employed through the posterior cul-de-sac in those without a uterus. Again, caution should be used for those with a history of abdominal surgery, bowel resection, pelvic inflammatory disease, endometriosis, or peritonitis, because adhesions may be present near the cul-de-sac.

The left upper quadrant site is usually free of adhesions and provides an excellent panoramic view of the pelvis if there is a large pelvic mass. It is important that after intubation, an orogastric or nasogastric tube is placed to empty the stomach. The primary trocar is inserted at a 45-degree angle to the abdominal wall in the sagittal plane. Once intra-abdominal placement is confirmed, a pneumoperitoneum is obtained.

Techniques for Primary Trocar Insertion

There are four common techniques used to insert the primary trocar: open or Hasson, Veress needle, direct, and optical trocar–assisted. The open technique was developed in 1971 as a method to decrease the inherent risk involved in blind insertion of a sharp object through the umbilicus. The technique involves making a small umbilical or infraumbilical incision and carrying this incision down to the fascia, essentially performing a mini-laparotomy. After incision of the fascia, most surgeons prefer to tag these edges with a suture to assist in fascial closure and also to secure the umbilical port after insufflation. The peritoneum is identified and entered sharply under direct visualization. A blunt-tipped cannula is inserted into the umbilicus and the fascial sutures are attached to the cannula to maintain a seal during insufflation and surgery. The open technique should eliminate the risk for vascular injury, but there is still a risk of bowel injury.

The Veress needle is a long, thin needle that can be used to gain entry into the peritoneum through the umbilicus, left upper quadrant, uterine fundus, or cul-de-sac. At the umbilicus, it is recommended that the anterior abdominal wall be elevated and the needle be inserted at either a 45-degree or 90-degree angle, depending on the patient's BMI. Patients who are not obese have the shortest distance between the skin and intraperitoneal cavity. In these subjects, elevation of the anterior abdominal wall and insertion of the Veress needle at 45 degrees will maximize the chance of intraperitoneal placement of the Veress and reduce the risk of injury to underlying vessels. Obese patients require placement of the Veress needle at or close to 90 degrees and also at the base of the umbilicus rather than its lower margin to decrease the chance of preperitoneal placement. After placement of the Veress needle, the most reliable indicator of intraperitoneal placement is initial CO_2 insufflation pressure, which should be less than 10 mm Hg (Vilos 2006).

Direct trocar insertion involves placing the trocar through the umbilicus prior to insufflation (Figure 3-6). It is the fastest method for insertion of the trocar and eliminates the use of the Veress needle. Three randomized controlled trials have shown that there are fewer minor complications with direct entry as compared to closed entry with the Veress needle. In these studies, there were no major complications with either method. These trials, however, were not powered to detect differences in complications and were primarily to evaluate the feasibility and ease of each technique.

Optical trocars allow for visualization of the layers that are being penetrated during entry. The trocars have a small laparoscope in the cannula that allows for this visualization. Theoretically, these trocars should be able to reduce the risk of injury during entry since the process is no longer blind. However, bowel and vascular injuries are still reported with these trocars. The advantage may be that seeing the injury will prompt recognition and repair and decrease complications that occur when recognition and repair is delayed.

Figure 3-6. Elevation of the anterior abdominal wall and insertion of the umbilical trocar.

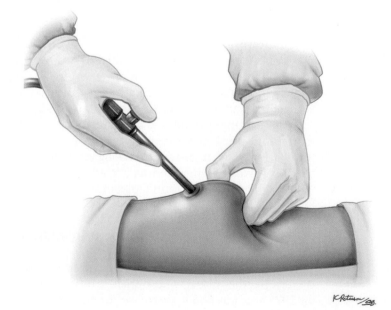

Types of Trocars

The available trocar tips are mainly divided into cutting or dilating types. Within these two divisions the tips can be further subdivided into sharp, blunt, radial, and conical tips, and may be disposable or reusable. These tips differ in the size and shape of the fascial defect that is produced upon entry. The cutting tips will have a sharp tip that cuts the tissue as it passes. The dilating tips will have a blunt tip that requires a greater degree of force to separate the tissues as it passes. Blunt tips can potentially lead to a greater risk for injury due to the greater force required to insert them. The combination of the blunt and radial expanding tip trocar has been shown to result in lower pain, less bleeding at the trocar site, and smaller wounds. An animal study comparing six different 12-mm trocars found that the cutting tips cause the largest fascial defects, and the blunt tips create the smallest defects. The sizes of the fascial defects ranged from 10.6 mm to 14.0 mm (Figure 3-7).

(See Video 3-3)

Case 1: Midline Adhesions

 View DVD: Video 3-3

A 42-year-old woman presents with cyclic pelvic pain and dyspareunia. She has a prior midline abdominal incision for a bowel resection related to Crohn disease. A left upper quadrant primary trocar insertion site is selected. An incision is made two fingerbreadths below the costal margin at the midclavicular line. A 5-mm trocar is advanced directly into the abdomen. Its placement is confirmed with the laparoscope and a pneumoperitoneum is obtained. The left upper quadrant site proves an ideal panoramic view of the pelvis for lysis of midline adhesions.

Case 2: Pelvic Mass S/P Renal Transplant

 View DVD: Video 3-3

A 45-year-old woman presents to the emergency department with acute abdominal pain. A large ovarian cyst is diagnosed by ultrasound. She has undergone an allograft renal transplant in the left iliac fossa. A primary left upper quadrant trocar insertion site is used. The cyst is drained and both ovaries are removed through a small umbilical incision.

Case 3: 13 Weeks Pregnant with Large Ovarian Cyst

View DVD: Video 3-3

A 27-year-old woman presents at 13 weeks, gestation with a 17-cm ovarian cyst. The gravid uterus complicates possible umbilical trocar insertion. A primary left upper quadrant trocar insertion site is used. The cyst is drained, excised from the ovary, and removed through an umbilical port site.

Complications

Meta-analysis comparing laparoscopy and laparotomy for benign gynecological procedures found that risk for any complication after laparoscopy is 8.9% and 15.2% for laparotomy. The overall risk for major complications was not different for laparoscopy and laparotomy (RR: 1.0, 95% confidence interval: 0.6-1.7). Mean risk for complications for laparoscopic gynecologic surgery is 3.2 per 1000 procedures. Given the rare occur-

Figure 3-7. Various trocar tips available. There are two basic types: cutting and dilating tips.

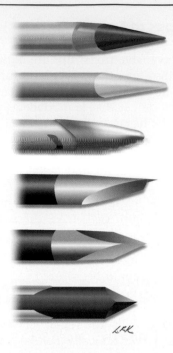

rence of major complications, a randomized controlled trial would need over 10,000 subjects in each treatment arm to achieve a 90% power to detect a difference in complications. This is why most studies about laparoscopic surgery complications are limited to case series and retrospective reviews.

Significant morbidity can occur when complications from trocar insertion are not recognized and addressed at the time of surgery. The potential sites for injury include bowel, bladder, major vessels, and nerves. Comparisons from meta-analysis of open versus closed insertion techniques have revealed that most trials have a poor study design and pooled results do not afford sufficient power to detect a difference in complication rates between the two techniques. The rate of major complications for the Hasson insertion technique is from 0% to 2% as compared to 0% to 4 % for the Veress needle insertion technique. Minor complications for all techniques range from 0% to 2.6% (Merlin 2003).

The incidence of bowel injuries is reported to be approximately 0.06% overall, being approximately 0.083% with the Veress or direct insertion techniques and 0.05% with the Hasson insertion technique (Munro 2002). The data may be biased due to heterogeneous populations for studies and the fact that risks are overestimated in retrospective studies because they compare high-risk subjects to low-risk subjects. Additionally, the Hasson technique is used more frequently for those with a history of abdominal surgery as well as in general surgery, in other words, for patients that are at higher risk for bowel adhesions. The incidence of major vascular injury is estimated to be between 0.07% and 0.05%. Vascular injuries tend to be more common for Veress needle insertion technique as compared to Hasson technique. There are few data about complications of direct trocar insertion and so it is difficult to say whether this technique has lower complications than the Hasson or Veress needle insertion techniques (Merlin 2003).

Management of Trocar Injuries

Depending on the site and type of injury, bowel injuries may be repaired through the laparoscope or by pulling the loop up through the incision and repairing it at the skin. Bowel injuries are typically repaired parallel to the long axis of the bowel so the lumen is not constricted. Patients who have minor laparoscopic surgery often do not have a bowel preparation in advance. Depending on the site and size of the injury, bowel contents may spill out. In this setting some surgeons recommend lavage of the peritoneal cavity and broad spectrum antibiotics for 24 to 48 hours. In some instances, a diverting stoma may be used to protect the site of the repair.

A hole through the stomach during insertion of the left upper quadrant ports usually does not have to be repaired since the stomach heals fairly quickly. The patient should have nasogastric tube suction left in place and be observed for 24 to 48 hours.

Bleeding from trocar sites, often from injury to the superficial or inferior epigastric arteries, can be managed by extending the skin incision and placing a suture to ligate the artery. A fascial closure device can also be used to place sutures on either side of the bleeding artery to achieve hemostasis. If there is only a small amount of bleeding, a bipolar instrument from another port site can be used to achieve hemostasis. Another option is placement of a Foley catheter into the trocar site and inflating the balloon intraperitoneally to tamponade the bleeding vessel. We have used this technique for temporary compression of a bleeding vessel, but recommend placing a suture around any vessel with significant bleeding. Always release the pneumoperitoneum and reassess for hemostasis prior to removing the trocars.

Bladder perforations can occur during trocar insertion, especially if one has not drained the bladder before inserting trocars. Small extraperitoneal injuries to the bladder can be managed with Foley catheter drainage for 5 to 7 days. Intraperitoneal injuries should be sutured closed in two layers. Cystoscopy should be performed to confirm a watertight seal and rule out any ureteral injury. A closed drain should be placed, depending on the size of the injury. Depending on the surgeon's laparoscopic suturing skills, the repair of intraperitoneal injuries can be performed using the laparoscope. We typically perform a cystogram 7 to 14 days after surgery to assure our repair is intact, then remove the catheter in the office.

Trocar sites that create a fascial defect that is greater than 5 mm in size should be closed so as to prevent hernia formation. The Carter-Thomason, along with the Endoclose device or Grice needle can be used to facilitate closure of the fascia (Figure 3-8). For the Hasson insertion technique, the umbilical port can be closed using the

Figure 3-8. Fascial closure technique: The Carter-Thomason device (cone-shaped) is placed through the fascial defect. Suture is passed through one of the openings with the Endoclose needle and then grasped by reinserting the needle through the other through the opening. The device and suture are removed and the suture is tied down.

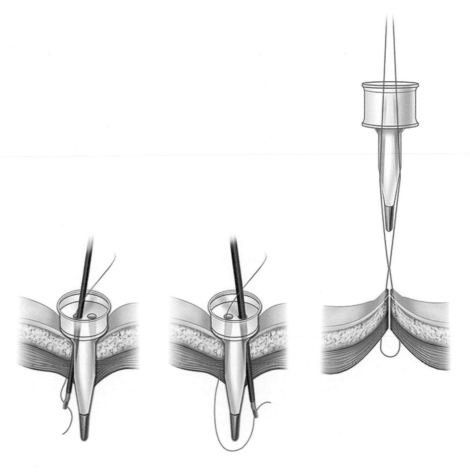

sutures that have been placed to hold the umbilical trocar in place. If the fascia has not been tagged, the fascia can bc grasped and closed under direct visualization after removal of all trocars and gas from the abdomen. This is generally easier to perform in thinner patients.

Conclusions

Laparoscopy has been shown to provide a safe, minimally invasive approach to performing most surgery that was traditionally performed via laparotomy. Trocar insertion is an important step in laparoscopy since it provides access to the surgical field and is also associated with much of the morbidity of laparoscopy. Based on the limited data on techniques for trocar insertion, the left upper quadrant insertion appears to be the best approach for initial trocar insertion for those with suspected adhesions, especially near the umbilicus. The Hasson insertion technique may decrease the risk for vascular injury but has not been shown to be superior or inferior to Veress needle or direct trocar insertion. Direct trocar insertion is the fastest approach for entry and appears to have similar rates of complications to closed Veress needle entry. Intraperitoneal placement of the Veress needle is best confirmed with insufflation pressures below 10 mm Hg. After insertion of the first trocar, the entry site should be inspected closely to check for injuries to underlying structures. The key to management of injuries due to laparoscopic trocars is to recognize and repair them at the time of surgery.

Suggested Reading

Borgatta L, Gruss L, Barad D, Kaali SG: Direct trocar insertion vs. Veress needle use for laparoscopic sterilization, *J Reprod Med* 35:891-894, 1990.

Byron JW, Markenson G, Miyazawa K: A randomized comparison of Veress needle and direct trocar insertion for laparoscopy, *Surg Gynecol Obstet* 177:259-262, 1993.

Chapron C, Fauconnier A, Goffinet F, Bréart G, Dubuisson JB: Laparoscopic surgery is not inherently dangerous for patients presenting with benign gynaecologic pathology: results of a meta-analysis, *Hum Reprod* 17:1334-1342, 2002.

Hasson HM: A modified instrument and method for laparoscopy, *Am J Obstet Gynecol* 110:886-887, 1971.

Hurd WH, Bude RO, DeLancey JO, Gauvin JM, Aisen AM: Abdominal wall characterization with magnetic resonance imaging and computed tomography: the effect of obesity on the laparoscopic approach, *J Reprod Med* 36:473-476, 1991.

Hurd WW, Bude RO, DeLancey JO, Newman JS: The location of the abdominal wall blood vessels in relationship to the abdominal landmarks apparent at laparoscopy, *Am J Obstet Gynecol,* 171:642-646, 1994.

Hurd WW, Bude RO, DeLancey JO, Pearl ML: The relationship of the umbilicus to the aortic bifurcation: implications for laparoscopic technique, *Obstet Gynecol* 80:48-51, 1992.

Lam TY, Lee SW, So HS, Kwok SP: Radially expanding trocar: a less painful alternative for laparoscopic surgery, *J Laparoendosc Adv Surg Tech A* 5:269-273, 2000.

Merlin TL, Hiller JE, Maddern GJ, Jamieson GG, Brown AR, Kolbe A: Pneumoperitoneum in laparoscopic surgery, *Br J Surg* 90:668-679, 2003.

Munro MG: Laparoscopic access: complications, technologies and techniques, *Curr Opin Obstet Gynecol* 14:365-374, 2002.

Nezhat FR, Silfen SL, Evans D, Nezhat C: Comparison of direct insertion of disposable and standard reusable laparoscopic trocars and previous pneumoperitoneum with Veress needle, *Obstet Gynecol* 78:148-150, 1991.

Santala M, Jarvel I, Kauppila A: Transfundal insertion of Veress needle in laparoscopy of obese subjects: a practical alternative, *Hum Reprod* 14:2277-2278, 1999.

Tarnay CM, Glass KB, Munro MG: Entry force and intra-abdominal pressure associated with six laparoscopic trocar-cannula systems, *Obstet Gynecol* 94:83-87, 1999.

Tarnay CM, Glass KB, Munro MG: Incision characteristics associated with six laparoscopic trocar-cannula systems, *Obstet Gynecol* 94:89-93, 1999.

Tulikangas PK, Nicklas A, Falcone T, Price LL: Anatomy of the left upper quadrant for cannula insertion, *J Am Assoc Gynecol Laparosc* 7:211-214, 2000.

Vilos AG, Vilos GA, Abu-Rafea B, Hollett-Caines J, Al-Omran M: Effect of body habitus and parity on initial Veress intraperitoneal CO_2 insufflation pressure during laparoscopic access in women, *J Minim Invasive Gynecol* 13:108-113, 2006.

Vilos GA, Ternamian A, Dempster J, Laberge PY, the Society of Obstetricians and Gynaecologists of Canada: Laparoscopic entry: a review of techniques, technologies and complications, *J Obstet Gynaecol Can* 29:433-465, 2007.

Whiteside JL, Barber MD, Walters MD, Falcone T: Anatomy of ilioinguinal and iliohypogastric nerves in relation to trocar placement and low transverse incisions, *Am J Obstet Gynecol* 189:1574-1578, 2003.

Yim SF, Yuen PM: Randomized double-masked comparison of radially expanding access device and conventional cutting tip trocar in laparoscopy, *Obstet Gynecol* 97:435-438, 2001.

Instrumentation and Energy Sources Utilized during Laparoscopic Procedures

Jeffrey M. Goldberg M.D.
Andrew I. Brill M.D.

Successful laparoscopic procedures not only require good surgical skills, but also proper instrumentation and operating suite set-up. This chapter reviews an example of an operating room set-up and some of the basic instruments used to accomplish most gynecologic laparoscopic procedures.

Operating Room Set-up

The operating room (OR) should be set up based on the surgeon's preference and the available equipment. An example of a standard set-up is shown in Figure 4-1. The OR table should be electric to facilitate changing patient position and should be capable of steep Trendelenburg position. Stirrups, such as Allens or Yellofins, are necessary for placing the patient's legs in a neutral position. A Mayo stand is used for the vaginal instruments needed for inserting a uterine manipulator and Foley catheter, as well as a hysteroscope if needed. The scrub nurse and laparoscopic instrument table are located between the patient's legs. The video processor, light source, insufflator, main monitor, and recording devices may be on a mobile cart or mounted on movable arms suspended from ceiling booms. (Figures 4-2 to 4-4) Separate video monitors are required for the surgeon and assistant on all but the shortest cases. The monitors are placed directly across from the operators so they can look straight ahead without twisting.

Camera, Monitor, and Recording System

Current endoscopic video cameras are three-chip, with dedicated chips for red, green, and blue for better color fidelity. The video camera head is connected to the laparoscope, and the camera cable is attached to the camera control unit (CCU). The image passes through the camera lens and is converted by a charge-coupled device (CCD) sensor to an electronic signal which is transmitted to the CCU. The CCU directs the signal to the monitors and recording systems. The monitors convert the electronic signals back to an analog image for viewing. The incorporation of high-definition technology is now being used for the laparoscopic camera systems and monitors for better image resolution. Images are also relayed by a cable from the CCU to a VCR, DVD, printer, or other digital recording device. Most video camera heads have buttons for controlling functions such as white balance (for color correction) and light intensity, as well as for activating image capture (Figure 4-5).

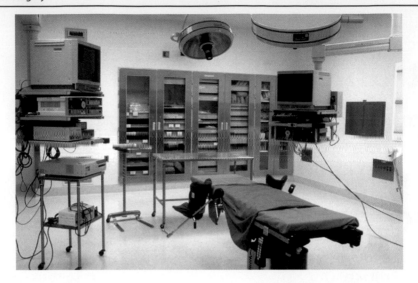

Figure 4-1. This is a typical endoscopy suite with ceiling-mounted equipment.

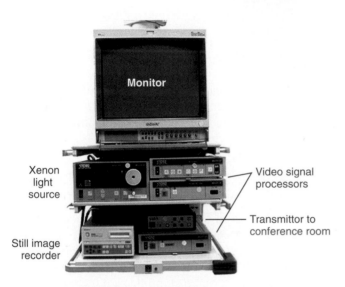

Figure 4-2. The ceiling-mounted instrument holds a high-resolution monitor, CCU, xenon light source, and digital image recorder.

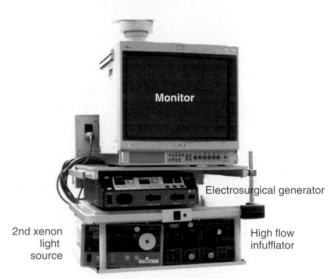

Figure 4-3. The second ceiling-mounted instrument cart has a monitor for the assistant, the electrosurgical generator, a second light source, and a high-flow insufflator.

The Light Source

A bright light source is essential to good image quality. Current light sources utilize xenon, halogen, or mercury bulbs. Xenon is most commonly used for laparoscopic surgery, as it yields higher light intensity and lasts longer; however, it is more expensive to replace. Two types of cables transmit light from the source to the laparoscope: fiber optic and liquid crystal gel cables. Both are fragile and must be handled with care. Damaged cables significantly reduce the amount of light transmitted. Gel cables are capable of transmitting more light to the abdomen but are more expensive and deliver more heat than the fiber optic cables. They are made more rigid by a metal sheath that makes them more difficult both to maintain and to store, and they are only available in 6-foot lengths.

Documentation

Printers and digital capture devices can be connected between the CCU and monitor. Still images can be printed directly from a thermal or ink jet printer or saved to a digital image recorder on a CD or DVD, a flash memory card, or a removable hard drive such as a minidisk. Video can also be recorded on a CD or DVD.

Figure 4-4. All of the electronic equipment can also be housed in a portable cart.

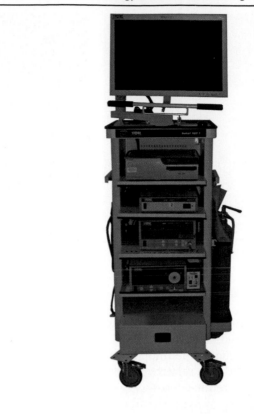

Figure 4-5. The video camera head enables the surgeon to control image size, focus, white balance, and light intensity, as well as to capture images.

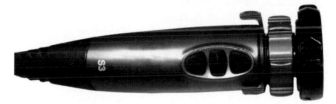

Laparoscopes

The laparoscope consists of a fiberoptic bundle to deliver the light and a quartz rod lens. Recently, digital scopes have been developed that replace the optical lens with a digital sensor at the tip of the scope. A variety of different scope diameters and viewing angles are available to suit the surgeon's preference and the specific tasks to be performed. Scope diameters range from 2 to 12 mm and viewing angles from 0 to 90 degrees (Figure 4-6). Most gynecologic laparoscopic procedures are performed with 5- or 10-mm 0-degree scopes, which afford a straight-ahead panoramic view. Angled scopes of 30 or 45 degrees may be useful to see around a large uterus. Additionally, operative laparoscopes have an offset eyepiece and an operative channel for placing instruments or delivering laser energy. The operative channel necessitates reduction in the size of the lens and fiber optic bundle, compromising image quality.

Insufflators

Insufflators deliver carbon dioxide (CO_2) gas at a controlled rate and pressure to create and maintain the pneumoperitoneum. It is important to understand these controls in order to trouble shoot when the pneumoperitoneum is lost. High pressure and low flow readings on the insufflator are due to obstruction to air flow such as the valve at the trocar sleeve being turned off or the gas tubing being kinked or stepped on. High flow with low pressure indicates a leak. Look for an open valve or cracked gasket on an trocar sleeve or disconnected gas tubing from the trocar sleeve or insufflator. Low flow with low pressure is a sign of an empty CO_2 tank.

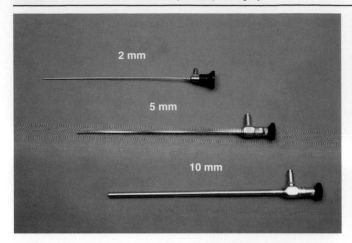

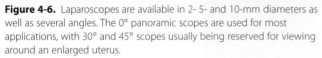

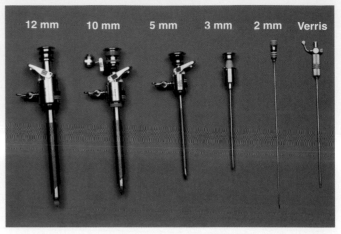

Figure 4-6. Laparoscopes are available in 2- 5- and 10-mm diameters as well as several angles. The 0° panoramic scopes are used for most applications, with 30° and 45° scopes usually being reserved for viewing around an enlarged uterus.

Figure 4-7. Reusable trocars from 2 to 12 mm are shown compared to a Veress needle. Disposable trocars of various diameters are also available.

Extensive operative laparoscopic procedures with multiple ports, frequent instrument exchanges, and use of suction require high-flow insufflators in order to maintain an adequate pneumoperitoneum. The CO_2 is delivered into the peritoneal cavity at 21°C with 0% relative humidity. Two meta-analyses have shown that warmed, humidified gas reduces postoperative pain and analgesia usage. Warmed gas also reduces the incidence of hypothermia. Animal studies have demonstrated that cold, dry CO_2 causes peritoneal desiccation, desquamation of mesothelial cells, and an inflammatory response leading to postoperative peritoneal adhesions. Adhesions did not occur in the group that received warmed, humidified CO_2. The Insuflow system (Lexicon Med, St Paul, MN) consists of a small heating unit and a fluid reservoir at the end of the tubing that connects to the port to provide the humidity.

Trocars

Trocars come in a range in sizes to accommodate laparoscopes and instruments from 2 mm to 15 mm (Figure 4-7). They may be disposable or reusable, and they have various mechanisms, such as trumpet or flapper valves, for preventing loss of the pneumoperitoneum during instrument exchanges. Sharp trocar tips may be conical or pyramidal, and disposable trocars may come with safety shields that slide over the trocar tip as it enters the peritoneal cavity. However, in clinical trials these have not been shown to reduce the risk of injury. Blunt-tip (Hasson-type) trocars are used for open laparoscopy. The trocar sleeve may be sutured to the fascia or held in place by a balloon within the peritoneal cavity.

Newer trocar designs, to try to limit injury from trocar insertion, include an optical trocar and a radially expanding sleeve. The optical trocar has a hollow obturator with a clear plastic conical tip. The laparoscope is placed in the obturator to the base of the plastic tip, enabling the surgeon to perform the initial trocar insertion under direct visualization. The Step trocar (Innerdyne Inc, Sunnyvale, CA) has a radially expanding sleeve that is inserted using a Veress needle as the trocar. The small diameter decreases the risk of injury as does the reduced force required to enter the peritoneal cavity. The Veress needle is removed and a blunt dilator enlarges the sleeve to accommodate 10-mm instruments. An additional benefit is that the fascial defect is claimed to be much smaller than those resulting from conventional sharp trocars making fascial closure unnecessary and reducing the possibility of incisional hernias.

Vaginal Instruments

The main function of the vaginal instruments is to facilitate insertion of the uterine manipulator and/or diagnostic hysteroscope (Figure 4-8). An open-sided bivalve specu-

Figure 4-8. These are the instruments on the vaginal tray. The open-sided Graves speculum facilitates its removal once the uterine manipulator is placed. The Rumi, Cohen, and Hulka uterine manipulators are available depending on the degree of uterine manipulation needed as well as whether chromotubation will be required.

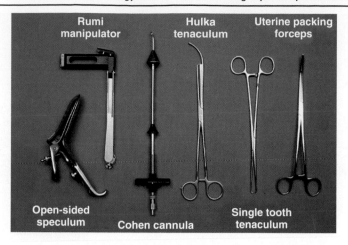

lum is easier to remove once the uterine manipulator is in place. A single-tooth tenaculum on the anterior lip of the cervix provides stability and straightens the uterine axis during cervical dilation or insertion of the uterine manipulator or hysteroscope. We use a uterine packing forceps as a dilator, as well as to assist in the placement of a pediatric Foley catheter into the uterus in select cases for chromotubation or in an attempt to reduce intrauterine adhesions following significant operative hysteroscopic adhesiolysis or myomectomy. A uterine sound or small diameter dilators may also be useful on the vaginal tray.

There are several types of uterine manipulators. The simplest is the Hulka tenaculum, which is essentially a combination of a uterine sound and a single-tooth tenaculum (see Figure 4-8). It provides minimal manipulation and no ability to perform chromopertubation. Jarcho, Rubin, and Cohen-Eder cannulas are hollow metal cannulas with tapered "acorn" tips of various sizes to occlude the cervix. They are held in place with a single-tooth tenaculum. Although they allow for chromotubation, uterine manipulation is limited. Other reusable uterine manipulators, such as the Valtchev or Pelosi, have interchangeable tips to accommodate the size of the uterus and external cervical os. The handle can rotate the tip within the uterus from 0 to 90 degrees of anteflexion, and chromotubation can also be performed.

The disposable HUMI, ZUMI, and Zannati uterine manipulators are hollow plastic tubes with an inflatable balloon at the distal end to keep the device in the uterus and prevent backflow of dye through the cervix during chromotubation (Figure 4-9). Uterine manipulation with these products is usually adequate for most cases. Our preferred device is the RUMI uterine manipulator. It has a reusable handle which may be rotated to provide up to 90 degrees of anteflexion and 60 degrees of retroflexion (Figure 4-10). The handle is ratcheted so the uterine position is maintained without having to hold it in place. Disposable tips of various sizes attach to the handle and are inserted into the uterine cavity. A distal balloon keeps it in place and occludes the cervix for chromotubation. The Koh colpotomizer attachment may be used for laparoscopic hysterectomy.

Suction and Irrigator System

A hollow probe connected to a syringe may be adequate to perform suction and irrigation for minor laparoscopic procedures with minimal bleeding. For more extensive procedures, a battery-operated suction and irrigation device is essential to maintain a clear field of view. The suction tubing is connected to standard OR suction and the irrigation tubing is spiked into a 1- or 3-L bag of lactated Ringer's solution or saline. In addition to its uses for lavage and for smoke and fluid evacuation, the suction-irrigator is extremely useful for blunt dissection and hydrodissection, and can also serve as a backstop for the CO_2 laser. Several types of 5- and 10-mm suction-irrigator probes are available, some of which allow a monopolar instrument to be placed down them.

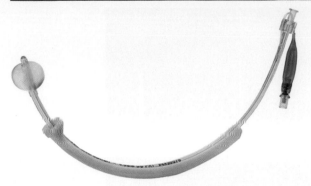

Figure 4-9. The HUMI-type disposable uterine manipulator is a curved plastic tube with a distal balloon to keep the device in place and occlude the cervix during chromotubation.

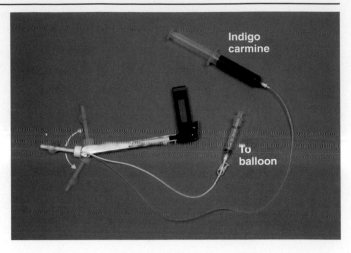

Figure 4-10. The RUMI manipulator consists of a reusable handle with a locking mechanism to maintain the uterus in up to 90 degrees of anteversion and 60 degrees of retroversion; a disposable tip is attached to the handle. The tip comes in several sizes and has a balloon to keep the tip in the uterine cavity and seal the cervix during chromotubation.

Basic Laparoscopic Instruments

Graspers

A variety of graspers are available, ranging from 2 to 10 mm in diameter. The handles may have a locking mechanism and/or a connector for an electrocautery cord (Figure 4-11). A 5-mm atraumatic grasper is employed for most grasping tasks. The Allis grasper is utilized when a more secure purchase of tissue is required for traction, such as for excising pelvic sidewall peritoneal lesions and for ovarian cystectomy. The Maryland grasper is selected for fine tissue dissection and grasping. It also has monopolar cautery capability, allowing for grasping and coagulating bleeding tissue.

Biopsy forceps are used for obtaining small superficial samples from the peritoneum or ovary. The bowel grasper is used for atraumatic manipulation and retraction of bowel as well as to cross-clamp the rectosigmoid colon during the underwater test for rectal integrity (Figure 4-12). The myoma screw and laparoscopic tenaculum serve to manipulate myomas to facilitate their removal. The laparoscopic tenaculum is also useful for manipulating the uterus at hysterectomy (Figure 4-13).

Instruments for Cutting and Coagulation

Reusable and disposable straight and curved Metzenbaum-type scissors with monopolar connection allow both cold cutting and cutting with monopolar current with the scissor tips. Coagulating current can also be delivered to fulgurate and coagulate tissue. Hook scissors are better suited for cutting thick and dense tissue (Figure 4-14). The monopolar hook is used for incising and coagulating tissue. It works well for incising the myometrium over myomas during myomectomy and for dividing the cervix from the vagina at hysterectomy. The unipolar needle is useful when more precise control is needed (Figure 4-15).

A Kleppinger-type bipolar forceps should be available to obtain hemostasis if bleeding is encountered. It is also used to coagulate endometriosis implants (Figure 4-16). The Tripolar device incorporates a cutting blade with bipolar tips to facilitate the coagulation and division of tissue without requiring instrument exchanges (Figure 4-17).

Ligasure technology uses the combination of pressure and energy to create the seal by melting the collagen and elastin in the vessel walls and reforming it into a permanent, plastic-like seal. The tissue is then divided using an internal blade. The Ligasure

Figure 4-11. Laparoscopic handles may be locking or nonlocking and may also have a post for connecting a cord to the electrosurgical generator.

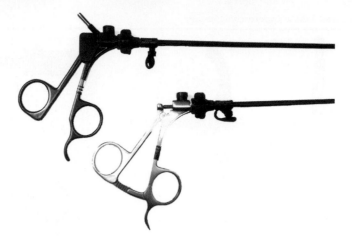

Figure 4-12. The following graspers are commonly employed: **A,** Maryland dissector for fine grasping and dissecting tissue planes. **B,** Allis graspers for a secure hold during ovarian cystectomy and excision of pelvic side-wall peritoneum endometriosis. **C,** General use grasper. **D,** Bowel grasper for atraumatic manipulation of the bowel. **E,** Biopsy forceps for obtaining tissue biopsy specimens.

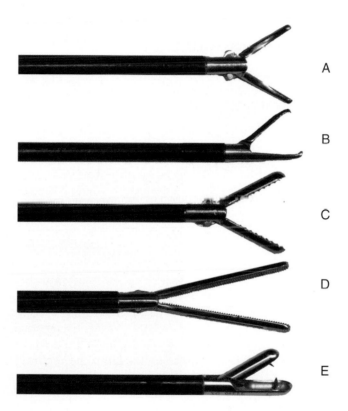

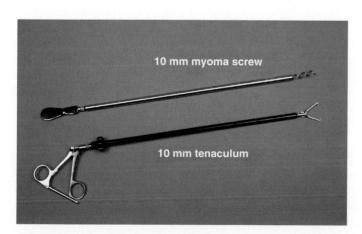

Figure 4-13. The myoma screw is screwed into the myoma, allowing it to be manipulated. The single-tooth tenaculum is used for traction and manipulation of a myoma to be removed or the uterus for hysterectomy. It is also used to grasp tissue to be morcellated.

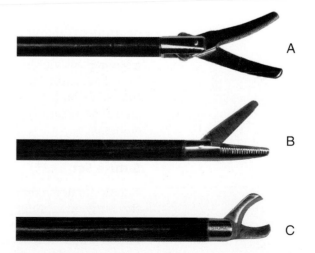

Figure 4-14. Scissors may be reusable or disposable and come with the following tips. They may also have cautery capability for cutting and coagulation of tissue. **A,** Curved Metzenbaum scissors. **B,** Straight scissors. **C,** Hook scissors.

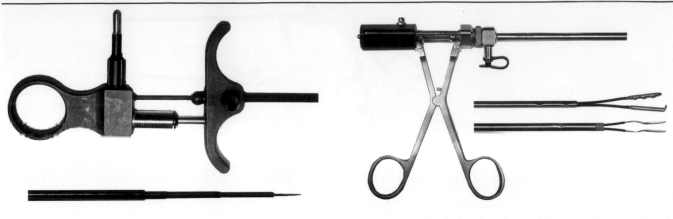

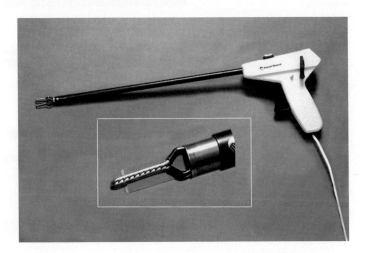

Figure 4-16. The bipolar handle with two of the inserts. The upper insert is better for grasping tissue or bleeding vessels, while the lower insert is better for cauterizing superficial lesions or oozing.

Figure 4-15. The monopolar needle handle (top) serves to deploy and retract the needle tip (center). The needle delivers a high power density for precise cutting with minimal thermal injury. The distal end of the unipolar hook is shown (bottom).

Figure 4-17. The tripolar is a disposable bipolar forceps with a cutting blade to divide the cauterized tissue.

instruments minimize thermal spread to approximately 2 mm. The Harmonic scalpel technology uses ultrasonic energy for both cutting and controlled coagulation. The grasping tips vibrate at 55,500 Hz which causes protein denaturation, forming a coagulum that seals small vessels. When the effect is prolonged, secondary heat is produced that seals larger vessels. Cutting is also possible without generating either smoke or char. The vibration of the ultrasonic scalpel is thought to generate low heat at the incision site.

Suture Set

Needle holders come with a variety of handle styles that may be chosen according to the surgeon's preference. The tips may be curved or straight. Some prefer a "self-righting" tip that facilitates grasping the needle in a position ready to suture while others would rather have the ability to grasp the needle at different angles. Needle holders are preferable to laparoscopic graspers such as Maryland dissectors, because the suture has a tendency to get caught in the instrument jaws of the latter during intracorporeal knot-tying (Figure 4-18).

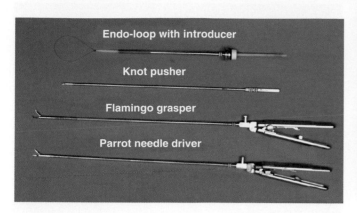

Figure 4-18. The basic suture set contains a needle driver and a grasper to assist with intracorporeal knot tying. The knot pusher slides the extracorporeally tied knot down to the tissue. The Endoloop with introducer is used to place a suture ligature around the tissue, then the preformed slip knot is tightened.

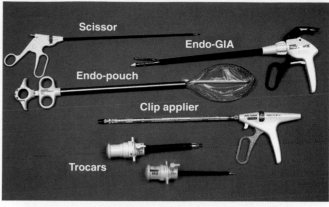

Figure 4-19. This is just a small sample of available disposable instrumentation for laparoscopic surgery. While reusable trocars and scissors are preferred for financial and ecological reasons, their disposable counterparts have the advantage of always being sharp. The Endopouch, automatic clip applier, and Endo-GIA stapling and cutting device have no reusable equivalents.

A knot pusher is used to slide extracorporeally tied knots down to the tissue (see Figure 4-18). The tip of the knot pusher may be open or closed. An EndoLoop is a preformed ligature loop with a slip knot; it is available with different suture materials and sizes. The suture is delivered through a plastic knot pusher. The EndoLoop is back-loaded into an introducer, which is then placed through a 5-mm port. A grasper picks up the tissue to be ligated and draws it through the loop. The end of the plastic knot pusher opposite from the loop is snapped off at a prescored area, and the suture is pulled back, tightening the slip knot.

Clips and Staplers

While not part of the laparoscopy set, clip appliers and staplers may also be used to achieve hemostasis and ligate tissue without cautery or suturing (Figure 4-19). Reusable clip appliers require that each clip be loaded prior to use, whereas disposable automatic clip appliers enable multiple applications without reloading. The Endo-GIA is loaded with a cartridge that delivers rows of staples. The device then cuts the tissue between the rows.

Other Basic Instruments

Solid and hollow blunt probes are used for tissue manipulation. The hollow probe may also be used for suction and irrigation on minor cases.

A laparoscopic needle is used to inject vasopressin for hemostasis as well as to aspirate simple cysts. Conventional laparotomy instruments are also part of the laparoscopy set-up for performing open trocar insertion, closing the fascia of larger port sites, and to be available in the event that conversion to laparotomy becomes necessary.

Tissue Removal Options

The 10-mm claw forceps is ideal for removing excised specimens such as the appendix, fallopian tube, or myoma fragments. It causes a great deal of trauma to tissue and should not be used on viable tissue. The 10-mm spoon forceps is used to remove blood clots, the products of conception following linear salpingostomy for ectopic pregnancy, and hard specimens that are not easy to grasp such as teeth from dermoid cysts or gallstones (Figure 4-20).

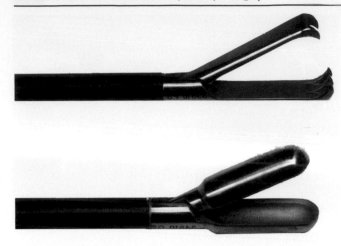

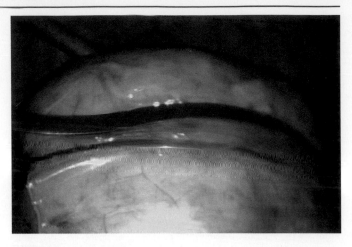

Figure 4-20. The 10-mm claw forceps *(top)*, is used for grasping excised tissue for removal. It should never be used on viable tissue. The 10-mm spoon forceps *(bottom)* is good for scooping up blood clots as well as products of conception from ectopic pregnancies. It is also ideal for removing hard specimens that are difficult to grasp, such as teeth from dermoid cysts or gallstones spilled during cholecystectomy.

Figure 4-21. A large enucleated ovarian cyst is being placed in an Endopouch. The metal rim at top holds the bag in an open position to facilitate depositing the specimen in the pouch. The drawstring below it is then tightened to close the pouch.

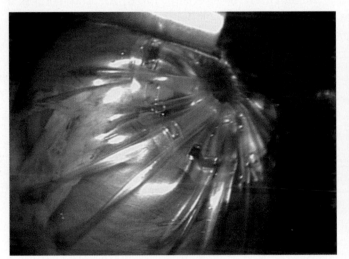

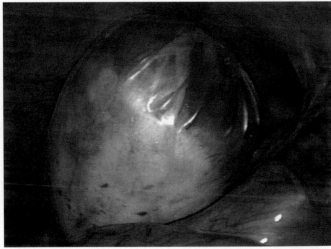

Figure 4-22. The specimen is completely within the bag and the drawstring is closed.

Figure 4-23. The Endopouch device and the 10-mm trocar are removed, and the opening of the bag is brought out through the incision. The specimen is then removed from the bag without spilling its contents into the peritoneal cavity.

Specimen Retrieval Bags

An Endopouch is a disposable plastic bag used for removing specimens while avoiding contamination of the peritoneal cavity or abdominal incision. Examples of specimens that are best removed this way include dermoid, mucinous, and malignant ovarian cysts; tubo-ovarian abscesses; and products of conception (Figures 4-21 to 4-23). Endopouches are available in different sizes and are placed through 10-mm or 15-mm ports. Most have a metal rim that is deployed to hold the pouch in the open position, to assist with placing the specimen in the bag. When the tissue is in the bag, a drawstring closes the bag, and the entire device is withdrawn while bringing the pouch opening outside the incision. Aspirating cyst contents prior to closing the bag facilitates specimen removal. The drawstring is then cut to open the bag and the specimen is removed from the bag with conventional graspers such as Kocher forceps.

Morcellators

Powered morcellators have significantly reduced operating time as well as surgeon fatigue during the removal of large specimens. The morcellator is essentially a hollow tube with a rotating cylindrical blade at the end which is activated by a foot pedal (Figure 4-24). A 10-mm tenaculum is placed through the morcellator sleeve to grasp the specimen and draw it through the rotating blade, thus removing a core of tissue (Figure 4-25). It is vitally important that the rotating blade be kept in full view at all times and that the morcellator never be advanced toward the specimen when the device is activated.

Colpotomy

A colpotomy incision may be used for tissue removal when the specimen is too large for an Endo-pouch, a morcellator is unavailable, and creating a larger skin incision is undesirable. The colpotomy can be made vaginally or laparoscopically, using a mono-polar hook or needle over a sponge stick in the vagina (Figures 4-26 to 4-28). It can be

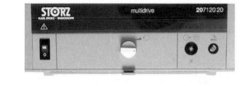

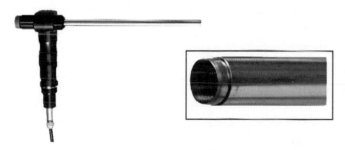

Figure 4-24. The powered morcellator is a hollow metal tube with a cylindrical rotating cutting blade which is activated by a foot switch. A 10-mm tenaculum is placed through the tube. The tissue is grasped and drawn up through the cutting blade.

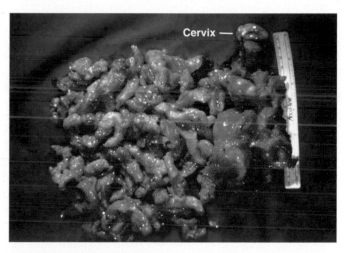

Figure 4-25. The morcellator removes a core of tissue with each pass. This is a large myomatous uterus which has been morcellated.

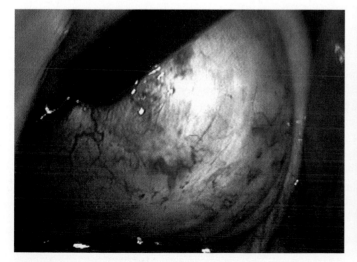

Figure 4-26. A colpotomy incision may be made laparoscopically for tissue removal. A sponge stick in the posterior vaginal fornix indicates where the monopolar hook will make the incision.

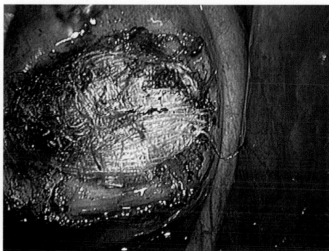

Figure 4-27. The sponge stick is seen in the vagina.

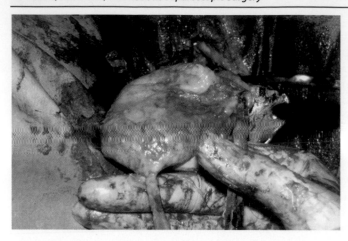

Figure 4-28. A dermoid cyst that was too large for an Endopouch was drained and removed through the colpotomy incision without intraperitoneal spill.

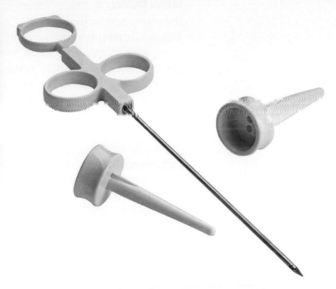

Figure 4-29. The Endoclose needle with 5- and 10-mm Carter-Thomason needle-assist devices facilitate closing the fascia of the port sites.

closed vaginally or laparoscopically using a suture such as 0 Vicryl or PDS with extracorporeal knot tying.

Port Closure

Chernias through 5-mm ports are essentially unheard of, it is only necessary to close the skin. However, the fascia should be repaired on all larger incisions. On thinner patients, S-retractors help to expose the fascial edges, which are closed with a 0 Vicryl suture on a UR-6 needle. A Grice-type EndoClose needle is an easier way to close the fascia on most patients. It looks similar to a Veress needle, but the tip functions as a grasper for holding suture (Figure 4-29). The end of the suture is held with the Endo-Close needle, which is then placed under the skin and through the fascia and peritoneum while observing though the scope in another port. The end of the suture is left in the abdominal cavity while the needle is withdrawn and replaced though the opposite side of the fascial defect. The free end of the suture is picked up with the EndoClose needle and brought out, and the ends are then tied. The Carter-Thomason device facilitates the placement of the EndoClose needle (see Figure 4-29).

Energy Sources

As they do for the laparotomic or vaginal surgeon, energy modalities encompass a key part of the laparoscopic surgeon's armamentarium. These energy-based surgical devices are utilized to attain a number of endpoints including hemostasis and the ability to decisively mobilize, secure, incise, and devitalize tissues. The primary goals of energy-assisted surgery are to conduct hemostatic dissection while producing the least amount of unintended thermal necrosis and subsequent scarification. Excessive thermal injury can be significantly reduced by sound surgical technique borne by a clear understanding of the applied energy-based device and the capacity to distinguish anatomical structures within the surgical field.

Electrosurgery

Household current is low-frequency alternating current (60 Hz [cycles per second]) which on inadvertent contact causes neuromuscular contraction by unremitting nerve depolarization. Much higher frequencies of alternating current produced by contemporary electrosurgical generators (300 to 600 kHz range) prevent this untoward phenomenon.

Electrosurgery is accomplished by the delivery of high-frequency alternating current (AC) from an electrosurgical generator (ESU) into tissue by a smaller active electrode; it is then conducted via low-resistance pathways to a significantly larger dispersive electrode. The electrical current is driven by electromotive force, termed voltage (V), that acts to complete the tissue circuit between these two electrodes. Although electrons are just couriers of charge, their conduction through the resistance (impedance) of living tissue creates significant tissue heating. The ability of electricity to achieve work in the form of heat is called resistive heating. If heated to 100°C, cellular water evaporates (desiccation), hemostasis occurs from blood vessel contraction and the surrounding tissue (coagulation), and collagens convert to glucose, which causes an adhesive effect between the tissue and electrode. Above 200°C, tissue undergoes carbonization and then charring.

Fundamentally, the rate of tissue temperature change will determine whether cutting (vaporization), fulguration, or desiccation (coagulation) occurs during electrosurgery. The rate of tissue heating is moderated by changing current density at the active electrode by manipulation of its surface area (e.g., flat vs. edge).

Electrosurgery is generally governed by Ohm's Law: $V = I \times R$. Power settings keyed into the ESU as watts (W) correspond to the rate of work being done. Since $W = I \times V$, using Ohm's Law $W = I^2 \times R$ and $W = V^2/R$. Consequently, the higher resistance of desiccated or carbonized tissues will cause correspondingly higher output voltages from the electrosurgical generator.

Monopolar Electrosurgery

Monopolar electrosurgery delivers an electrical current via an active electrode (e.g., needle, spatula, and hook) that is conducted via a multiplicity of tissue pathways to the dispersive (return) electrode. Although equal quantities of current are conducted through each electrode, the thermal effects are restricted to the active electrode due to its markedly smaller surface area. Ultimately, the rate of heat production or burn in living tissue is primarily governed by the current density (i.e., surface area). Thermal change by resistive heating is also significantly linked to the application time of energy, called dwell-time.

Electrosurgical Outputs

The labels on a typical electrosurgical generator, "cut," "blend," and "coag," are not uniquely related to specific tissue endpoints. Rather, changing these settings simply varies the output current and voltage in relation to time, called waveforms. The "cut" waveform is continuous and has the lowest peak voltage, while switching to "blend" and then "coag" progressively interrupts current with corresponding higher peak voltages. Since force and voltage are one and the same during electrosurgery, the zone of thermal damage is greater from higher peak voltages associated with blend and then coag waveforms. Newer automatic feedback electrosurgical generators are able to keep the output voltage relatively constant over a wide range of tissue impedance making thermal damage independent of the waveform setting.

Noncontact Electrosurgery

Electrosurgical cutting (vaporization) occurs whenever voltage is enough to ionize the air gap between an active electrode and tissue to cause sparking; this is more apt to occur if arcing remains continuous. At the tissue strike point, cellular water is superheated, causing vaporization by production of highly disruptive steam. Because cut, blend, and coag outputs all deliver sufficient voltage, cutting can be created with any of these waveforms. The width of thermal damage occurring at the margins of these cuts is determined by the peak voltage; it is predictably greatest with the coag waveform. The propensity for wider hemostasis with "blend" or "coag" output can be selectively used for incision during myomectomy, down the broad ligament and along the vaginal fornices during hysterectomy, and across vascular adhesions. Higher-voltage waveforms can also be used to smooth the progress through higher resistance tissues like omentum, subcutaneous fat, and adhesions.

Fulguration is the use of sparking, typically with the "coag" waveform, to coagulate an open surface of small bleeders where tamponade is not practicable. Spark coagulation is limited by a wet surgical field, due to diffusion of current by conduction. Higher peak voltages cause high tissue temperatures resulting in a superficial coagulum that is carbonized and hence easily dislodged.

Some electrosurgical generators (argon beam coagulators) use argon, an inert and noncombustible gas, as part of the current delivery system. At the active electrode, the emitted current is surrounded by argon gas. As the current ionizes the gas, it becomes more conductive than air and provides an efficient pathway to the tissue. This technology is argon-enhanced fulguration. Because the beam concentrates the electrosurgical current, a potentially smoother, more pliable eschar is produced. At the same time, the gas disperses the blood, ostensibly improving visualization.

Contact Electrosurgery

Whenever an active electrode comes into contact with tissue, current density is significantly reduced. Tissue is consequently heated more slowly resulting in more gradual cellular dehydration. As tissue water content is slowly evaporated, the depth of thermal damage is predictably deeper during contact desiccation. Unsurprisingly, the rapid surface heating from higher peak voltages associated with the blend and coag waveforms precludes deeper current penetration and results in more superficial zones of thermal change. Penetration is predictably deepest using the low-voltage cut waveform.

Problems During Laparoscopic Monopolar Electrosurgery

The potential for unrecognized injury to the viscera during monopolar laparoscopic electrosurgery is amplified by the fact that most of the potential conductors are out of the surgeon's field of view. These conductors include the abdominal wall, all metallic trocar sheaths and instruments, somatic and visceral tissues, and the active electrode.

Insulation Failure   Any breach in the insulation along the shaft of an active electrode can provide an alternate pathway for the flow of current. On activation, an electric arc can bridge directly from the electrode to the viscera. Significant thermal damage will occur if the current density is high enough to overheat the tissue. This type of injury is typically unrecognized at the time of surgery.

Direct Coupling   Current becomes directly coupled to another conductor on inadvertent contact, such as with a suction-irrigator or laparoscopic instrument. These currents are safely dispersed into the abdominal wall as long as the instruments are passed through an all-metal cannula. However, a nonconductive plastic cannula will isolate this current, which may take an alternative pathway through adjacent tissue such as bowel. Depending upon current density at the point of contact, a clinically significant burn may evolve.

Capacitive Coupling   Capacitive coupling is the induction of current to a nearby conductor such as a metal trocar through the insulation around an active electrode. This induced current will be conducted and then safely dispersed through the abdominal wall. If the metal trocar sheath is secured to the abdominal wall by a plastic device, the induced current is isolated from the abdominal wall. Accidental contact between the metal cannula and viscera can create an alternate pathway. If the current density is sufficiently concentrated, thermal damage can occur.

Bipolar Electrosurgery

Bipolar instrumentation combines the active and dispersive electrodes, which are separated by a small distance. As opposed to monopolar electrosurgery, the intervening tissue is part of the electrical circuit rather than the patient.

The ability to tamponade tissue between two closely spaced electrodes provides a number of benefits, including the ability to occlude sizable arteries and veins as well as the capability to sufficiently heat tissue despite immersion in fluid. Despite the isolation of current to a discrete volume of tissue, unintended thermal damage may occur beyond its confines. The unmoderated application of current can potentiate a large thermal bloom that spreads steam bubbles through neighboring parenchyma. Excessive thermal spread during bipolar electrosurgery is reduced by ending the current application on tissue blanching and when steam is no longer seen. The use of an in-line ammeter, which meters the flow of current between the tissue and the jaws of the bipolar grasper, may promote overdesiccation of tissue. Because the heating of larger tissue mass generates more heat, excessive thermal damage can be further minimized by using the sides or tips of a slightly open bipolar device to directly tamponade and then desiccate tissue.

More recent innovations in bipolar electrosurgery reflect the development of solid-state, impedance-feedback technology that is capable of delivering either pulsed or continuous output with relatively constant low voltage. These novel electrosurgical generators are paired with an assortment of innovative ligating-cutting devices designed to provide immediate feedback about tissue impedance (resistance) at the tissue site. As the tissue impedance rises with heating and desiccation, power output is maintained by increasing the amount of current rather than by raising the output voltage. Consequently, total energy delivery is substantially less than with conventional bipolar systems. Lower energy deposition predictably reduces carbonization, sticking, smoke, and the lateral zone of thermal necrosis. The paired generator automatically signals complete desiccation (maximal tissue impedance) of the tissue bundle by tonal feedback, which can then be incised by advancing a centrally-set mechanical blade. All of these devices are more effective vessel sealers if the tissue tension is reduced during the application of electrical energy and they can reliably secure blood vessels that are 7 or less in diameter.

To date, there are three bipolar ligating-cutting devices that incorporate low-voltage, impedance-feedback technology for laparoscopic electrosurgery. The LigaSure Vessel Sealing Device (Covidien, Boulder, CO) applies a very high coaptive pressure to the tissue, while generating lower tissue temperatures that are under 100°C. This ruptures the hydrogen cross-links of the triple helical molecules of collagen and elastin which then renature on cooling to form a vascular seal that has high elasticity and can withstand supraphysiologic burst pressures. The second device, the Plasmakinetics Cutting Forceps (Gyrus-ACMI, Minneapolis, MN) delivers the electrical current in pulses that are moderated using impedance feedback. A third device, the EnSeal Laparoscopic Vessel Fusion System (Ethicon, Cincinnati, OH) employs a set of plastic elastomeric jaws embedded with nanometer-sized spherules of carbon that can locally regulate the current. In this device, the centrally set mechanical blade both cuts and squeezes the tissue bundle under extremely high pressure to accomplish vessel sealing and to minimize the lateral thermal bloom associated with steam formation from tissue water.

The clinical utility of new electrosurgical devices is beyond their ability to coagulate and cut tissue. These devices should also be critically evaluated for their propensity to produce smoke and tissue sticking, as well as their ability to perform under varying conditions including fatty and desiccated tissue under variable tissue tension. Each new energy device should also be carefully assessed as a multifunctional laparoscopic instrument for its capacity to grasp, elevate, dissect, and secure tissues of different mass and density.

Ultrasonic Energy

Using the active tissue effects of mechanical energy, ultrasonic blades of the harmonic scalpel can be used to efficiently coagulate and cut tissue using a number of technical maneuvers that correspondingly alter tissue density. Tissue effects from ultrasonic energy are produced by a titanium blade that vibrates nearly 60,000 times per second from an in-line piezoelectric crystal housed in the handle of the device. The high-frequency vibration causes a low-temperature protein denaturation by rupturing the hydrogen bonds of tissue proteins. Tissue is inevitably cut by a process of cavitational fragmentation that naturally evolves from the mechanical vibration and percussive effects of steam emanating through the adjacent tissue. Differing from the volumetric diffusion of thermal spread during electrosurgery, the lateral thermal damage during ultrasonic incision is more limited by the linear nature of energy propagation directed through the tip of the blade. Available ultrasonic blade configurations include a 5-mm curved or hook blade and 5-mm ligating-cutting shears that desiccate and cut tissue after it is secured between a grooved plastic pad and the vibrating blade. This technology is able to reliably secure blood vessels that are 5 mm or less in diameter.

By employing various combinations of blade shape, blade excursion (power setting, 1 through 5), and tissue tension (density), a variety of tissue endpoints can be readily accomplished. Cutting velocity with ultrasonic energy is directly related to blade excursion, tissue traction, and blade surface area (energy density), and is inversely related to tissue density. Thus, the most efficient cutting with the least amount of thermal damage occurs when tissue is placed on tension and lifted or rotated with the edge of a blade set at maximum excursion (setting 5). Coagulation is predictably the inverse of cutting: greatest during tissue relaxation, larger blade surface area, and lowest excursion (setting 1). Therefore, coagulation is best achieved by relaxing tension, minimizing blade excursion, and using a blunt edge or flattened blade surface. Incision of vascular tissue before complete desiccation and coagulation with ultrasonic energy is best avoided by carefully watching the evolution of tissue dehydration, while preventing the natural tendency to lift, rotate, or place forward traction on a coapted tissue pedicle.

Suggested Reading

Amaral JF, Chrostek C: Depth of thermal injury: ultrasonically activated scalpel vs electrosurgery, *Surg Endosc* 9:226, 1995.

Bhoyrul S, Payne J, Steffes B, Swanstrom L, Way LW: A randomized prospective study of radially expanding trocars in laparoscopic surgery, *J Gastrointest Surg* 4:392-397, 2000.

Brill AI: Energy systems for operative laparoscopy, *J Am Assoc Gynecol Laparosc* 5(4):333-349, 1998.

Friedman J: The technical aspects of electrosurgery, *Oral Surg* 36:177-187, 1973.

Honig WM: The mechanism of cutting in electrosurgery, *IEEE Trans Biomed Eng* 22:58-62, 1975.

Luciano A, Soderstrom R, Martin D: Essential principles of electrosurgery in operative laparoscopy, *J Am Assoc Gynecol Laparosc* 1:189-195, 1994.

McCarus SD: Physiologic mechanism of the ultrasonically activated scalpel, *J Am Assoc Gynecol Laparosc* 3:601-608, 1996.

Neudecker J, Sauerland S, Neugebauer E, Bergamaschi R, Bonjer HJ, Cuschieri A, et al: The European Association for Endoscopic Surgery clinical practice guideline on the pneumoperitoneum for laparoscopic surgery, *Surg Endosc* 16:1121-1143, 2002.

Odell RC: Pearls, pitfalls, and advancement in the delivery of electrosurgical energy during laparoscopy, *Probl Gen Surg* 19(2):5-17, 2002.

Peng Y, Zheng M, Ye Q, Chen X, Yu B, Liu B: Heated and humidified CO_2 prevents hypothermia, peritoneal injury, and intra-abdominal adhesions during prolonged laparoscopic insufflations, *J Surg Res* 151:40-47, 2009.

Phipps JH: Thermometry studies with bipolar diathermy during hysterectomy, *Gynaecol Laparosc* 3:5-7, 1994.

Sajid MS, Mallick AS, Rimpel J, Bokari SA, Cheek E, Baig MK: Effect of heated and humidified carbon dioxide on patients after laparoscopic procedures. A meta-analysis, *Surg Laparosc Endosc Percutan Tech* 18:539-546, 2008.

Sammour T, Kahokehr A, Hill AG: Meta-analysis of the effect of warm humidified insufflation on pain after laparoscopy, *Brit J Surg* 95:950-956, 2008.

Sigel B, Dunn MR: The mechanism of blood vessel closure by high frequency electrocoagulation, *Surg Gynecol Obstet* 121:823-831, 1965.

Soderstrom RM: Electrosurgical injuries during laparoscopy: prevention and management, *Curr Opin Obstet Gynecol* 6:248-250, 1994.

Tulandi T, Chan KL, Arseneau J: Histopathological and adhesion formation after incision using ultrasonic vibrating scalpel and regular scalpel in the rat, *Fertil Steril* 61:548–560, 1994.

Vancaillie TG: Electrosurgery at laparoscopy: guidelines to avoid complications, *Gyn Endosc* 3:1143-1150, 1994.

Wu MP, Ou CS, Chen SL, Yen YET, Rowbotham R: Complications and recommended practices for electrosurgery in laparoscopy, *Am J Surg* 179(1):67-73, 2000.

Techniques for Laparoscopic Suturing

Kevin J. Stepp M.D.
Sarah Kane M.D.

 Video Clips on DVD

5-1 Principles and Techniques of Laparoscopic
Suturing (8 minutes/0 seconds)

Introduction

Over the past 30 years, the popularity and application of laparoscopy has revolutionized the field of gynecologic surgery. Many, if not all, abdominal and pelvic procedures have been attempted by laparoscopy. The surgeon should attempt to replicate an open procedure exactly to maximize the success rates and minimize complications while still taking advantage of the decreased morbidity of laparoscopy. With the advent of electrosurgical and other laparoscopic instruments, efficiency can be improved, but the need for suturing in certain situations cannot be ignored. Laparoscopy for major and reconstructive procedures, with or without robotic assistance, has played a role in highlighting the importance of laparoscopic suturing.

Suturing and knot-tying are typically considered the most difficult of the laparoscopic skills to master. The ability to suture proficiently is sometimes all that separates a good laparoscopic surgeon from an expert laparoscopic surgeon. In this chapter we illustrate techniques to develop the skills necessary to form a foundation for proper laparoscopic suturing technique.

Preparation

Trainers

We cannot overemphasize the importance of practice using a laparoscopic trainer prior to attempting suturing skills in patients. There are different options for training; the choice depends both upon their availability at one's institution and upon one's budget.

Laparoscopic box trainers have been a staple of surgical education for the past several decades (Figure 5-1). Box trainers are an affordable option and offer the opportunity to practice positioning, suturing, and knot-tying with real-life tactile feedback, and use of an assistant. High-fidelity computer simulation trainers with or without haptic (tactile) feedback are also now available (Figure 5-2). In addition to teaching basic fundamentals of laparoscopy, these newer virtual-reality training systems can be programmed for gynecology-specific cases such as tubal ligation, ectopic pregnancy, or oophorectomy. Furthermore, many offer specific modules for laparoscopic suturing and knot-tying. They also offer a detailed assessment of performance and improvement, realistic visualization, and some do have tactile feedback. They do not offer use

Figure 5-1. Laparoscopic box trainer.

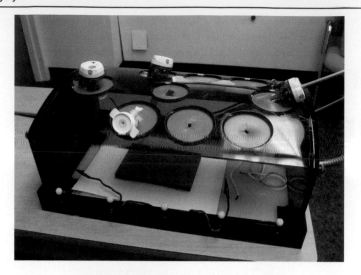

Figure 5-2. High-fidelity laparoscopic simulator. Image provided by Immersion Medical, Inc. Image may not be copied without permission from Immersion Medical, Inc.

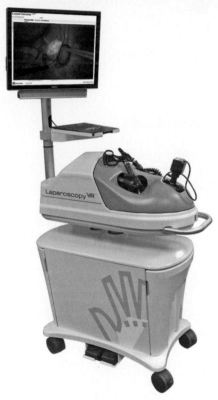

of assistants and do not have the universal affordability and portability of box trainers, but they are becoming more popular where available. Either choice is acceptable for the development of necessary skills prior to experience in the operating room. Ideally, a comprehensive training program would include a combination of the box trainers, animal modules, and high-fidelity simulation.

Surgeon Positioning

Depending on the type of port placement you prefer and the availability of skilled assistants, your positioning may vary slightly. In general, the surgeon should stand facing the patient with no obstructions to a full range of motion. The height of the patient should be adjusted so that the surgeon's arms are comfortably positioned with elbows flexed in a natural position (Figure 5-3). Monitors should be positioned so that the surgeon has a clear forward view without rotation of the body or neck (Figure 5-4). Frequently, when operating in the pelvis, the surgeon will be standing at or above the level of the patient's shoulder. Therefore it is necessary that the patient's arms be

Figure 5-3. Proper surgeon positioning with elbows flexed in a natural position.

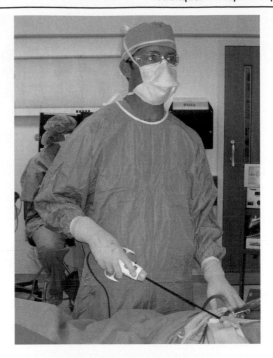

Figure 5-4. Surgical team and patient position.

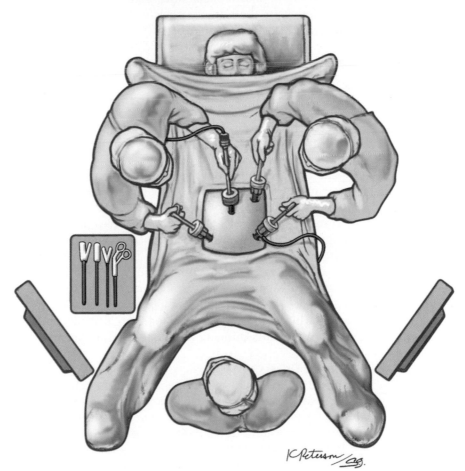

tucked safely at her sides. Supportive slings or "sleds" can accommodate even the most obese patient's arms on the operating table. This provides a more ergonomic and less fatiguing position for the surgeon during laparoscopic suturing.

The choice of port placement is important to reduce fatigue and the need to contort one's body during suturing. Medial or central port locations do not provide for an effective suturing position. Lateral port locations are the most ergonomic and effective.

Figure 5-5. Laparoscopic port positions.

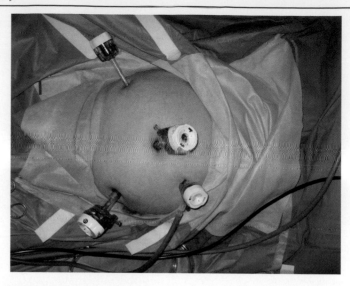

In cases where suturing is required, it is most efficient if the primary surgeon uses two hands. Two ipsilateral ports are easiest and are often preferred. We commonly use a 5-mm left upper quadrant port and a 5-mm port or 10- to 12-mm port in the lower quadrant for suture placement (Figure 5-5). Although cosmesis is a concern, safety and efficiency are the primary measures that allow us to avoid a larger laparotomy incision. Regardless of the number of ports placed, postoperative pain is minor and scarring is minimal. Additional ports should be placed to accomplish the surgery in an efficient manner. As experience is gained, alternative port placement and fewer ports may be considered to improve cosmesis.

Equipment

Ports

When laparoscopic suturing is anticipated, at least one 10-mm port is ideal for introducing suture. A standard 10-mm port will admit a CT-1 needle into the abdomen without difficulty and allow for extracorporeal knot-tying. In many cases the port can be placed in the right or left lower quadrant. However, placement in the umbilicus or suprapubic region is an alternative. In situations when no 10-mm or larger ports are available, alternate techniques to introduce the needle are available and are described later. The type of valve system within the port is important if extracorporeal knot-tying is planned. A flap-valve system, found on most reusable and some disposable ports, will allow the intraperitoneal gas to escape if tension is kept on the suture when tying. To avoid this, a conical valve mechanism is available on many disposable ports. These are better at maintaining an adequate pneumoperitoneum.

Needle Drivers

There are several types of needle drivers. They vary in handle style, type of grasping tip, weight, and right- or left-handedness; a few are pictured here (Figure 5-6). There are also several commercially available suturing devices that are promoted as making suturing easier. But we believe that once you master the techniques illustrated in this book, you will have the skills that allow you to suture with confidence, just as you would in open surgery. Which drivers you choose is a matter of personal preference.

Some needle drivers are self-righting. Self-righting needle drivers have the advantage of presenting the needle perpendicularly to the shaft of the driver quickly and accurately. However, they lack the ability to vary the angle of the needle tip. Some tasks are easier when one can do this. In the video and illustrations we use non–self-righting drivers to demonstrate the ability of perfect positioning (see Video 5-1). A needle driver may have a curved or straight grasping tip. A curved tip increases the mechanical advantage when driving the needle, as well as helping to facilitate intracorporeal

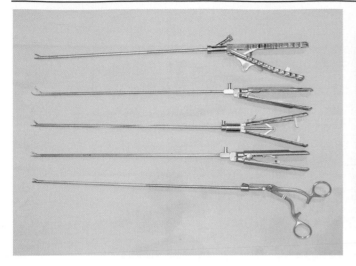

Figure 5-6. Laparoscopic needle drivers.

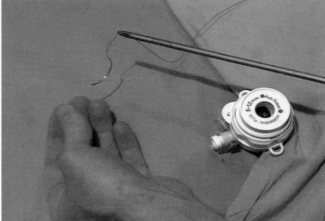

Figure 5-7. Introducing the needle.

tying. A straight tip is useful in either hand and on either side of the patient, and can also be used for intracorporeal or extracorporeal tying.

The use of instruments not specifically designed for suturing, such as graspers or Maryland dissectors, is not recommended. Grasping may not be adequate and the suture can be easily caught in the exposed hinges of these instruments.

Techniques

View DVD: Video 5-1

Introducing the Needle

There are a few techniques for getting the needle into the abdomen. First, the surgeon or the assistant can grasp the suture approximately 3 to 5 cm from the needle and introduce the driver and needle into the abdomen through the 10-mm port (Figure 5-7). The needle is then placed safely in the abdomen and can be grasped for final positioning of the needle. If a full-length suture is used, place a clamp on the end of the suture to prevent it from being pulled into the abdomen.

Another method may improve efficiency by setting the needle up for easy positioning on the driver once in the abdomen. With a needle driver in your nondominant hand, grasp the heel of the needle with the tip of the driver and place the point of the needle along the side of the driver (Figure 5-8). The needle is then placed into the abdomen where it can be easily grasped with another needle driver. This technique can also be used with an assistant introducing the needle from the other side of the patient.

Other methods of needle introduction are available. Sutures with a "ski needle" will pass through a 5-mm port. However, intracorporeal tying must be used when no 10-mm port is available. In certain situations when a small amount of unexpected suturing is required, there is a "back-loading" technique to deliver the suture into the abdomen. A 5-mm port is removed. Outside the body, the needle driver is placed through the port and the suture is grasped a few centimeters away from the needle. The driver and needle are then advanced into the abdomen through the port incision with the port to follow. The port is then replaced into the abdominal wall and the suture does not pass through the port. The suture is pulled completely into the abdomen and the needle and suture are now ready for use. With this technique, intracorporeal tying is necessary.

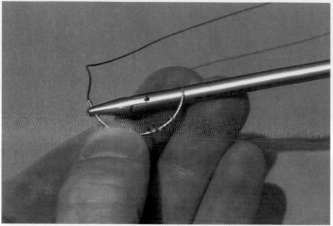

Figure 5-8. Introducing the needle on the driver.

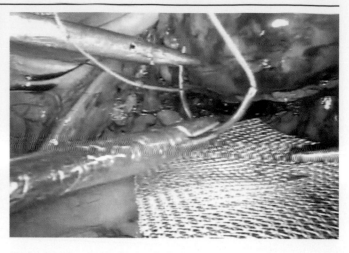

Figure 5-9. Positioning the needle for suturing.

Loading and Positioning the Needle

View DVD: Video 5-1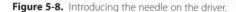

Needle position is perhaps the most important element that can make the suturing process easier or much more difficult. Spending a few extra seconds in positioning will reward the surgeon with a smooth pass and a well-placed suture in the tissue. Depending on the method of getting the needle into the abdomen, there are a few techniques to ensure proper positioning. In the associated video, these methods are demonstrated with non–self-righting drivers.

The free needle technique starts with the needle free in the abdomen. Using the nondominant hand, grasp the point of the needle loosely but securely. With another needle driver in the dominant hand, grasp the suture approximately 3 cm from the heel of the needle. The needle can then be rotated 360 degrees in any plane and positioned perfectly. Release the suture with the dominant hand and load the needle approximately halfway between the heel and point of the needle (Figure 5-9). The position of the needle can be rechecked at this point. If the position is not perfect, regrasp the needle tip with the nondominant hand and repeat the procedure. Alternatively, in cases where the needle is free in the abdomen, the needle may be grasped at its midpoint with the dominant hand and rotated using the suture in a similar fashion as previously described. If an assistant is used, he or she can perform the steps as described for the surgeon's nondominant hand.

The loaded technique is used if the needle is passed into the abdomen preloaded for easy presentation to the surgeon's dominant hand instrument. First grasp the needle approximately halfway between the heel and point of the needle (Figure 5-10). Depending on port placement and the surgeon's needs, this may be all that is needed for proper positioning. Place the tip on the far side of the driver to increase the final angle away from the surgeon. Most likely, small adjustments will need to be made once the needle is transferred to the dominant hand instrument. Using the nondominant hand and grasping the suture approximately 3 cm from the heel of the needle, the needle is positioned properly with gentle traction (Figure 5-11).

The limitations of two-dimensional vision in laparoscopy can make it difficult to visualize the exact position of the needle in relation to the driver. This can be overcome by bringing the laparoscope lens closer to the needle while slowly rotating the driver. This will reveal the needle position.

Suture Choice and Techniques

With a properly loaded needle, the tissue can be approximated in an efficient manner. Either with the nondominant hand or using an assistant, the tissue to be sutured should

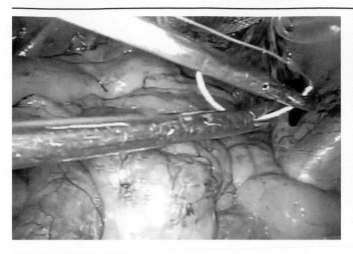

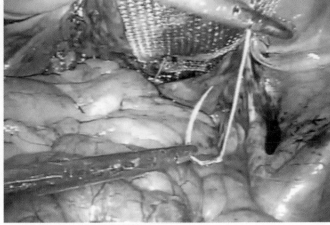

Figure 5-10. Positioning the needle.

Figure 5-11. Positioning the needle.

be elevated and stabilized as the suture is placed. Proper positioning of the needle perpendicular to the tissue is essential, as it is difficult to compensate for improper alignment. Standard laparoscopic instruments do not articulate like the human wrist or robotic instrumentation.

As with open procedures, laparoscopic suturing can be performed with either simple or running suture technique. We usually use simple interrupted sutures. For most applications this type of suture is all that is needed, and it avoids potential difficulties with tangled suture material.

When running suture is indicated, it can be facilitated by first tying a simple interrupted suture at the end closest to the surgeon, either extracorporeally or intracorporeally. The suture is trimmed leaving one end longer. Begin suturing at the opposite end and proceed with the running suture toward the previously tied suture. The assistant is responsible for keeping tension on the suture and preventing entanglement. Once the end of the suture line is reached, the suture can be tied intracorporeally to the tail of the previous suture.

We have found that a monofilament or lubricated braided suture 20 to 30 cm in length works best for running sutures and facilitates pulling the suture through the tissue. Monofilament or braided suture can be used for simple suturing. We recommend a suture approximately 12 to 15 cm in length for intracorporeal tying and 36 cm for extracorporeal tying. For ease of visualization with either suture or tying method, use of dyed suture is imperative.

Tying the Knot

View DVD: Video 5-1

Once the suture is placed to the surgeon's satisfaction, it must be secured. Here we illustrate the techniques of intracorporeal and extracorporeal knot-tying.

Extracorporeal

Extracorporeal knot-tying is performed with a full-length suture and a knot pusher. There are two different types of knot pushers open: and closed end (Figure 5-12 A and B). Which one is used is a matter of surgeon preference; both are described here.

The closed-end knot pusher has a hole at the end of the instrument through which the suture must be threaded before the knot can be pushed down. One end of the suture is threaded through the eye of the knot pusher (Figure 5-13). The needle can be used to ease visualization of this step prior to cutting the needle off. A hemostat or clamp is then placed on the free end to prevent the knot pusher from coming off between throws. Lay the knot pusher aside while keeping slight tension on suture with the one hand holding the clamp. The first throw of the knot is then performed below

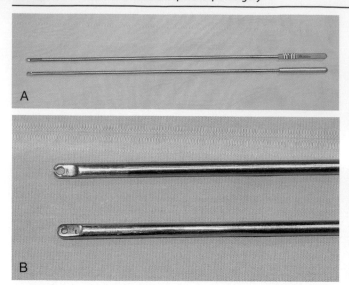

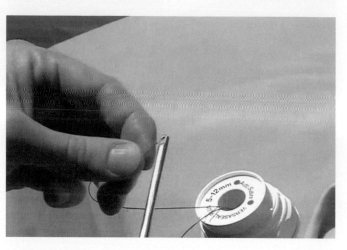

Figure 5-12. A and B, Laparoscopic knot pushers.

Figure 5-13. Extracorporeal knot-tying with a closed-end knot pusher.

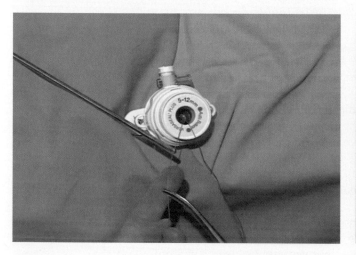

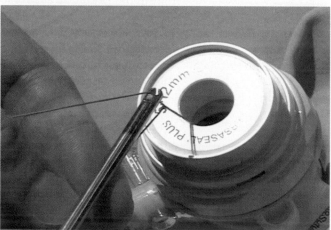

Figure 5-14. Extracorporeal knot-tying with a closed-end knot pusher.

Figure 5-15. Extracorporeal knot-tying with an open-end knot pusher.

the knot pusher. Then, using the knot pusher, slide the knot free of tension gently into the port and into the pelvis to approximate the tissue. Take care that the knot lies down flat. Do not use a surgeon's knot for extracorporeal tying because it makes it difficult to slide down properly. Rather, two half-hitches in the same direction will secure the knot without slipping.

The knot pusher is then pulled back, but not removed from the suture. Lay it aside and keep slight tension on the suture with one hand holding the clamp (Figure 5-14). Each successive knot can then be thrown and pushed down with alternating directions of each throw to produce square knots. Excessive tension on the suture between throws will allow gas to escape.

When the open-end knot pusher is used, the technique is much the same except that the knot pusher is attached to the suture between each throw. This allows the surgeon to place the knot pusher on different ends of the suture if necessary.

In this technique, the clamp is attached to one end of the suture. The surgeon makes the first throw of the suture and holds both ends in one hand. While keeping tension with one hand, the open-end knot pusher is applied to the suture above the knot (Figure 5-15) and the knot is then pushed down into the pelvis and laid flat. The procedure is repeated until the appropriate knot is complete.

When using the open-end knot pusher, it may occasionally slip off the suture before the knot is completely down. This can be remedied in one of two ways. The knot pusher can be reapplied above the knot by zooming the camera in on the knot. If this is too difficult, a closed-end knot pusher can be placed to push down the knot.

Intracorporeal

Intracorporeal knot-tying can be a bit more challenging, but with a few basic techniques and some practice, it can be performed efficiently. Preparation and positioning are keys to performing these techniques successfully. Techniques vary when using a single surgeon or an assistant, so we describe both.

When a single surgeon is preparing for the first throw, we recommend a shorter length of suture than is required for extracorporeal tying. Generally, lengths of 12 to 15 cm will do. Once the suture is passed through the tissue, prepare by grasping the tip of the needle with the nondominant hand so that the heel of the needle and/or suture is parallel with the shaft of the needle driver that the suture will be wrapped around (Figures 5-16 and 5-17). This will form a space through which the needle driver in the dominant hand can pass. Alternatively, positioning the needle so that it forms a "smile-up" position will also provide for adequate space to wrap the suture around the assistant needle driver (Figure 5-17B). Next, position the free end of the suture so it can be easily grasped after the first throw of the suture (Figure 5-18A). If the free end of the suture is not positioned correctly or is too long, the suture may slide off the needle driver, decreasing efficiency (Figure 5-18B). A surgeon's knot is used, similar to an instrument tie in open surgery. By moving the needle driver in the dominant

Figure 5-16. Positioning the needle and suture for intracorporeal knot-tying.

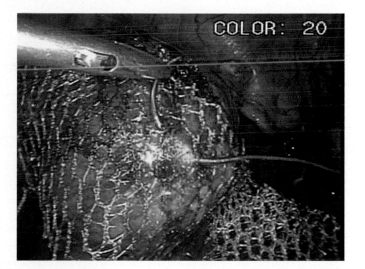

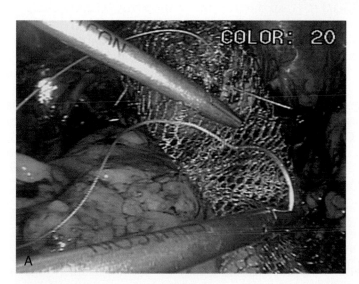

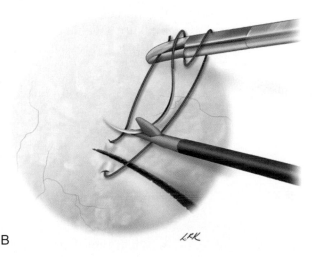

Figure 5-17 A, Positioning needle so the suture is parallel to the assistant needle driver. B, Positioning the needle for intracorporeal tying using the "smile-up" technique.

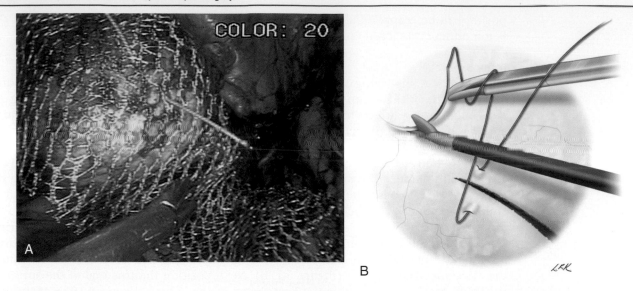

Figure 5-18 A and B. Position the free end of the suture for easy grasping. Improper position of the free end of the suture makes it difficult to grasp after the suture is wrapped.

Figure 5-19. Performing a surgeon's knot—ready for the first wrap.

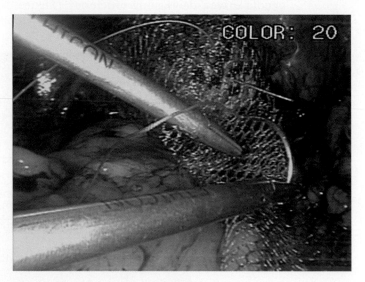

hand, two passes are made to wrap the suture around the driver (Figures 5-19 through 5-21). The driver is then advanced to grasp the free end of the suture (Figure 5-22). As the knot is tightened, pull primarily with the needle end to maintain adequate length for the next throw and leave a short tail for tying (Figures 5-23, 5-24A and B). Again, the knot should lie flat on the tissue. This procedure is repeated, alternating directions with each throw and laying the knots flat, until the knot is complete (Figures 5-25 through 5-29).

When an assistant is present, the key is to alternate each throw between surgeons to maintain square knots. Assistants can be useful to expose and present tissue or to help manipulate the needle. One surgeon should present the needle so that the suture is coming off parallel to the other's needle driver and the first throw is made. Then grasp the free end and tighten the knot, taking care to maintain an adequate length for future knots. The surgeons switch roles and the procedure is repeated.

Clinical Pearls

We can offer some tips that may help when beginning in laparoscopic suturing.

- When tying extracorporeally, pneumoperitoneum may be lost if too much tension is placed on the suture or a flap-valve port is used. This can be remedied by technique or by port choice.

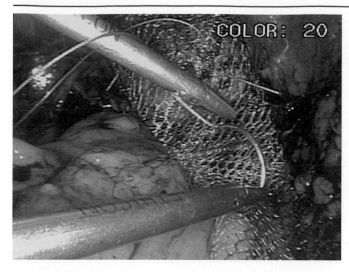

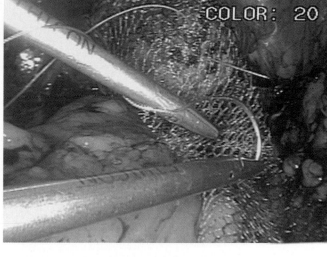

Figure 5-20. Performing a surgeon's knot—complete the first wrap.

Figure 5-21. Performing a surgeon's knot—complete the second wrap.

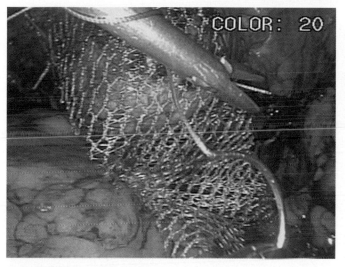

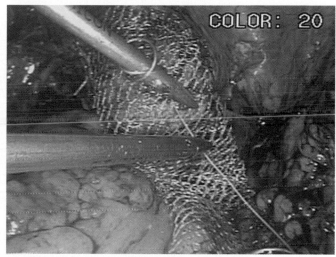

Figure 5-22. Intracorporeal tying—grasp the free end.

Figure 5-23. Intracorporeal tying—tighten the knot.

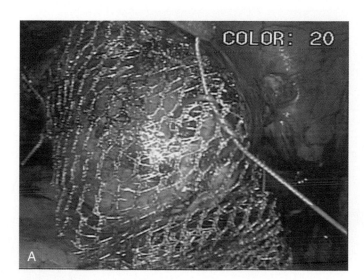

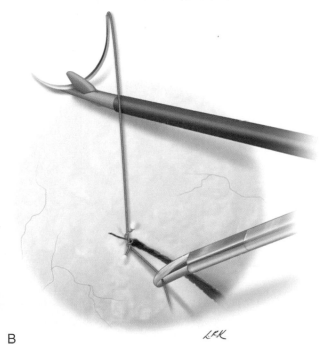

Figure 5-24. A and B, Surgeon's knot lies flat.

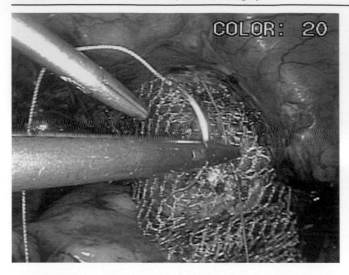

Figure 5-25. Intracorporeal tying—performing the second throw in the opposite direction.

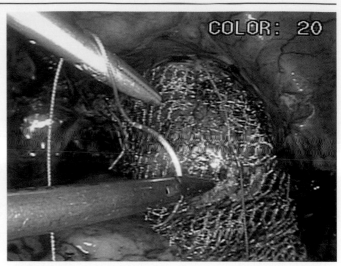

Figure 5-26. Intracorporeal tying—performing the second throw in the opposite direction.

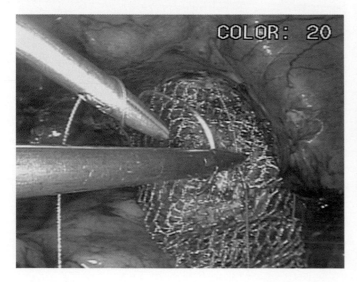

Figure 5-27. Intracorporeal tying—performing the second throw in the opposite direction.

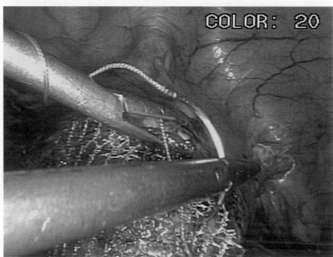

Figure 5-28. Intracorporeal tying—grasp the free end.

Figure 5-29. Intracorporeal tying—the knot lies flat.

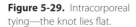

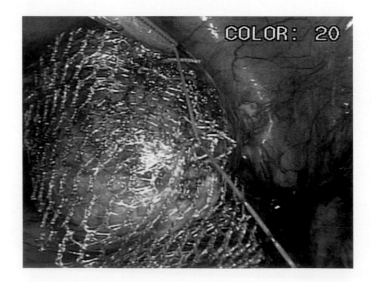

- If the suture becomes twisted and does not lie flat, it can be untwisted by rotating a knot pusher around the knot until the twist is removed.

- It may be necessary to navigate around structures and corners within the pelvis. Care can be taken to prevent the suture from getting caught on or damaging an adjacent tissue. As the knot is pushed down, push it in a direction away from the structure to be avoided. Once the knot is beyond the obstacle, it can then be slid down gently by keeping tension on the suture and angling the knot pusher as it is advanced.

- Granny knots may also be used with extracorporeal or intracorporeal tying. Making each of the first two throws in the same direction will create a sliding knot allowing the suture to be free of tension as the next throw is made.

Conclusion

The present and future of gynecologic surgery lies in laparoscopy, and the need for surgeons to develop skill in laparoscopic suturing techniques has become more evident. Although surgical techniques are constantly evolving with development of robotic-assisted laparoscopy, reticulating instruments, and laparoendoscopic single-site (LESS) surgery utilizing only a single laparoscopic port, the basic techniques of suturing remain unchanged. After identifying important preoperative factors such as proper positioning, equipment choice, and use of assistants, laparoscopic suturing is a skill that can be learned with patience and practice.

Suggested Reading

Koh C: *Laparoscopic Suturing in the Vertical Zone Karl Storz*, Tuttingen, Germany, 2004

Laparoscopic Management of Adnexal Masses

Richard D. Drake M.D.
Tommaso Falcone M.D.

 Video Clips on DVD

6-1 Laparoscopic Management of a Variety of Adnexal Masses including Laparoscopic Removal of a Dermoid Cyst, Removal of an Adnexal Mass in a Pregnant Patient, and a Laparoscopic Cystectomy of a Benign Cyst (8 minutes/ 4 seconds)

6-2 Laparoscopic Management of an Adnexal Mass in a Kidney Transplant Patient (7 minutes/57 seconds)

6-3 Laparoscopic Management of an Ovarian Remnant (8 minutes/28 seconds)

Introduction

Adnexal masses of both benign and malignant etiologies can be found in women of all ages. Studies predict that up to 10% of women will undergo surgical management of an adnexal mass for suspected malignancy at some point in their lives. The various etiologies found during surgical evaluation are listed in Table 6-1. These masses/cysts may cause severe symptoms of pelvic pain, pressure, or fullness, or they may remain completely asymptomatic and only be found serendipitously, either on examination or on imaging studies ordered for another indication. With the advent of laparoscopy and advancements in surgical techniques, we have been able to add minimally invasive surgery into the realm of evaluation and treatment of these lesions with decreased morbidity. Several randomized clinical trials have shown that laparoscopic management of benign adnexal disease is associated with faster recovery, decreased pain, and less analgesic use, fewer wound complications and, possibly, fewer de novo adhesions compared with laparotomy. However, proper patient selection is necessary to utilize this diagnostic and often therapeutic tool appropriately.

The incidence of malignant adnexal masses varies with the different stages of a woman's reproductive life. In the prereproductive and early reproductive years, ages 10 through 19, an adnexal mass has up to an 8.2% to 35% risk of malignancy. In reproductive and postmenopausal women, the risk of cancer is 5% to 18% and 30% to 60%, respectively. In general, a mass that is highly suspicious for cancer should be treated by laparotomy. An adnexal mass, whether found on physical examination or on radiologic imaging, usually requires further assessment for a definitive diagnosis. Several imaging modalities (ultrasound [US], MRI, CT, and even PET scans) and laboratory assays (CA-125, most commonly) have attempted, with varying results of accuracy, to identify factors which would discern the potential for malignancy. The underlying thought process when assessing an adnexal mass is: what is the potential for cancer? The Society of Gynecologic Oncologists (SGO) and the American College of Obstetricians and Gynecologists (ACOG) have developed recommendations/guidelines for those masses at a higher risk of malignancy that will need surgical evaluation; these are listed in Table 6-2.

Table 6-1 Etiologies of Pelvic Masses

Ovary	*Uterus*
Functional cysts • Follicular • Corpus luteum • Hemorrhagic corpus luteum Endometrioma Polycystic ovaries Torsion Neoplasm (benign and malignant) • Epithelial • Germ cell (i.e., benign teratoma) • Stromal	Cornual pregnancy (ectopic) Myoma • Degenerative • Pedunculated • Parasitic Sarcomas Müllerian abnormalities
Gastrointestinal	*Fallopian Tubes*
Appendicitis Abscess Carcinoma Endometriosis Feces Diverticulosis Inflammatory bowel disease	Ectopic Hydrosalpinx Pyosalpinx Tubo-ovarian abscess Cancer Paratubal cyst
	Genitourinary
	Bladder—neurogenic Pelvic kidney Urachal cyst
Metastatic lesions	*Miscellaneous*
Breast GI Endometrial	Hematoma Retroperitoneal lesion (sarcoma) Lymphoma Inclusion cyst Hernias Lymphocele Tuberculosis

Table 6-2 Recommendations for Referral to Gynecologic Oncologist for Possible Ovarian Cancer Mass (Society of Gynecologic Oncologists and American College of Obstetricians and Gynecologists)

Premenopausal Women (typically younger than 50 years of age)	Postmenopausal Women
CA 125 > 200 IU/mL	CA 125 > 35 IU/mL (any elevation above the normal range)
Ascites	Ascites
Metastatic lesions	Metastatic lesions
Family history of ovarian or breast cancer in a first-degree relative	Family history of ovarian or breast cancer in a first-degree relative
	Nodular or fixed pelvic mass

Preoperative Work-up

A thorough work-up, and sometimes, conservative management, can prevent unnecessary surgery that may lead to early menopause or surgical complications. High-risk symptoms such as new-onset abdominal bloating, early satiety, or abdominal and pelvic pain require investigation. A thorough work-up should include a history, physical examination, imaging studies, and laboratory studies.

A thorough history should include questions about:

Symptoms (pain, abdominal distention, early satiety, bloating, pelvic fullness)

Surgical history (laparotomies, endometriosis surgery, complications)

Family history (ovarian, breast, GI cancers)

A physical examination should evaluate the chest for pleural effusions, the breasts for masses or discharge, and the abdomen for ascites; a good pelvic exam should be performed to assess for masses, nodularity, or tenderness. Imaging of suspected/presumed adnexal masses to enhance the pelvic exam may include pelvic US evaluation, CT scan of abdomen and pelvis if suspicion of ovarian cancer is high, MRI, and PET scan. Laboratory studies to assess the adnexal mass should include CA-125 for all patients, and if the patient is younger than 30 years of age, alpha-fetoprotein (AFP), lactate dehydrogenase (LDH), human chorionic gonadotropin (HCG), inhibin, and carcinoembryonic antigen (CEA).

In asymptomatic women, vaginal ultrasound is the imaging modality of choice. CA-125 is still the only consistently accepted standard tumor marker. It is elevated in approximately 50% to 60% of stage 1 ovarian cancers. It is increased in benign conditions and difficult to interpret in premenopausal women. Premenopausal women with markedly elevated levels (CA-125 > 200 IU/mL) should have a consultation with a gynecologic oncologist (Table 6-2). Any CA-125 elevation in a postmenopausal woman with a pelvic mass is highly suspicious for malignancy and should be referred to a gynecologic oncologist.

Most adnexal masses in pregnancy can be managed without intervention. There is a low risk for malignancy and acute complications. If surgery is required for symptomatic or suspicious adnexal masses, the second trimester of pregnancy offers the lowest risk.

Patient Selection and Basic Laparoscopic Techniques

While most adnexal masses in reproductive-age women will be benign, to fully assess the actual etiology, surgical intervention is often necessary, especially if the mass is enlarging, symptomatic, or worrisome for malignancy based on imaging, lab results, or physical examination. Simple cysts up to 10 cm in diameter in asymptomatic women can be followed without intervention in all women. The options for surgical assessment include either an exploratory laparotomy or laparoscopy.

Roman and coauthors evaluated the probability of diagnosing pelvic malignancy by US pelvic exam, and CA-125 criteria to determine the most appropriate surgical management (Table 6-3). The decision as to which avenue to pursue will depend largely on the degree of suspicion of underlying cancer, the patient's medical and surgical history, and the skill of the surgeon. In general, laparoscopic surgery could be considered in adnexal masses which have a low to intermediate risk of malignancy, and in selected cases of high risk where it seems possible from radiologic exam that the etiology of the lesion may be a dermoid, an endometrioma, or a metastasis from another

---

Table 6-3 Risk Assessment

Low-risk features of adnexal masses—Can be managed by laparoscopy
- Unilocular cyst less than 10 cm
- CA-125
  - Less than 200 IU in premenopausal women
  - Normal range in postmenopausal women

Intermediate risk—Can be assessed and potentially managed by laparoscopy
- Ultrasound characteristics
  - Thin septations
  - Dermoid features
  - Endometrioma
- CA-125
  - Less than 200 IU in premenopausal women
  - Normal range in postmenopausal women

High risk—Should be managed by laparotomy
- High-risk ultrasound features
  - Solid components
  - Thick septa
  - Mural nodularity
- Any elevation of CA-125 in postmenopausal women
- CA-125 over 200 IU/mL in premenopausal women

source. Laparotomy should be considered in all patients with a high index of suspicion for malignancy (see Table 6-3) (i.e., ascites, carcinomatosis of the abdomen on CT, large [>10 cm] solid masses) or if the mass will be technically difficult to remove safely laparoscopically (e.g., 25-cm pelvic mass).

Laparoscopy allows smaller, more cosmetic incisions when exploring a mass. This technique also allows magnification of the pelvic area to further assess issues such as endometriosis and to dissect these areas more fully. Minimally invasive surgical techniques can shorten hospital stay and recovery time. Careful abdominal entry, with meticulous surgical dissection and mass removal (preferably intact without intra-abdominal rupture) can limit potential risks of the laparoscopic approach in women with a final diagnosis of cancer.

The general principles that should be followed with all cases of adnexal disease if there is a suspicion of malignancy include:

- Examination under anesthesia
- Inspection, biopsy, and frozen section
- Pelvic and abdominal washings
- Be prepared to convert to laparotomy if malignancy is confirmed
- Do not rupture a cyst in the peritoneal cavity
- Place specimens in a bag before removal

Case 1: Unilateral Salpingo-oophorectomy, Retroperitoneal Approach

A 45-year-old woman, gravida 2 para 2, presented for her annual physical examination. Pelvic examination revealed a fullness in the right adnexa. She was asymptomatic and her Pap tests were normal. She had completed her family. A pelvic ultrasonogram revealed a 5 cm cyst with a thin septum in the center. A CA-125 level was normal. The patient had no medical problems and no history of past surgery. After informed consent was obtained, it was decided to proceed to unilateral salpingo-oophorectomy with possible conversion to laparotomy if malignancy was identified.

Surgical Techniques

1. Step 1 as above.
2. In this case, a direct trocar insertion through the umbilicus was used. After injection of Marcaine (bupivacaine) 0.25%, an incision was made in the umbilicus and a 5-mm trocar was inserted. Pneumoperitoneum was established after confirming intraperitoneal location. After inspection of the insertion site showed no evidence of complications, additional trocars were placed in the left and right lower quadrant areas under direct laparoscopic visualization in order to avoid any trauma to the underlying organs. The left ovary was normal.
3. Pelvic washings were taken with normal saline, and inspection of the entire abdomen and pelvis was performed, paying careful attention for possible metastasis, adhesions, and aberrant structures.
4. The peritoneum lateral to the right ovary and tube was incised (Figure 6-1) and the retroperitoneum entered. The ureter was identified on the medial leaf of the broad ligament (Figure 6-2).
5. An additional opening was made in the peritoneum below the ovarian vessels (Figure 6-3).
6. In this case, the ovarian vessels were doubly ligated with Vicryl using extracorporeal knot-tying technique (Figure 6-4). The vessels were then cut between the sutures (Figure 6-5). Bipolar cautery can also be used for this step.
7. At the level of the uterus, the utero-ovarian ligament was coagulated using bipolar cautery and cut. The resected ovary was then collected in a 10-mm endoscopic bag for removal (Figure 6-6).

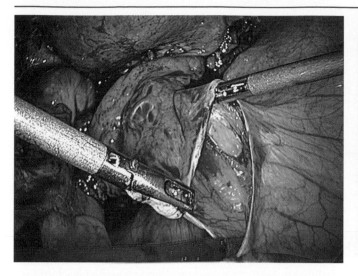

Figure 6-1. The peritoneum lateral to the right ovary and tube is incised and the retroperitoneum entered.

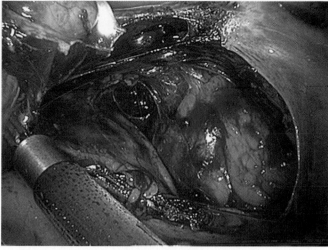

Figure 6-2. The right ureter is identified on the medial leaf of the broad ligament.

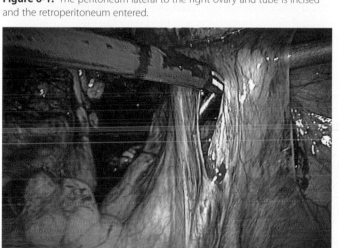

Figure 6-3. An additional opening is made in the peritoneum below the right ovarian vessels.

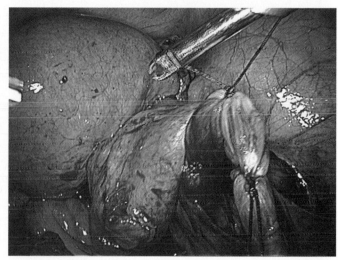

Figure 6-4. The ovarian vessels are doubly ligated with Vicryl, using extracorporeal knot-tying technique.

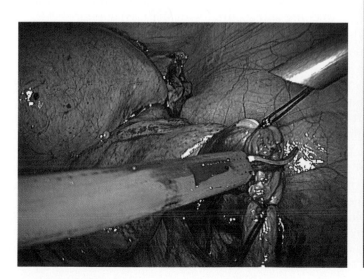

Figure 6-5. The vessels are then cut between the sutures.

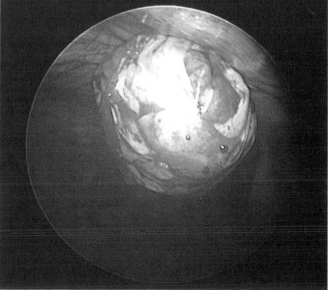

Figure 6-6. The resected ovary is then collected in a 10-mm endoscopic bag for removal. This is a view under the right lower quadrant port.

8. Dry towels were placed on the abdomen around the bag opening to absorb any spillage. The cyst was ruptured and drained while still in the bag. The bag with the decompressed cyst was delivered through the 10-mm incision without any intra-abdominal spillage.

9. After removal of the other ovary, the areas of dissection were inspected for hemostasis, both with normal insufflation and with reduction of the pneumoperitoneum. Hemostasis was obtained, and the 10 mm port site fascia was closed with an endofascial closure device under direct laparoscopic visualization without any complications. The port site skin was closed with a subcuticular stitch using 4-0 suture.

The patient was sent home after surgery with narcotic analgesics and had no complications in the postoperative period.

Case 2: Complex Mass in a Pregnant Patient

 View DVD: Video 6-1

The patient is a 42-year-old pregnant female at 14 weeks with a persistent complex right pelvic mass, 10 cm in size. She was noted to have the cyst since her first ultrasound at 7 weeks' gestation and it has persisted to 14 weeks. The persistence and complexity of the cyst warranted further investigation. Therefore the proposed plan was to manage the cyst laparoscopically in order to minimize surgical recovery, decrease the potential for adhesive disease, and to potentially decrease stimulation of the uterus.

A thorough understanding of previous surgeries (i.e., previous cesarean sections, cholecystectomy, any left upper quadrant surgeries), any anatomic/medical problems which could effect insertion (i.e., situs inversus, splenomegaly, hepatomegaly, cirrhosis) is paramount for planning surgical strategy. This patient had no anatomic or medical problems, no previous surgeries, and therefore no contraindications to laparoscopy. Prophylactic antibiotics, consisting of a cephalosporin, were given just before surgery. The patient gave consent for possible open approach if cancer was identified, with the plan for surgical staging with no interruption of the pregnancy; gynecologic oncology standby was available for surgery.

Surgical Techniques

1. The decision was made in this case to use an open laparoscopic technique to place the umbilical trocar, to decrease the risk of uterine trauma with initial insertion. The umbilical area was injected with 0.25% Marcaine for additional analgesia. A scalpel was used to make a 10-mm incision, and dissection was continued down to the fascia. The fascia was then sutured with 0 Vicryl suture, both to hold the trocar in place and to close the defect at the end of the case. A 10-mm blunt trocar was then inserted through the opening and secured with the fascial sutures.

2. After proper insertion of the umbilical trocar with no evidence of trauma to the surrounding structures noted, the accessory trocars were placed under direct laparoscopic visualization, one in the left mid-quadrant area lateral to the epigastric vessels, and one opposite it in the right mid-quadrant. Pelvic washing with normal saline solution was performed and collected in case this was a cancerous lesion. The abdomen and pelvis were then inspected for any possible excrescences, nodularity, or metastasis. The pelvic mass was also inspected for excrescences or nodularity, because they may be signs of more advanced malignancy. Seeing no high-risk features, the oophorectomy was continued.

3. Laparoscopic surgery in pregnancy requires more attention to the peritoneal insufflation pressure. It should be kept at less than 15 mm Hg usually around 13 mm Hg. The anesthesiologist should adjust minute ventilation to keep the partial pressure of CO_2 lower than usual to reflect the compensated respiratory alkalosis of pregnancy. This adjustment is important to prevent fetal acidosis from transperitoneal absorption of the CO_2 pneumoperitoneum.

4. The ureter was identified transperitoneally, as was the infundibulopelvic (IP) ligament (Figure 6-7). The IP ligament was then cauterized (in this case with bipolar

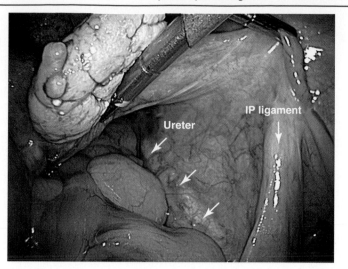

Figure 6-7. The right ureter visualized at the pelvic brim through the peritoneum. IP, infundibulopelvic ligament.

cautery) and transected. Serial dissection was then performed up to the utero-ovarian ligament. This ligament was also cauterized and transected to completely mobilize the adnexa. Once mobilized, the ovary and tube were collected in a 10-cm endoscopic bag through the 10-mm trocar.

5. The 10-mm trocar was removed and the bag opening was pulled up through the 10-mm trocar site. The bag was surrounded with absorbable towels and was grasped with clamps to prevent inadvertent loss of the bag back into the abdomen. The cyst was then drained and the ovary and tube were delivered out of the abdomen while still inside the endoscopic bag. The specimen was sent to pathology to determine the etiology of the cyst. The pathology report returned with the diagnosis being a benign serous cystadenoma.

6. The area of dissection was reinspected for hemostasis, while reducing the insufflation pressure to around 5 mm Hg. With hemostasis noted, the 10-mm umbilical port was removed under laparoscopic visualization and the fascia was closed with the previously placed Vicryl sutures. The left and right 5-mm lateral trocars were removed under direct laparoscopic visualization in order to identify any bleeding from injured vessels. The incision areas were irrigated and hemostasis noted. The skin at the trocar sites was closed with 4-0 Monocryl in subcuticular fashion and adhesive strips were placed over this for additional support. The fetal heart tones were confirmed by Doppler at the end of the case to confirm viability and the patient was taken to the recovery room.

Case 3: Cystectomy for a Dermoid Cyst

 View DVD: Video 6-1

This patient is a 27-year-old nulliparous female who presented for evaluation of a 10 cm × 8 cm right adnexal mass identified on bimanual examination. An ultrasonographic evaluation was most consistent with a dermoid cyst. Because the characteristics were most consistent with a benign dermoid cyst, a laparoscopic approach was a reasonable option. She had no previous surgeries and desired to preserve fertility. Preoperative evaluation included serum CA-125, AFP, LDH, and HCG levels, all of which were within normal limits.

The technique for a similar case will be presented; it differs only in that there was a left-sided dermoid cyst.

Surgical Techniques

1. The patient was placed in the dorsal low lithotomy position and prepped. A third-generation cephalosporin was given for prophylaxis. The intraumbilical area was injected with 0.25% Marcaine for additional analgesia and a 5-mm incision was made. A 5-mm optical trocar was then inserted into the abdomen under direct visualization through the trocar. No complications were noted with inspection of the entry site. Additional Marcaine was infiltrated at the sites where the ancillary trocars were inserted in the left and right lower quadrants under direct laparoscopic visualization. Pelvic washings were taken, and the pelvis and upper abdomen were inspected.

2. After identifying the affected left ovary and seeing no other obvious sources of malignancy, an ovarian cystectomy was performed. The ovarian cortex over the cyst was incised with monopolar cautery (Figure 6-8) at low voltage, 15 W. Higher voltage has a higher probability of cyst rupture. Alternatively, scissors can be used.

3. The dissection plane can be identified by hydrodissection (Figure 6-9) with a suction-irrigator device, being careful not to rupture the cyst. Once the plane between the ovarian cortex and the cyst base is developed, it can be sharply and bluntly dissected (Figure 6-10).

4. The cyst was collected in a laparoscopic bag brought up to the body surface (Figures 6-11 and 6-12). While still in the bag, the cyst was opened, drained, and delivered out of the abdomen (Figure 6-13).

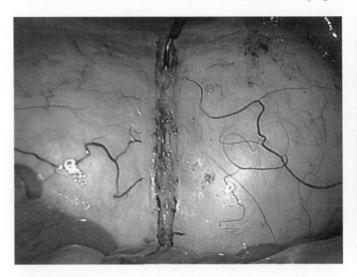

Figure 6-8. At the start of a cystectomy, the ovarian cortex over the cyst is incised with monopolar cautery at low voltage, 15 W.

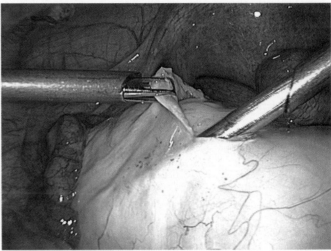

Figure 6-9. A dissection plane can be identified by hydrodissection using a suction-irrigator device. It is important to be careful not to rupture the cyst.

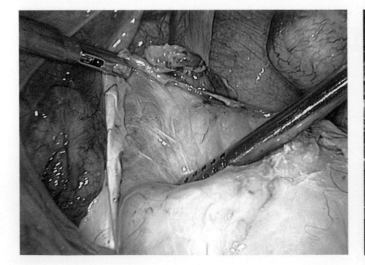

Figure 6-10. Once the plane between the ovarian cortex and the cyst base is developed, it can be sharply and bluntly dissected.

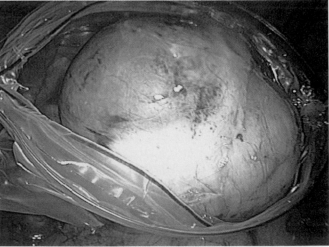

Figure 6-11. The cyst is collected in a laparoscopic bag.

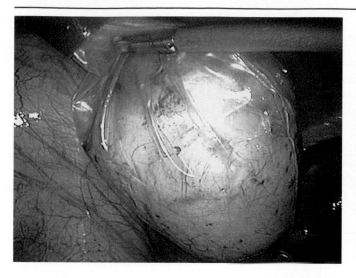

Figure 6-12. The cyst is brought up to the port site.

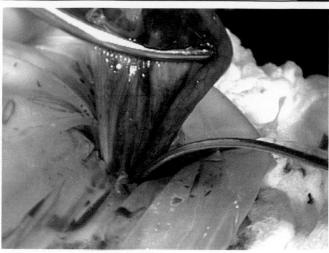

Figure 6-13. While still in the bag, the cyst is opened, drained, and delivered out of the abdomen.

Figure 6-14. The left ovary is reinspected for hemostasis, and finding no bleeding

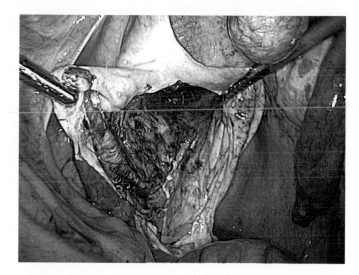

5. The left ovary was reinspected for hemostasis, and with no bleeding found (Figure 6-14), the trocars were taken out under direct laparoscopic visualization to identify any bleeding at the insertion sites.

6. The fascia at the 10-mm trocar sites was closed with interrupted Vicryl suture. The subcutaneous areas were irrigated, and the overlying skin was closed with 4-0 Monocryl in a subcuticular technique. The patient was discharged home that day with postoperative narcotics and instructions for care.

Case 4: Bilateral Salpingo-oophorectomy in a Transplant Patient

 View DVD: Video 6-2

The patient is a 54-year-old female who presented with a history of acute abdominal pain. She has a history of hypertension, chronic renal failure, and kidney transplant. She is on immunosuppressive medication. On physical examination, her body mass index was 28 and she had a surgical incision from the previous transplant. She had no range-of-motion limitations of the extremities. A mobile mass with no nodularity was palpated in the posterior cul-de-sac on pelvic exam, and the uterus was 6-week-sized, nontender, and mobile. CA-125 was normal. Upon ultrasound evaluation, she was found to have a 17 × 13 cm simple cyst in the left adnexal mass, which was confirmed on a CT scan. There were no worrisome features of the cyst nor was there ascites present. After this assessment, the patient consented to a laparoscopic bilateral salpingo-oophorectomy, with possible conversion to laparotomy if malignancy was identified.

Surgical Techniques

1. In the operating room, the patient was placed in low lithotomy position. Preoperative antibiotics with a second-generation cephalosporin (cefazolin) were given within 30 minutes of first incision. Pneumatic sequential compression stockings were placed on the patient before starting the case. A uterine manipulator was placed transcervically for additional control during the procedure.

2. An exam under anesthesia revealed a mass that reached the umbilicus. For this reason a left upper quadrant approach was utilized so as not to rupture the mass. All incision areas were pre-injected with 0.25% Marcaine for additional analgesic effect. After confirming intraperitoneal access, a pneumoperitoneuem was established. A 10-mm trocar was then placed at the umbilicus, under direct vision. After inspection of the insertion site showed no evidence of complication, additional trocars were placed in the left and right lower quadrants under direct laparoscopic visualization in order to avoid any trauma to the underlying organs. The transplanted kidney was seen in the right iliac fossa as a retroperitoneal mass. The right ovary was normal.

3. Pelvic washings were taken with normal saline, and inspection of the entire abdomen and pelvis was performed, paying careful attention for possible metastasis, adhesions, and aberrant structures. The left ovary was identified and brought into view. Typically the cyst should not be ruptured. However in this case there was no suspicion for malignancy and the cyst was being removed for symptom control. The cyst was therefore punctured and all the fluid aspirated without intraperitoneal spill.

4. An incision was made in the peritoneum lateral to the left ovary and ovarian vessels and the retroperitoneal space was entered. It was not necessary in this case to identify the ureter since the kidney was nonfunctional.

5. Bipolar cautery was then used across the infundibulopelvic and broad ligaments in a sequential fashion and the coagulated areas were then cut with laparoscopic scissors.

6. This patient wished to have the other ovary removed at the same time, so the resection process was repeated. Both adnexae were placed in an endoscopic bag and brought out through a lower quadrant trocar incision. Typically the incision requires some extension. Do not pull on the bag because it will rupture. The incision should be extended to accommodate the size of the adnexal lesion or the cyst can be morcellated in the bag at the surface of the skin. Frozen section revealed a benign cystadenoma of the ovary.

7. After removal of the other ovary, the areas of dissection were inspected for hemostasis, both with normal insufflation and with reduction of the pneumoperitoneum. Hemostasis was obtained, and the 10-mm port site fascia was closed with an endofascial closure device under direct laparoscopic visualization without any complications. The skin at the port sites was closed with subcuticular stitch using 4-0 suture.

Endometriomas and Residual Ovary Syndrome

View DVD: Video 6-3

Excision of endometriomas is more difficult than removal of dermoid cysts or cystadenomas, because endometriomas frequently rupture and the dissection planes are not evident. The edge of the normal cortex and the cyst are held with Allis graspers, which are gently pulled in opposite directions to peel the cyst out (Figure 6-15). This must be performed without excessive traction, or parts of the ovarian cortex will tear off and/or the cyst will rupture. Chapter 11 goes into more detail on management of endometriomas.

Ovarian remnant syndrome is associated with chronic pelvic pain in some patients. This is a poorly defined syndrome. The surgical intervention is especially difficult since many of these patients have had several surgeries including a hysterectomy and

Figure 6-15. Excision of endometriomas is more difficult. The edges of the normal cortex and the cyst are held with Allis graspers that are gently pulled in opposite directions to peel the cyst out.

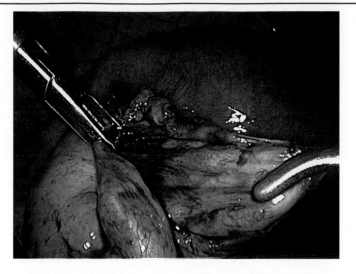

bilateral salpingo-oophorectomy. Case #5 presents a 34-year-old woman with chronic pelvic pain after removal of the uterus and both ovaries. A pelvic ultrasound reveals bilateral 2-cm adnexal masses. The patient has failed all modes of conservative therapy and desires an attempt at surgical correction. Her pain is consistent with ovarian remnant syndrome, so she is scheduled for laparoscopic removal of bilateral adnexal masses with the understanding that these cases all require a retroperitoneal approach because the ovarian tissue is often in the retroperitoneal space adherent to the ureter.

Complications of Laparoscopic Adnexal Surgery

Complications of laparoscopic surgery are covered in Chapter 15. There are two specific complications that may be unique to adnexal surgery. First is the potential for intraoperative rupture of a malignant cyst. Randomized clinical trials have demonstrated that, in most cases, the frequency of rupture is the same by laparoscopy and by laparotomy. Intraoperative rupture of a stage 1A malignant cyst may commit the patient to chemotherapy which she may not have otherwise received. Spillage of dermoid, mucinous, or endometriosis cyst contents is not associated with increased morbidity, as long as extensive peritoneal lavage is used to thoroughly remove the cyst contents. A second feature that is a possibility with spill of a malignant cyst is port site implantation. Prevention of spill of a malignant cyst will prevent most of these occurrences.

Conclusion

Laparoscopy offers an alternative to standard laparotomy, because most adnexal masses will have benign pathologic findings. Even some women with malignant masses can be managed via laparoscopy, if the principles of oncologic surgery are followed (no intra-abdominal rupture of cyst, appropriate staging procedures if no extrapelvic disease is noted). Knowledge of the retroperitoneum along the pelvic sidewall and the steps needed to mobilize the ureter will allow difficult masses to be removed intact and can avoid leaving residual ovarian epithelium that can lead to an ovarian remnant. Preoperative referral of all high-risk and probably all intermediate-risk women to a gynecologic oncologist should be considered for complete surgical staging, if needed. Additionally, all women should be counseled thoroughly with regard to the potential of a malignancy being found at the time of frozen section and the need for more extensive surgical procedures to be performed either laparoscopically or via laparotomy. This will allow efficient surgical management of those women at the time of initial surgery and not worsen their prognosis.

Suggested Reading

American College of Obstetricians and Gynecologists: ACOG committee opinion: the role of the generalist obstetrician-gynecologist in the early detection of ovarian cancer, *Obstet Gynecol* 100(6):1413-1416, 2002.

American College of Obstetricians and Gynecologists: ACOG practice bulletin: management of adnexal masses, *Obstet Gynecol* 110(1):201-214, 2007.

Alcazar JL, Merce LT, Laparte C, Jurado M, Lopez-Garcia G: A new scoring system to differentiate benign from malignant adnexal masses, *Am J Obstet Gynecol* 188.605-602, 2003.

Bakkum-Gamez JN, Richardson DL, Seamon LG, Aletti GD, Powless CA, Keeney GL, O'Malley DM, Cliby WA: Influence of intraoperative capsule rupture on outcomes in stage I epithelial ovarian cancer, *Obstet Gynecol* 113:11-17, 2009.

Breen JL, Maxson WS: Ovarian tumors in children and adolescents, *Clin Obstet Gynecol* 20:607-623, 1997.

Bristow RE, Nugent AC, Zahurak ML, Khouzami V, Fox HE: Impact of surgeon specialty on ovarian-conserving surgery in young females with an adnexal mass, *J Adolesc Health* 39(3):411-416, 2006.

Deckardt R, Saks M, Graeff H: Comparison of minimally invasive surgery and laparotomy in the treatment of adnexal masses, *J Am Assoc Gynecol Laparosc* 1:333-338, 1994.

Fanfani F, Fagotti A, Ercoli A, Bifulco G, Longo R, Mancuso S, Scambia G: A prospective randomized study of laparoscopy and minilaparotomy in the management of benign adnexal masses, *Hum Reprod* 19:2367-2371, 2004.

Goff BA, Mandel LS, Melancon CH, Muntz HG: Frequency of symptoms of ovarian cancer in women presenting to primary care clinics, *JAMA* 291:2705-2712, 2004.

Goff BA, Mandel LS, Drescher CW, et al: Development of an ovarian cancer symptom index: possibilities for earlier detection, *Cancer* 109:221-227, 2007.

Lehner R, Wenzl R, Heinzl H, Husslein P, Sevelda P: Influence of delayed staging laparotomy after laparoscopic removal of ovarian masses later found malignant, *Obstet Gynecol* 92:967-971, 1998

Maggino T, Gadducci A, D'Addario V, et al: Prospective multicenter study on CA 125 in postmenopausal pelvic masses, *Gynecol Oncol* 54:117-123, 1994.

Malkasian Jr GD, Knapp RC, Lavin PT, et al: Preoperative evaluation of serum CA 125 levels in premenopausal and postmenopausal patients with pelvic masses: discrimination of benign from malignant disease, *Am J Obstet Gynecol* 159:341-346, 1988.

Ramirez PT, Wolf JK, Levenback C: Laparoscopic port-site metastases: etiology and prevention, *Gynecol Oncol* 91:179-189, 2003.

Roman DL, Muderspach LI, Stein SM, Laifer-Narin S, Groshen S, Morrow CP: Pelvic exam, tumor marker level, and gray scale and Doppler sonography in the prediction of pelvic cancer, *Obstet Gynecol* 89:493-500, 1997.

Society of Gynecologic Oncologists: Consensus opinion for adnexal mass, *Gynecol Oncol* 78:S1-13, 2000.

Stepp KJ, Tulikangas PK, Goldberg JM, Attaran M, Falcone T: Laparoscopy for adnexal masses in the second trimester of pregnancy, *J Am Assoc Gynecol Laparosc* 10:55-59, 2003.

Yuen PM, Yu KM, Yip SK, Lau WC, Rogers MS, Chang A: A randomized prospective study of laparoscopy and laparotomy in the management of benign ovarian masses, *Am J Obstet Gynecol* 177:109-114, 1997.

Indications and Techniques for Laparoscopic Myomectomy

7

Devorah Wieder M.D., M.P.H.
Jeffrey M. Goldberg M.D.
Tommaso Falcone M.D.

 Video Clips on DVD

7-1 Laparoscopic Myomectomy of Large Intramural Fibroids (6 minutes/57 seconds)

7-2 Laparoscopic Myomectomy for a Pedunculated Fibroid (7 minutes/34 seconds)

7-3 Criteria for Planning Optimal Myometrial Incision during Laparoscopic Myomectomy (6 minutes/29 seconds)

Introduction

Advancements in surgical technology, combined with changing reproductive patterns, have made myomectomy an increasingly attractive procedure for both patients and physicians. For many years, open myomectomy by laparotomy was the only option for women desiring uterine conservation and treatment of fibroids. Today, women have more choices than ever before. Each patient must be individually evaluated to determine the optimal treatment approach. Presenting complaint, myoma number, size, and location, as well as medical comorbidities should determine the method of resection. Improved laparoscopic instrumentation and refinements of technique have made minimally invasive myomectomy feasible for an increasing proportion of patients. Despite the expanding popularity of the procedure, many controversies still remain as to patient selection and operative method.

Estimates of the prevalence of uterine fibroids vary by method of diagnosis. Disparate rates are found with radiologic, surgical, or pathologic evaluation. Additionally, the clinical relevance of the presence of leiomyomas can be highly variable. The estimated prevalence of myomas, in asymptomatic reproductive-age United States women screened by ultrasound, is 5% to 10%. By the age of 50, this rate increases to almost 70% for Caucasian women and 80% for African-Americans. Among symptomatic women in the Nurses' Health Study, however, the overall incidence rate of fibroids diagnosed was 12.8 per 1000 woman-years among women aged 25-44, rising exponentially with advancing age. Rates vary by ethnic groups; African-Americans are notable for multiple and larger fibroids that are often diagnosed at a younger age. These various presentations may reflect underlying genetic differences among populations, with fibroid growth representing a common end response of the uterine smooth muscle to a variety of inciting factors. Half of women with fibroids are symptomatic, and present for care complaining of menorrhagia, pelvic pain or pressure, urinary or gastrointestinal symptoms, dyspareunia, infertility, and pregnancy complications. The burden of this disease is great, as symptomatic fibroids are the fifth leading cause of hospitaliza-

81

Figure 7-1. Myoma Size and location result in various reproductive effects:
- Menorrhagia or menometrorrhagia
- Pelvic pain, dyspareunia, bloating
- Urinary obstruction, constipation and hydronephrosis
- Deformation of normal anatomy
- Interference with sperm and ovum transport
- Decreased implantation. Reprinted with the permission of the Cleveland Clinic Center for Medical Art & Photography © 2008. All rights reserved.

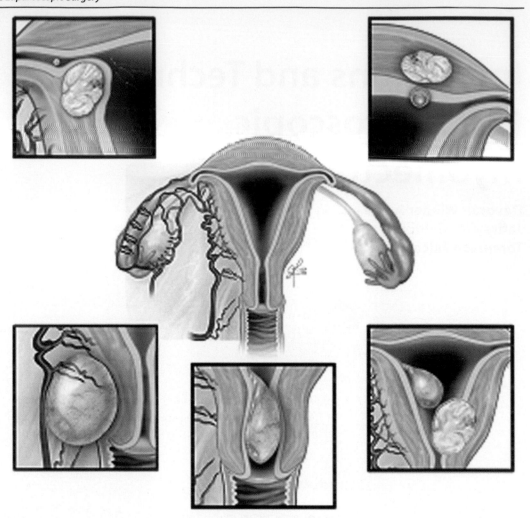

tion for gynecologic disorders among American women. Fibroids still represent the primary indication for hysterectomy.

By definition, leiomyomas are benign monoclonal tumors of smooth muscle that show various cytogenetic abnormalities. These growths have a characteristic pearly white appearance with bundles of smooth muscle fibers creating a whorled appearance. Uterine leiomyomas are hormonally responsive and have an increased number of estrogen and progesterone receptors that are likely responsible for the higher incidence among reproductive-age women. The most common symptoms of uterine myomas are bleeding, chronic pelvic pain, and reproductive concerns (Figure 7-1). In pregnancy, most myomas will remain stable in size, but they may cause complications such as preterm delivery, uterine atony, hemorrhage, and abnormal placentation including placenta previa. If present in the lower uterine segment, cesarean section may be indicated due to obstruction. This can potentially complicate exposure during the surgery.

Nonsurgical Management of Fibroids

Medical treatment serves to improve symptoms and avoid surgery. However, oral contraceptive pills and nonsteroidal antiinflammatory drugs do not affect myoma size. Myoma size can be reduced by 30% to 65% within 3 months of therapy by treatment with a gonadotropin releasing hormone (GnRH) agonist. There is, however, a rapid return to pretreatment size with cessation of therapy. GnRH agonists have also been used as a preoperative adjuvant. Other agents such as raloxifene, GnRH antagonists, mifepristone, gestrinone, levonorgestrel IUD, and aromatase inhibitors are under investigation. Alternative procedures such as endometrial ablation, uterine artery embolization, laparoscopic uterine artery ligation, and endoscopic myolysis via laser, diathermy, cryomyolysis, or high-intensity ultrasound are increasingly employed to treat menometrorrhagia in selected patients, but as yet have limited application in women desiring future fertility.

Preoperative Evaluation and Patient Selection

Patients with symptomatic fibroids may describe pelvic pain or pressure, abnormal uterine bleeding, and a history of infertility. Indications for treatment of uterine fibroids include anemia, pelvic pain and pressure, urinary frequency or hydroureter, increasing abdominal girth, and rapid or postmenopausal growth of fibroids. The indications for myomectomy per the American College of Obstetricians and Gynecologists and the American Society for Reproductive Medicine are:

1. Patients with infertility or recurrent pregnancy loss after excluding all other causes or the presence of a markedly distorted cavity

2. Symptomatic patients desiring to maintain fertility

Preoperative evaluation should include a thorough history and physical examination, and possibly, assessment for anemia and uterine malignancy. Patients should be made aware of the risks of recurrence of leiomyomas after surgery. Imaging by transvaginal ultrasound and hysterosalpingogram may be helpful, although more precise imaging of fibroids that impinge on the uterine cavity can be obtained via a saline infusion sonohysterogram (Figure 7-2). In patients with multiple fibroids difficult to characterize via ultrasound, pelvic magnetic resonance imaging may be helpful for preoperative counseling and planning, to more precisely locate the myomas and to rule out adenomyosis (Figure 7-3).

GnRH agonists are thought to increase difficulty of dissection by disrupting natural cleavage planes. However, this treatment can still play a role in improving preoperative hematocrit in severely anemic patients. Increased recurrence after pretreatment has been observed when the now smaller fibroids are not located and removed. Erythropoietin alfa has also been suggested in patients with low hematocrit related to chronic menometrorrhagia. Some patients may be offered autologous blood donation prior to surgery if locally available.

The number of fibroids as well as fibroid size and location are the primary factors to consider when choosing the route of surgery (laparoscopic vs. abdominal). To some degree, fibroid size criteria will depend on the surgeon's skill and level of comfort. Case

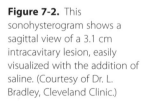

Figure 7-2. This sonohysterogram shows a sagittal view of a 3.1 cm intracavitary lesion, easily visualized with the addition of saline. (Courtesy of Dr. L. Bradley, Cleveland Clinic.)

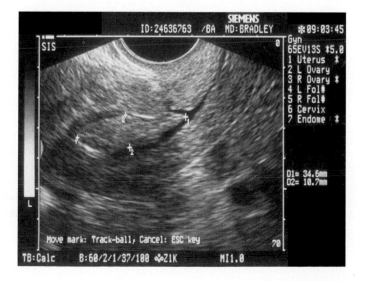

Figure 7-3. MRI T$_2$-weighted sagittal (A) and axial (B) images of multiple uterine fibroids, of low signal relative to the myometrium, throughout the uterus in multiple locations, including: submucosal (sm), myometrial (m), and exophytic (exo). (Courtesy of Dr. A. Magen, Cleveland Clinic.)

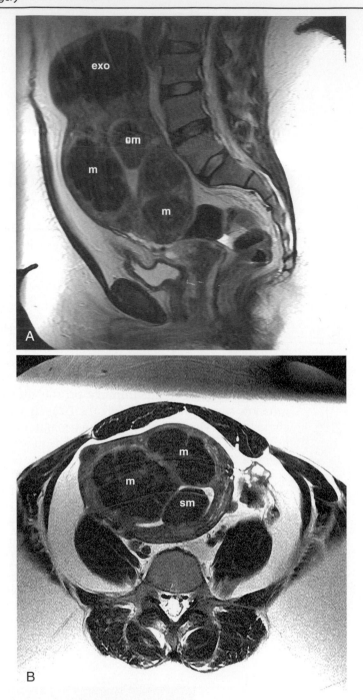

series, describing risk factors and rates for conversion to laparotomy, are helpful in establishing broad guidelines and evaluating current regional practice patterns. Generally, laparoscopic myomectomy can be attempted in patients with an overall uterine size less than 16 weeks, with a dominant fibroid less than 15 cm in greatest dimension. Fibroids should be fewer than five in number. Larger, more numerous fibroids, and those that involve the broad ligament, uterine cornua, or uterine vasculature should only be attempted by highly skilled and experienced laparoscopic surgeons. Strong suspicion of uterine sarcoma should prompt an open approach with an oncologist available for complete staging.

To demonstrate the surgical technique of laparoscopic myomectomy, three cases are be presented, demonstrated (videoclips), and discussed:

Case 1: Abnormal Uterine Bleeding

 View DVD: Video 7-1

SB is a 45-year-old woman, gravida 3 para 2104, who presents complaining of worsening, increased uterine bleeding and pelvic pressure. She states that her menses last 8 to 9 days. During the first several days, she changes a pad every 1 to 2 hours. She is constantly concerned about soiling her clothes. She reports significant pelvic pressure and low back pain. She has tried medical management with continuous oral contraceptive pills and the levonorgestrol intrauterine device without success. Her laboratory studies are unremarkable aside from a hematocrit of 28.5%. She denies shortness of breath or dizziness. She works full time in a demanding field and has been researching minimally invasive surgery on the internet to avoid taking an extended medical leave. MRI findings reveal an enlarged uterus measuring 16 cm. A single large homogeneously enhancing fibroid is present in the fundus and measures 12 cm × 7.6 cm × 8.1 cm.

After a thorough discussion of the risks and benefits of laparoscopic myomectomy, including risk of conversion to an open myomectomy, informed consent is obtained. SB then relates that she has just been promoted and cannot take time off for any surgery for the next 6 months. In the interim, she is placed on a 3-month course of leuprolide acetate to induce amenorrhea. She subsequently requests add-back therapy for severe hot flashes.

Discussion of Case: Abnormal Uterine Bleeding

The most common symptom reported by women with myomas is abnormal bleeding. More specifically, frequent, heavy menses are described, which are often associated with submucosal or intramural fibroids. A history of light spotting between menses may represent an intracavitary or intracervical myoma but warrants investigation for other endometrial abnormalities. The spectrum of menorrhagia can range greatly with some women requiring evaluation in the emergency department, multiple blood transfusions, and intravenous iron therapy. In otherwise healthy patients, the degree of adaptation to profound anemia can be quite remarkable and therefore, subjective patient assessment of the extent of bleeding should always be correlated with a complete blood count. Bleeding episodes greater than 7 days have the greatest clinical predictive value for anemia. Frequency of pad changes, dizziness, and tachycardia should also be routinely assessed. Episodes of bleeding can cause significant disruption to daily routine, lost work or school time, and embarrassment related to soiling of clothes.

Surgical Techniques

1. The patient is placed in lithotomy position with arms tucked at her sides. The patient's legs are placed in stirrups that maintain the hips in a neutral position with the weight of the legs on the bottom of the feet, such as Yellofins by Allen Medical Systems. Pneumatic compression stockings are placed on the calves to reduce the risk of venous thromboembolism. A uterine manipulator through which chromotubation may be performed is placed in the uterine cavity. This is important not only for manipulation of the uterus but also to facilitate recognition of entry into the uterine cavity during surgery by the instillation of indigo carmine dye via the manipulator and observing the blue dye leaking through the suspected entry point.

2. Trocar placement: A 5-mm intraumbilical port can be used for the laparoscope. Right and left lower quadrant ports are placed medial and superior to the anterior superior iliac spine taking care to avoid the inferior epigastric arteries. The right- or left-sided port can later be enlarged to enable suturing. These ports may be placed slightly more caudad if the uterus is very large. An additional 5-mm port can be placed at the level of the umbilicus to facilitate suturing. A final 10-mm suprapubic port is placed in the midline for manipulation of the myoma and for morcellation. In some cases a 30-degree laparoscope may be useful in obtaining adequate visualization (Figure 7-4).

3. Dilute vasopressin (20 units per 100 mL saline) is injected into the myometrium over the myoma to enhance hemostasis. Intraoperative use of vasopressin helps to reduce blood loss and operative time. The creation of a cleavage plane is also aided by hydrodissection. The addition of bupivicaine may further decrease postoperative pain. Vasopressin is contraindicated in patients with hypertension (Figure 7-5).

Figure 7-4. Trocar placement. A 5-mm intraumbilical port can be used for the laparoscope, followed by right and left lower quadrant ports, with an additional left port for suturing. A 10-mm suprapubic port can be placed in the midline for manipulation of the myoma and for morcellation.

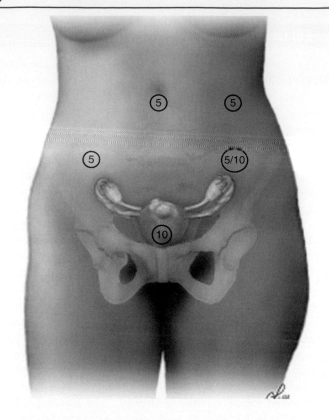

Figure 7-5. Vasopressin is injected into the myometrium overlying the myoma and into the myoma itself.

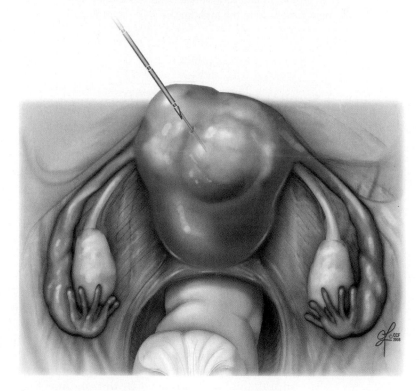

4. The serosa and myometrium may be incised with a monopolar hook, harmonic scalpel, or laser (Figure 7-6). Figure 7-6 shows a horizontal incision. A vertical incision can also be made. The debate on horizontal versus vertical incision is discussed in Video 7-3.

5. The myoma is grasped with a 10-mm tenaculum or myoma screw through the suprapubic port. The overlying myometrium is then pushed toward the base of the myoma with countertraction on the myoma (Figure 7-7).

Figure 7-6. The uterine incision is made with the monopolar hook. In this case a horizontal incision is made. Reprinted with the permission of the Cleveland Clinic Center for Medical Art & Photography © 2008. All rights reserved.

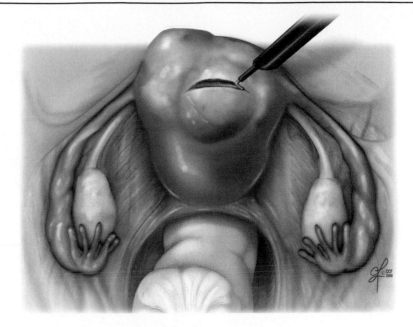

Figure 7-7. The myoma is dissected bluntly and any bleeding is cauterized Reprinted with the permission of the Cleveland Clinic Center for Medical Art & Photography © 2000. All rights reserved.

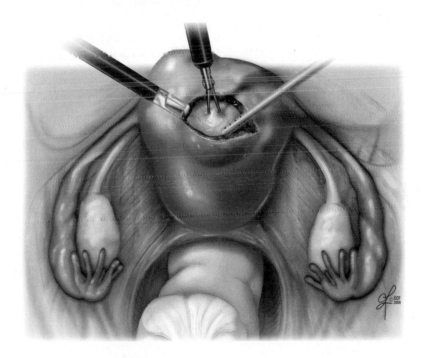

6. A monopolar hook is used to divide fibers connecting the myoma base to the myometrium.

7. Hemostasis is achieved with bipolar electrocautery. Uncontrolled bleeding is the primary reason for conversion to laparotomy. An interval step may be to perform laparoscopic uterine artery ligation to decrease bleeding.

8. The myometrial defect is closed with number 0 interrupted delayed absorbable sutures in layers for hemostasis and to obliterate the dead space. Redundant myometrium and serosa may be excised. Sutures may be tied intracorporeally or extracorporeally. Figures 7-8, 7-9, and 7-10 show closure of a horizontal incision. (Video 7-1 shows closure of a vertical incision and Video 7-3 closure of a horizontal incision.)

9. The myoma is then grasped with a tenaculum and drawn through a motorized morcellator. During morcellation, the blade should only be activated when in use.

Figure 7-8. The myoma bed is reapproximated in layers to ensure hemostasis. Reprinted with the permission of the Cleveland Clinic Center for Medical Art & Photography © 2008. All rights reserved.

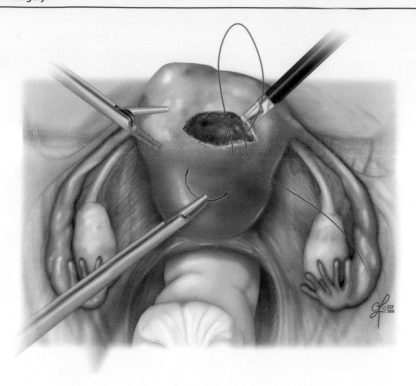

Figure 7-9. The serosa is then closed after multiple myometrial layers. Reprinted with the permission of the Cleveland Clinic Center for Medical Art & Photography © 2008. All rights reserved.

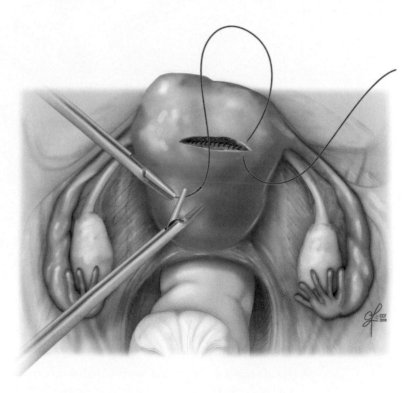

It should be held in a fixed position under direct visualization at all times. A surgical assistant can facilitate morcellation. The tissue should be excised in a circumferential manner to maximize the size of the fragments and the efficiency of removal. A complete survey of the abdomen should be performed to locate and remove all fragments, to avoid parasitic implantation of fibroid remnants (Figure 7-11). (See Video 7-1 📹)

10. After closing the serosal layer with 3-0 delayed absorbable suture, adhesion barriers may be placed over the suture line after complete hemostasis is achieved, to reduce postoperative adhesion formation.

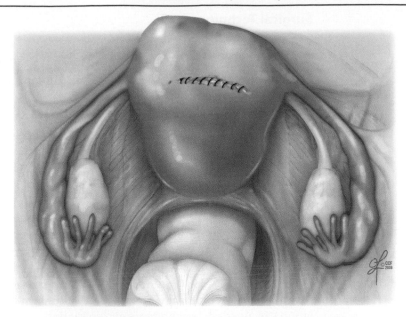

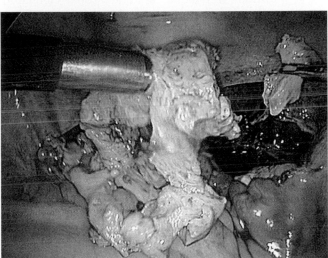

Figure 7-11. The myoma is drawn through a motorized morcellator.

Case 2: Pedunculated Myoma

 View DVD: Video 7-2

CL is a 47-year-old woman, gravida 2 para 2002, who complains of increasing pelvic pressure and abdominal girth. She reports daily episodes of urgency and frequency, and occasional dyspareunia. She has recently noted that she has been shopping for larger-sized pants than in years past despite a stable weight. Her pelvic ultrasound reveals an 8-cm myoma that appears to be pedunculated. She had a recent episode of severe abdominal pain for which she was evaluated in the emergency department. She was told her symptoms were related to a torsed or necrotic fibroid and her pain alleviated with oral narcotics. As a generally healthy woman who engages in daily biking and fitness classes, CL was very alarmed by her hospitalization. Prior to this episode and to her ultrasound, she and her previous gynecologist had discussed observation until menopause. She now desires surgical management due to her increasing symptoms. CL desires to

resume her active lifestyle as soon as possible. Of note, she has a history of two prior cesarean sections and a previous laparotomy following an automobile accident as a young woman. After a detailed discussion of medical and surgical management, including discussion of laparoscopic and open techniques, she consents to laparoscopic myomectomy.

Discussion of Case: Pelvic Pain Secondary to a Pedunculated Myoma

Pelvic pain and pressure relates most to the position and size of the myoma. Symptoms may be unrelated to the menstrual cycle. Compression of related pelvic structures such as the bladder and rectum give rise to irritative bladder symptoms and bowel dysfunction. Dyspareunia may be related to both fibroid size and position. Pain may also be associated with ischemia and necrosis occurring when the fibroid grows beyond its vascular supply or when a pedunculated fibroid undergoes torsion.

Surgical Techniques

1. Trocars are placed as described in the Case 1, with placement of a left upper quadrant port, given the patient's history of previous surgeries.
2. Dilute vasopressin is injected into the fibroid stalk and bipolar cautery applied to aid in hemostasis (Figures 7-12 and 7-13).
3. The stalk is transected with a harmonic scalpel or monopolar hook (Figure 7-14).
4. Hemostasis is achieved by bipolar cautery. The defect may be sutured closed if needed.
5. The specimen is then removed in fragments after electronic morcellation.

Vaginal Removal of Myomas via Colpotomy

Myomas may also be retrieved through colpotomy incisions to avoid extensive morcellation or minilaparotomy. The myoma is positioned in the pelvis for ease of retrieval. The myoma may be bisected laparoscopically to facilitate removal. Colpotomy is performed with a monopolar hook between the uterosacral ligaments over a sponge stick or right-angle retractor tenting the posterior fornix, taking care not to damage the rectum. The myoma may be delivered vaginally, either intact or with further morcellation. If needed, an endoscopic collection bag may be introduced. Subsequently, pneumoperitoneum may be restored by packing the vagina. The colpotomy incision may be repaired laparoscopically or vaginally.

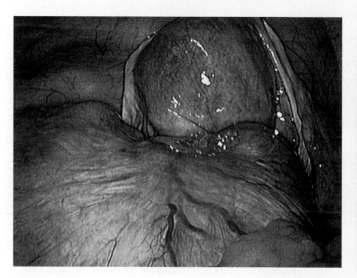

Figure 7-12. A large pedunculated myoma.

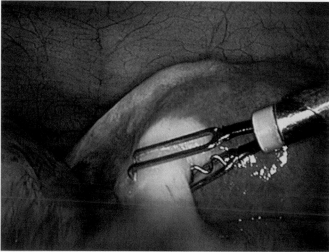

Figure 7-13. The stalk is cauterized with bipolar electrocautery.

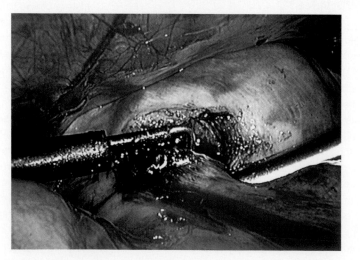

Figure 7-14. The stalk is incised.

Case 3: Infertility and Multiple Myomas

 View DVD: Video 7-3

AD is a 39-year-old woman, gravida 3 para 0030, now recently remarried, who presents with secondary infertility. Her past obstetrical history is significant for a remote therapeutic abortion and two first trimester spontaneous abortions during her first marriage. She reports a history of painful menses since menarche. AD now complains of gradually increasing menorrhagia and dysmenorrhea. Her evaluation for infertility reveals ovulatory cycles and no male factor concerns. She has undergone a hysterosalpingogram that showed tubal patency, but which was remarkable for a distorted uterine cavity. A follow-up sonohysterogram shows a 5 cm posterior intramural fibroid projecting into the uterine cavity and an adjacent 7-cm intramural fundal fibroid. An MRI confirms no other fibroids or adenomyosis. She presents with her husband, who is also childless, stating they have read multiple lay books on pregnancy and infertility. She asks for your center's pregnancy rates after myomectomy, whether or not she will require a cesarean section, and how soon she can attempt pregnancy after surgery. Her infertility concerns are discussed in detail including the effects of possible endometriosis and fibroids on fertility. She is advised that there is a strong possibility of entry into the uterine cavity during the procedure. If she undergoes an extensive myomectomy, cesarean section would be recommended. She is also advised of the possibility of minilaparotomy to ensure adequate closure of the uterine incision. She decides to proceed with laparoscopic myomectomy, possible minilaparotomy, lysis of adhesions, and excision of endometriosis.

Case Discussion: Laparoscopic Myomectomy for Infertility

Given the age-related incidence of fibroids, as well as current demographic trends of delaying childbearing, it is not surprising that an increasing number of patients presenting with infertility undergo evaluation and treatment for fibroids. When all other causes of infertility are excluded, fibroids have been estimated to cause infertility in 2% to 3% of cases. This rate is based on the work of Buttram and Reiter in 1981, who found that of surgeries performed for infertility, 2.4% were myomectomies. In this same study, a history of infertility was found in 27% of the patients operated on for fibroids. The medical literature related to the effects of fibroids on

fertility is expansive but lacks true randomized controlled trials. The true effect of fibroids on reproduction is difficult to pinpoint, but may be secondary to deformation of the uterine contour, tubal ostia, or cervix or alterations in uterine contractility may interfere with sperm and ovum transport (see Figure 7-1). An abnormal or inflamed endometrium overlying the fibroid with altered blood supply and/or growth factor expression may also have an impact on successful implantation.

Retrospective studies comparing fertility in women with and without fibroids show improved pregnancy and delivery rates in those without fibroids. Studies have also reported reduced in vitro fertilization (IVF) pregnancy rates in women with fibroids. Beneficial effects after surgery are seen in studies looking at pregnancy rates after myomectomy. Data from case series is confounded by the lack of control groups and cases drawn from a treatment-seeking group. Data from case-control and cohort studies have shown that there is a decreased risk of fibroids among parous women. These observational studies are confounded by samples selected from parous women leading to bias, as well as inability to establish causality.

In the absence of randomized controlled trials, data from IVF cycles in women with and without fibroids are illuminating. Meta-analyses have shown that submucosal fibroids greatly impact fertility, while intramural fibroids have a lesser but still detrimental effect. Most studies noted significant interference with fertility only when fibroids were greater than 4 cm. Studies on IVF outcomes after myomectomy are few in number and are limited by small sample size and variable inclusion criteria. These studies evaluate the effects of fibroids on embryo implantation, but do not address the effects of fibroids on gamete and embryo transport in natural cycles.

The presence of fibroids may also contribute to pregnancy complications such as spontaneous abortion, preterm delivery, malpresentation, outlet tract obstruction, abnormal placentation, and postpartum hemorrhage. The weight of recent evidence indicates that a submucosal, cavity-distorting, or large intramural myoma may have a negative effect on reproductive outcome. The attributable effect of fibroids on reproductive function and the precise mechanism of interference vary according to location, size, and number of fibroids. Thus, it is often difficult to accurately advise each individual patient on subsequent fertility rates.

Surgical Techniques: Laparoscopic Myomectomy for Infertility

1. Trocars are placed as described earlier.
2. The pelvic anatomy is carefully studied to determine the optimal incision placement (Figures 7-15 and 7-16). The orientation and location of the myometrial incision has implications for operative blood loss, ease of uterine reconstruction, and future adhesion risk (See Video 7-3). Postoperative adhesion formation is thought to be increased by posterior incisions and may adversely affect fertility. Criteria for planning the location and orientation of the myometrial incision include the location

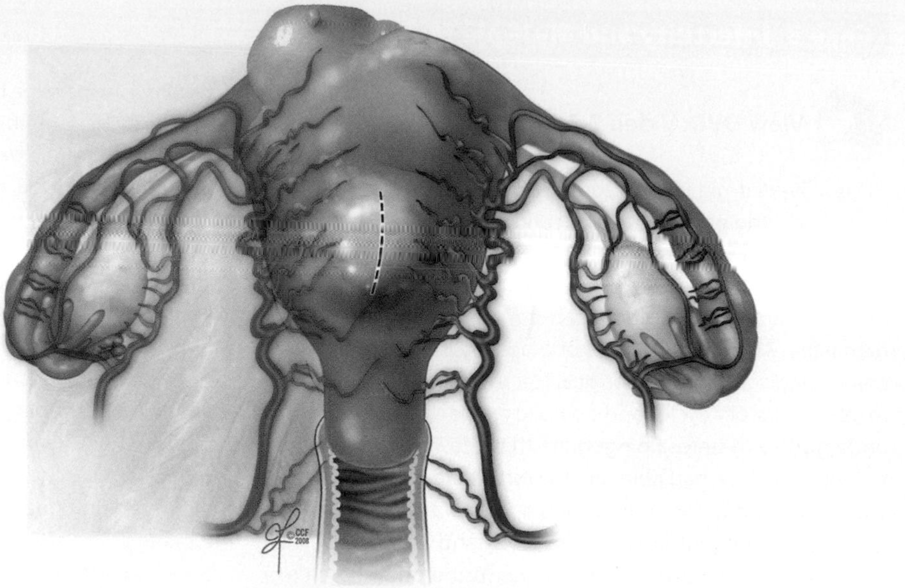

Figure 7-15. The direction of serosal incision is dictated by multiple considerations, such as vertical incisions avoid extension into the fallopian tubes or uterine arteries (Video clip 7-3). Reprinted with the permission of the Cleveland Clinic Center for Medical Art & Photography © 2008. All rights reserved.

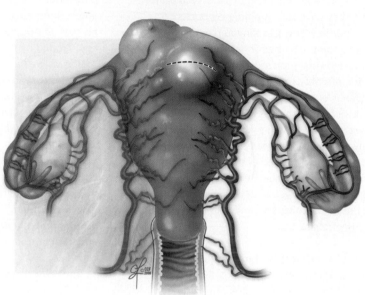

Figure 7-16. Horizontal incisions are easier to suture (Video clip 7-3). Reprinted with the permission of the Cleveland Clinic Center for Medical Art & Photography © 2008. All rights reserved.

and number of fibroids, with the goal of removing as many fibroids through as few incisions as possible. Even posterior fibroids can be removed through an anterior incision if the bulk of the fibroids are anterior. Consideration of the structural and vascular anatomy of the uterus would favor a vertical incision to avoid extension of the incision into the tube or uterine vessels. Factors favoring a horizontal incision include reduced blood loss and improved technical ease of uterine closure.

3. The serosa and myometrium over the myoma are incised with a monopolar hook and the fibroid is enucleated with sharp and blunt dissection. The fibroid bed is palpated via instruments to locate the underlying fibroid. Laparoscopic ultrasound may be used to delineate nearby fibroids. These ultrasound probes have been used in several specialties outside gynecology for some time. This technique has the potential to overcome the loss of tactile sensation during laparoscopy, and thus better characterize the extent of the lesion. Despite rigorous preoperative evaluation, including MRI, the exact location of the fibroid of interest may still be difficult to localize. Use of intraoperative ultrasound can serve to reduce the size of the hysterotomy incision and prevent recurrence related to undetected fibroids.

4. Based on fibroid location, entry into the uterine cavity may be unavoidable. If unclear, cavity entry can be confirmed by instillation of indigo carmine dye into the

uterine cavity and visualization of spill into the myomectomy bed. Incisions in the endometrial cavity may be closed with interrupted 4-0 suture.

5. The defect is usually easily repaired in several layers and subsequent cesarean section is usually recommended.

Other Surgical Techniques for Laparoscopic Myomectomy

Laparoscopic-Assisted Myomectomy

This hybrid procedure involves dissecting the myoma laparoscopically, then performing a minilaparotomy incision to remove the myoma from the abdomen and repair the uterine defect with conventional suturing techniques. It has the advantage of being quicker than laparoscopic suturing and morcellation. Further, the uterine repair may be more secure than laparoscopic closure, which may reduce the risk of uterine rupture during pregnancy. This approach may result in increased postoperative pain and length of recovery; however, both are less than with the conventional abdominal approach. After shelling out the myoma laparoscopically, a minilaparotomy is made by extending the suprapubic port incision. The myoma and uterine fundus are delivered to the incision and the myoma is excised, in fragments, if necessary. The uterus is repaired in layers and returned to the abdomen. The minilaparotomy skin incision is closed with a running stitch of 4-0 delayed absorbable suture (Figures 7-17 through 7-19).

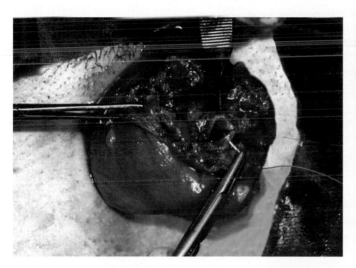

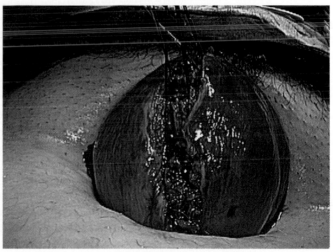

Figure 7-17. The myoma and fundus are delivered to the incision. Notice the cavity was entered and is being closed with 3-0 Vicryl suture.

Figure 7-18. The defect is repaired in layers.

Figure 7-19. Incisions after laparoscopic-assisted myomectomy.

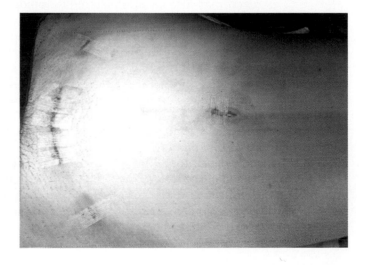

Hand-Assisted Myomectomy

The recent introduction of hand-assist ports for laparoscopy can further broaden the scope of laparoscopic myomectomy. Use of these ports can avoid a large abdominal incision in technically demanding cases where palpation is needed to assist dissection or exposure. The hand-assist port maintains the pneumoperitoneum, thus allowing for a laparoscopic view of the dissection. The fibroids may be removed via the hand-assist port (Gelport, Applied Medical), and then suturing may be completed laparoscopically. This option can be especially useful for posterior myomas that would be difficult to suture via minilaparotomy or when further laparoscopic procedures such as excision of endometriosis are planned.

Broad Ligament Fibroids

Despite thorough preoperative imaging, fibroids located within the broad ligament may not be diagnosed until the time of laparoscopy. This location is often associated with hydronephrosis, causing a diagnostic conundrum when present in patients who have had previous hysterectomy. Meticulous dissection may be required to clearly identify and avoid damage to important structures such as the ureter and uterine artery. Careful attention to hemostasis is vital to avoid uncontrolled bleeding.

Outcomes and Complications

The value of laparoscopic access as an alternative to laparotomy can be evaluated from clinical trials that show decreased intraoperative blood loss, less postoperative pain, shorter length of hospital stay, quicker recovery, improved cosmesis, and decreased adhesion formation. Studies have shown a comparable operative time and low rate of conversion to laparotomy. Postoperative change in hematocrit and need for transfusion do not vary between the laparoscopic and open approaches. Of note, pregnancy rates, abortion rates, preterm delivery, and the use of cesarean section are also comparable.

Limitations of the laparoscopic approach include loss of tactile sensation that is helpful in identifying intramural myomas, and time limitations due to large size and number of fibroids. Cases can by complicated by difficulty suturing the uterine defect, and time-consuming tissue removal. Some evidence also suggests that the inadequate closure of the uterine defect during laparoscopy can lead to increased rates of uterine rupture. Laparoscopic myomectomy should not be performed in women with diffuse myomas requiring extensive uterine reconstruction or in those with adenomyosis.

Intrauterine adhesions may occur if the uterine cavity is entered. Placement of an intrauterine balloon catheter or IUD after myomectomy with entry into the uterine cavity has been suggested to avoid postoperative Asherman syndrome; however, evidence for this practice is limited. If a balloon catheter is placed, prophylactic antibiotics are commonly given and the catheter is removed after 1 week. A regimen of high-dose estrogen may also be administered to rapidly proliferate the endometrium in an effort to reduce adhesions.

Laparoscopic access appears to decrease extrauterine adhesion formation compared with laparotomy. Adhesion formation may be increased by performing a posterior uterine incision, and by the presence of exposed suture and bulky knots. Interceed (Gynecare, Ethicon Inc.) or Gore-Tex adhesion barriers (Gore Medical, WL Gore & Associates) have been reported to decrease postoperative adhesion formation in a recent Cochrane review.

Studies have shown that risk of conversion to laparotomy is more likely in patients with a large number of myomas, myomas measuring more than 5 cm, anterior and intramural location, and preoperative use of GnRH agonists. Some surgeons believe that pretreatment with GnRH agonists will make the identification and dissection of a cleavage plane much harder. Other reasons for conversion to laparotomy are intraoperative hemorrhage and the presence of adenomyosis or uterine sarcoma.

Intraoperative discovery of unsuspected adenomyosis represents a unique challenge. Improvement in symptoms and successful pregnancy following cytoreduction of affected myometrium has been seen by some, while others recommend only myometrial biopsy to confirm the diagnosis.

If uterine sarcoma is truly suspected, an open technique may be advised to avoid morcellation. If benign pathology is more likely but some concern remains, the myoma can be delivered via minilaparotomy or colpotomy and sent for frozen pathologic section. Pathology results may then dictate conversion to open hysterectomy with staging.

Major complications include hemorrhage with or without hematoma formation in the uterus or pelvis, possibly requiring transfusion or repeat surgery. Bowel, ureter, and bladder injury have also been reported. A recent study at four Italian referral centers of 2050 laparoscopic myomectomy procedures found a rate of 9.1% for minor complications and 2% for major complications. Common complications after laparoscopic myomectomy include cystitis, fever, and anemia. "Myomectomy fever" of unknown origin resolving spontaneously is commonly reported.

The most challenging and vitally important technical aspect of laparoscopic myomectomy is proper suture closure of the myometrial defect. The suture should encompass the full depth of the edges and close the entire defect. Some defects require several layers because the main concern is the potential for uterine rupture during pregnancy. Inadequate healing may occur if the defect is not well approximated or space is left for a hematoma to form. The rate of uterine rupture after laparoscopic myomectomy is unknown; however, a series of 100 cases reported a rate of 1%. Further, no reliable rates of uterine rupture following conventional open myomectomy are available for comparison. Modifiable risks include: (1) not suturing a superficial myomectomy defect after the removal of subserosal myomas; (2) inadequate suturing (not suturing or suturing only the superficial layers); and (3) the excessive use of electrocautery. The essential observations from such reports and case series are that suturing technique is a critical determinant of uterine rupture and that some cases will occur even after myomectormy by laparotomy.

The recurrence of myomas has been reported to be higher after laparoscopic surgery than by laparotomy. However, recurrence after laparoscopic surgery was diagnosed by ultrasonography whereas the older laparotomy studies relied on less sensitive bimanual examination. More importantly, the need for further treatment is about 10% with both modalities. Generally, recurrence is reported in between 20% and 30% of cases. Increased recurrence is seen with pretreatment with gonadotropin-releasing hormone (GnRH) agonists, increasing numbers of myomas removed, and nulliparity. Most recurrences were reported between 10 and 30 months after surgery.

SUMMARY: Improvements in laparoscopic technology and the increased skill set of many clinicians have enabled an increase in the role of laparoscopy for myomectomy. As illustrated by the cases in this chapter, there are multiple applications for this technique and given an increasingly well-informed patient population, demand for minimally invasive techniques is likely to continue. The key steps of laparoscopic myomectomy remain unchanged. However, the many permutations of myoma size and distribution demand mastery of the aforementioned variations on these basic sequences. With careful patient selection and meticulous technique, many adverse outcomes can be avoided or optimally managed to ensure patient safety and successful completion of the planned laparoscopic procedure.

Suggested Reading

Amundson C, Silva B, Falcone T, Bradley L, Goldberg JM, Mascha E, Lindsey R, Stevens L: A case control study of laparoscopic versus abdominal myomectomy, *J Laparoendosc Adv Surg Tech A* 10:191-197, 2000.

Benecke C, Kruger TF, Siebert TI, Van der Merwe JP, Steyn DW: Effect of fibroids on fertility in patients undergoing assisted reproduction, *Gynecol Obstet Invest* 59:225-230, 2005.

Borgfeldt C, Andolf E: Transvaginal ultrasonographic findings in the uterus and the endometrium; low prevalence of leiomyoma in a random sample of women age 25-40 years, *Acta Obstet Gyn Scand* 79:202-207, 2000.

Buttram VC, Reiter RC, Uterine leiomyomata, *Fertil Steril* 36:433-445, 1981.

Cagnacci A, Pirillo D, Malmusi S, Arangino S, Alessandrini C, Volpe A: Early outcome of myomectomy by laparotomy, minilaparotomy and laparoscopically assisted minilaparotomy: a randomized prospective study, *Hum Reprod* 18(12):2590-2594, 2003.

Criniti A, Lin PC: Applications of intraoperative ultrasound in gynecological surgery, *Curr Opin Obstet Gynecol* 17:339-342, 2005.

Dubuisson JB, Fauconnier A, Fourchotte V, Babaki-Fard K, Coste J, Chapron C: Laparoscopic myomectomy: predicting the risk of conversion to an open procedure, *Hum Reprod* 16(8):1726-1731, 2001.

Dueholm M, Lundorf E, Hansen ES, Ledertoug S, Olesen F: Accuracy of magnetic resonance imaging and transvaginal ultrasonography in the diagnosis, mapping, and measurement of uterine myomas, *Am J Obstet Gynecol* 186(3):409-415, 2002.

Falcone T, Bedaiwy MA: Minimally invasive management of uterine fibroids, *Curr Opin Obstet Gynecol* 14:401-408, 2002.

Frishman GN, Jurema MW: Myomas and myomectomy. *J Minim Invasive Gynecol* 12:443-456, 2005.

Griffiths A, D'Angelo A, Amso N: Surgical treatment of fibroids for subfertility, *Cochrane Database Syst Rev* Issue 3: CD003857, 2006.

Holzer A, Jirecek ST, Illievich UM, Huber J, Wenzl RJ: Laparoscopic versus open myomectomy: a double-blind study to evaluate postoperative pain, *Anesth Analg* 102(5):1480-1484, 2006.

Horne AW, Critchley H: The effect of uterine fibroids on embryo implantation, *Semin Reprod Med* 25:483-490, 2007.

Hsu WC, Hwang JS, Chang WC, Huang SC, Sheu BC, Torng PL: Prediction of operation time for laparoscopic myomectomy by ultrasound measurements, *Surg Endosc* 21(9):1600-1606, 2007.

Kongnyuy EJ, Wiysonge CS: Interventions to reduce haemorrhage during myomectomy for fibroids. *Cochrane Database Syst Rev* Issue 1: CD005355, 2007.

Lethaby A, Vollenhoven B, Sowter M: Pre-operative GnRH analogue therapy before hysterectomy or myomectomy for uterine fibroids. *Cochrane Database Syst Rev* Issue 2: CD000547, 2001.

Lin PC, Thyer A, Soules MR: Intraoperative ultrasound during a laparoscopic myomectomy, *Fertil Steril* 81(6):1671-1674, 2004.

Marshall LM, Spiegelman D, Barbieri RL, et al: Variation in the incidence of uterine leiomyoma among premenopausal women by age and race, *Obstet Gynecol* 90:967-973, 1997.

Nezhat F, Seidman DS, Nezhat C, Nezhat CH: Laparoscopic myomectomy today: why, when and for whom? *Hum Reprod* 11(5):933-934, 1996.

Palomba S, Zupi E, Russo T, Falbo A, Marconi D, Tolino A, Manguso F, Mattei A, Zullo F: A multicenter randomized, controlled study comparing laparoscopic versus minilaparotomic myomectomy: short-term outcomes, *Fertil Steril* 88(4):942-951, 2007.

Palomba S, Zupi E, Falbo A, Russo T, Marconi D, Tolino A, Manguso F, Mattei A, Zullo F: A multicenter randomized, controlled study comparing laparoscopic versus minilaparotomic myomectomy: reproductive outcomes, *Fertil Steril* 88(4):933-941, 2007.

Paul PG, Koshy AK, Thomas T: Pregnancy outcomes following laparoscopic myomectomy and single-layer myometrial closure, *Hum Reprod* 21(12):3278-3281, 2006.

Payson M: Epidemiology of myomas, *Obstet Gynecol Clin North Am* 33(1):1-11, 2006.

Pelosi MA, Pelosi III, MA, Eim J: Hand-assisted laparoscopy for megamyomectomy: a case report, *J Reprod Med* 45(6):519-525, 2000.

Practice Committee of the American Society for Reproductive Medicine: Myomas and reproductive function, *Fertil Steril* 86(5 suppl):S194-S199, 2006.

Reed SD, Newton KM, Thompson LB, McCrummen BA, Warolin AK: The incidence of repeat uterine surgery following myomectomy, *J Womens Health* 15(9):1046-1052, 2006.

Rossetti A, Sizzi O, Soranna L, Cucinelli F, Mancuso S, Lanzone A: Long-term results of laparoscopic myomectomy: recurrence rate in comparison with abdominal myomectomy, *Hum Reprod* 16(4):770-774, 2001.

Somigliana E, Vercellini P, Daguati R, Pasin R, De Giorgi O, Crosignani PG: Fibroids and female reproduction: a critical analysis of the evidence, *Hum Reprod Update* 13(5):465-476, 2007.

Sizzi O, Rossetti A, Malzoni M, Minelli L, La Grotta F, Soranna L, Panunzi S, Spagnolo R, Imperato F, Landi S, Fiaccamento A, Stola E: Italian multicenter study on complications of laparoscopic myomectomy, *J Minim Invasive Gynecol* 14(4):453-462, 2007.

Velebil P, Wingo PA, Xia Z, Wilcox LS, Peterson HB: Rate of hospitalization for gynecologic disorders among reproductive age women in the United States, *Obstet Gynecol* 86:764-769, 1995.

Whiteman MK, Hillis SD, Jamieson DJ, Morrow B, Podgornik MN, Brett KM, Marchbanks PA: Inpatient hysterectomy surveillance in the United States, 2000-2004, *Am J Obstet Gynecol* 198(1):34.e1-34.e7, 2008.

Zullo F, Palomba S, Corea D, Pellicano M, Russo T, Falbo A, Barletta E, Saraco P, Doldo P, Zupi E: Bupivacaine plus epinephrine for laparoscopic myomectomy: a randomized placebo-controlled trial, *Obstet Gynecol* 104(2):243-249, 2004.

Indications and Techniques for Total and Subtotal Laparoscopic Hysterectomy

8

Beri Ridgeway M.D.
Tommaso Falcone M.D.

 Video Clips on DVD

8-1 Technique for Uterine Manipulation (3 minutes/46 seconds)

8-2 Techniques to Morcellate a Uterus (2 minutes/19 seconds)

8-3 Laparoscopic Vaginal Cuff Closure Using a Running Suture (3 minutes/56 seconds)

8-4 Laparoscopic Modified McCall Culdoplasty (1 minutes/36 seconds)

8-5 Laparoscopic Hysterectomy (10 minutes/39 seconds)

8-6 Laparoscopic Supracervical Hysterectomy after Failed Uterine Artery Embolization (6 minutes/59 seconds)

Introduction

Laparoscopic hysterectomy was first performed in 1989, and has gained significant popularity in the past two decades. This procedure was developed with the hope of decreasing the morbidity and mortality related to abdominal hysterectomy, one of the most commonly performed gynecologic surgeries. Laparoscopic hysterectomy encompasses total laparoscopic hysterectomy, which includes removing the uterus and cervix, and subtotal or supracervical laparoscopic hysterectomy, during which only the uterine corpus is removed. Laparoscopic hysterectomy is performed entirely laparoscopically, including all dissection, ligation, and transection of pedicles. Laparoscopic hysterectomy is to be distinguished from laparoscopic-assisted vaginal hysterectomy (LAVH). During LAVH, the first portion of the procedure, ligation and transection of the infundibulopelvic or utero-ovarian ligaments and possibly ligation and transection of the uterine vessels, is performed laparoscopically. The remainder of the procedure is performed vaginally, including colpotomy, dissection of the bladder, and ligation and transection of the uterosacral and cardinal ligaments (Table 8-1). According to the Cochrane Review, the term laparoscopic hysterectomy should be applied to any hysterectomy in which all vessels are occluded laparoscopically. When no portion of the procedure is performed vaginally, the term "total laparoscopic hysterectomy" should be employed. This chapter will discuss total and supracervical laparoscopic hysterectomies, which are considered stage 5 laparoscopic hysterectomies.

Despite the relative popularity of this procedure, in the year 2003, abdominal hysterectomy was still far more prevalent than laparoscopic hysterectomy for benign

Table 8-1 Staging of Laparoscopic Hysterectomy

Stage 0	Laparoscopy done, but no additional laparoscopic procedure performed before vaginal hysterectomy
Stage 1	Procedure includes both laparoscopic adhesiolysis and/or excision of endometriosis
Stage 2	Either or both adnexa freed laparoscopically
Stage 3	Laparoscopic dissection of bladder from uterus
Stage 4	Uterine artery transected laparoscopically
Stage 5	Anterior and/or posterior colpotomy or entire uterus freed laparoscopically

disease (66.1% versus 11.8%). These rates have been relatively constant, with database studies demonstrating similar rates of each procedure from 1990 through 1997. Interestingly, these studies include laparoscopic hysterectomy and LAVH in the same category and a shift between LAVH and total laparoscopic hysterectomy may be difficult to detect.

Indications

The indications for laparoscopic hysterectomy are controversial and have included symptomatic uterine leiomyoma, menstrual disorders, pelvic organ prolapse, and malignant and premalignant disease. Advantages to the laparoscopic approach to hysterectomy include: excellent anatomic view of the abdominal and pelvic cavities, superior tissue imaging, facilitation of hemostasis and reduction in the morbidity associated with laparotomy. Additionally, this approach allows adnexal surgery, adhesiolysis, ureterolysis, retroperitoneal dissections, and excision of endometriosis. According to the American College of Obstetrics and Gynecology Committee Opinion, the technique used for hysterectomy should be dictated by the indications for surgery, patient characteristics, and patient preference. Most patients requiring hysterectomy should be offered the vaginal approach when technically feasible and medically appropriate. If specific additional procedures that can be completed laparoscopically are anticipated before surgery, the laparoscopic approach to hysterectomy may be an appropriate alternative. These procedures include: lysis of adhesions, treatment of endometriosis, management of uterine leiomyomas that complicate the performance of vaginal hysterectomy, ligation of infundibulopelvic ligaments to facilitate difficult ovary removal, and evaluation of the pelvic and abdominal cavity before hysterectomy. However, the benefits of laparoscopic hysterectomy must be weighed against the risks and additional expense.

When hysterectomy is indicated in a patient where completion of a vaginal hysterectomy would be difficult, laparoscopic hysterectomy may offer advantages over abdominal hysterectomy. For example, access to the uterus from the vagina may be limited by a narrow pubic arch, adhesions, lack of uterine descensus, cervical elongation, low-lying uterine myomas, or bulky uterine pathology. Additionally, prior pelvic surgery or pelvic infections may predispose a patient to pelvic adhesions that may make a vaginal hysterectomy more difficult or increase the likelihood of complications. Laparoscopy can aid in visualization and lysis of adhesions in cases like these. Furthermore, a large, bulky uterus makes vaginal hysterectomy more difficult. In cases where the uterine vessels cannot be safely occluded vaginally prior to vaginal morcellation, laparoscopic or abdominal hysterectomy is indicated. In cases of deep infiltrating endometriosis when hysterectomy is also indicated, the laparoscopic approach allows concurrent excision thereby maximizing therapy. Some surgeons advocate the use of laparoscopy to safely perform concurrent oophorectomy, though many skilled vaginal surgeons are able to perform most oophorectomies vaginally. However, there are cases when laparoscopy eases oophorectomy, as in cases where the ovaries are densely adherent to the pelvic sidewall, requiring a retroperitoneal approach to identify the ureter.

The main limitations to a laparoscopic approach are medical or anesthetic disorders that do not allow adequate pneumoperitoneum or proper ventilation. Very dense pelvic abdominal adhesions from previous surgery and very large uterine size are relative contraindications, however, this is surgeon-dependent and the decision can be made after assessing the pelvis laparoscopically. If the uterine size or shape limits access to the uterine vessels, laparoscopic hysterectomy may not be possible. Obesity is not a contraindication to laparoscopic hysterectomy and may actually minimize the morbidity associated with laparotomy.

Total versus Subtotal Hysterectomy

In cases without cervical dysplasia, uterine hyperplasia, premalignancy, known or suspected malignancy, or cervical fibroids, patients may have the choice between total laparoscopic hysterectomy and subtotal hysterectomy. Subtotal hysterectomy is defined as the removal of the uterine corpus at or below the level of the internal cervical os and attempted ablation of the endocervical canal after removal of the corpus. In laparoscopic subtotal hysterectomy, morcellation of the uterine fundus is required to facilitate its removal through the port-site incisions. Historically, the supracervical or subtotal hysterectomy was abandoned in favor of total hysterectomy because of problems related to the retained cervix. However, subtotal hysterectomy has gained a renewed interest as one technique to reduce the effects of hysterectomy on urinary and sexual function. Unfortunately, to date, the possible benefits of supracervical hysterectomy with regard to perioperative morbidity and postoperative sexual and urinary function are not supported by research. In three randomized controlled trials that did not include laparoscopic hysterectomy, there were no differences in complication rates including infection, blood loss requiring transfusion, or urinary tract, bowel, or vascular injury. Reported rates of postoperative cyclical vaginal bleeding in women randomized to subtotal hysterectomy were 5% to 20%. Approximately 1.5% of these participants had a second operation within 3 months to remove the cervix. Additionally, choosing to preserve the cervix to conserve sexual and urinary function has not been supported by these studies. There were no differences in postoperative stress or urge urinary incontinence, urinary frequency, or incomplete bladder emptying in most studies. One European study did find a higher incidence of urinary incontinence after subtotal hysterectomy. In regard to sexual function, there was no difference in any outcome in any of the prospective studies. Retrospective studies comparing outcomes between laparoscopic total and subtotal hysterectomies demonstrate conflicting results. One study at a large managed care organization demonstrated longer operative time, but less blood loss, shorter hospital stay, and fewer major complications in laparoscopic subtotal hysterectomy compared to total abdominal hysterectomy. Despite the lack of data supporting superior outcomes for subtotal hysterectomy, the decision between total and subtotal hysterectomy is often highly personal. Many patients may have strong preexisting ideas about retaining the cervix and this should be discussed with the patient preoperatively in detail.

Candidates interested in subtotal hysterectomy must have normal results from a recent cytologic cervical examination and a normal gross appearance of the cervix documented before surgery. Clinicians should also consider testing for high-risk human papilloma virus strains. Morcellation of the uterine corpus is required in the laparoscopic subtotal hysterectomy. Because of this step, adequate preoperative assessment of the endometrial cavity to exclude neoplasm is necessary.

Case 1: Total Laparoscopic Hysterectomy to Treat Symptomatic Uterine Fibroids

 View DVD: Video 8-5

The patient is a 45-year-old woman, gravida 4 para 3, with a 6-year history of menometrorrhagia. Symptoms consist of heavy vaginal bleeding every 20 to 34 days. She typically bleeds for 7 days, noting clots on the first 2 days. She also complains of dysmenorrhea and pelvic heaviness. Her work-up included a detailed history and physical examination which revealed an enlarged, irregularly-shaped uterus. PAP smear and high-risk HPV DNA testing were negative. An ultrasonogram revealed an enlarged uterus measuring 14 × 7 cm, with multiple intramural fibroids. An endometrial biopsy demonstrated normal secretory endometrium. The patient was managed initially with oral contraceptives and Depot Lupron but did not note much improvement and did not tolerate the side effects.

Discussion of Case: Preoperative Preparation

As with any surgical procedure, assure that the patient meets criteria for surgical management, including failed attempts at medical therapy. Once operative management is deemed necessary, it is crucial that the patient understand the risks, benefits, and alternatives to the surgical procedure, as well as the expected recovery. In the specific case of laparoscopic hysterectomy, there must be an understanding between physician and patient on the surgical approach, type of hysterectomy (total versus subtotal), and whether concomitant oophorectomy is planned. Depending on the indication for hysterectomy and age of the patient, Pap screen testing, high-risk human papilloma virus strain testing, radiographic study (ultrasound or MRI) of the pelvis, and pathologic evaluation of the endometrial lining may be indicated. Preoperative work-up should include a detailed history and physical examination, baseline laboratory tests including complete blood count, basic metabolic panel, and type and screen. Referral to an internist may be necessary in patients with comorbidities such as heart disease. In premenopausal women, pregnancy should be ruled out on the day of surgery.

Prophylactic antibiotics decrease the risk of surgical site infections and their use is one of the most important steps to decrease surgical morbidity. The timing of antibiotic administration is critical to lowering the frequency of surgical site infection. The antibiotic should be given preoperatively to achieve minimal inhibitory concentrations in the skin and tissues by the time the incision is made. This typically means an intravenous injection within 60 minutes of incision with a first generation cephalosporin ACOG recommends cefazolin 1 g IV. For patients weighing greater than 100 kg or for those with a BMI >35, 2 g is indicated. For patients who have an allergy to penicillins or cephalosporins, they recommend clindamycin 600 mg IV AND gentamicin 1.5 mg/kg IV or quinolone 400mg IV or aztreonam 1 g IV. Alternatively, metronidazole 500mg IV AND gentamicin 1.5 mg/kg IV or quinolone 400 mg IV may be used. These antibiotics were chosen because the likely pathogens for hysterectomies are gram-negative bacilli, enterococci, group B streptococci, and anaerobes. Longer procedures require redosing at 3 hour intervals for cefazolin. Blood loss over 1500 mL also requires redosing. Prophylactic antibiotics should be discontinued within 24 hours.

In general, all patients undergoing hysterectomy require a prevention strategy for venous thromboembolism (VTE). In these patients, unfractionated heparin (5000 units every 12 hours) or low-molecular-weight heparin (e.g., enoxaparin 40 mg or dalteparin 2500 units) or intermittent pneumatic compression device is recommended. These treatment approaches should be continued until the patient is ambulatory. In patients older than 60 years age and in those with significant risks such as previous VTE, malignancy, or hypercoagulable state, unfractionated heparin (5000 units every 8 hours) or low-molecular-weight-heparin (enoxaparin 40mg or dalteparin 5000 units) and intermittent pneumatic compression devices should be used. In high risk patients, continuing prophylaxis for 2-4 weeks after discharge should be considered. Patients on oral contraceptives up to the time of hysterectomy should be considered for heparin therapy.

Surgical Techniques: Total Laparoscopic Hysterectomy

View DVD: Videos 8-1 through 8-5

1. After general anesthesia is induced and the patient is intubated, an orogastric tube should be introduced, and she should be positioned in the low lithotomy position using adjustable cushioned stirrups, such as Allen or Yellofin stirrups (Figure 8-1). The arms should be tucked and cushioned to prevent nerve injury. Arm sleds may be necessary in patients who are obese. Because steep Trendelenburg positioning is often used in total laparoscopic hysterectomy, it may be helpful to place an egg-crate cushion or shoulder braces to prevent sliding during the procedure. We often minimally shave the pubic hair in case laparotomy is necessary. An exam under anesthesia is performed. Careful attention should be paid to the uterine size, contour, and width, uterine mobility, cervical size and location, and evidence of masses or endometriosis.

2. The patient's abdomen, vagina, and upper thighs are prepared with Betadine or Hibiclens. A Foley catheter is inserted into the bladder. A uterine manipulator is

Figure 8-1. The patient is positioned in the low lithotomy position.

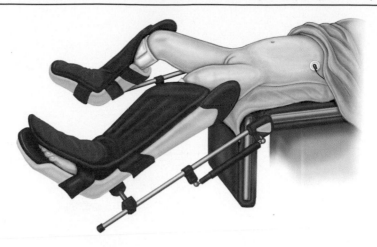

inserted into the uterine cavity. This is one of the most important steps, because uterine manipulation can can help to expose all pertinent anatomy and make the procedure safer. There are several types of uterine manipulators currently on the market. A sponge stick in the vagina can be used if a uterine manipulator is not available. We prefer the Koh colpotomizer (Cooper Surgical, Inc., Trumbull, CT) attached to the Rumi manipulator (Cooper Surgical, Inc., Trumbull, CT) with vaginal occluder sleeve (see Video 8-1). Though insertion of this device may take several minutes, its ability to manipulate the uterus in multiple directions often saves time in the end. We suture the Rumi manipulator and Koh colpotomizer into the cervix at 12 and 6 o'clock to prevent slippage and to facilitate removal of the specimen at the end of the case.

3. Once the manipulator is secured, gloves are changed, and attention is turned to the abdomen. The most important technical consideration for all laparoscopic surgery is port placement. The umbilical site is typically used in patients without a previous history of surgery or intra-abdominal infection. However, in cases of previous surgery where there was a midline incision or in patients with a history of pelvic-abdominal infection, an alternative site, usually the left upper quadrant, is chosen to introduce the primary trocar (Figure 8-2). Alternatively, an open laparoscopy, or minilaparotomy, at the umbilicus can be performed.

The standard closed technique involves the use of a pneumoperitoneum needle (Veress needle), insufflation, and then primary trocar insertion. Direct trocar insertion with no insufflation prior to trocar insertion may also be used. A meta-analysis showed no advantage of one technique over the other. The safest approach is likely the one with which the surgeon has the most experience. If the left upper quadrant approach is used, then the surgeon should be aware of the closest anatomic structures to the left costal margin. Typically, the cannula is introduced below the left costal margin in the midclavicular line. The closest structures to this area are the stomach and the left lobe of the liver. Therefore, an oro-gastric tube should be introduced to empty the stomach before starting the case.

Once insufflation is achieved, the patient is placed in steep Trendelenburg position because this allows the pelvic contents, specifically the bowel, to move cephalad. Additional ports are placed (see Figure 8-2). We prefer three additional ports, one in each lower quadrant and one in the left midclavicular line at the level of the umbilicus. Typically, we place the lower quadrant ports 2 cm superior and 2 cm medial to the anterior superior iliac spine. This trocar placement pattern avoids damage to the ilioinguinal and iliohypogastric nerves. However, in cases where the uterus is enlarged, placement of the lower quadrant ports must be adjusted cephalad, with the ports nearing the level of the umbilicus in cases of a very large uterus. With placement of each trocar, anatomic landmarks must be used to avoid visceral and vascular injury.

4. A general survey of the abdomen and pelvis is performed. At this point in the procedure, it is necessary to decide whether laparoscopic completion of the

Figure 8-2. Three to four ports are placed intra-abdominally. For a large uterus, the ports may be placed more cephalad.

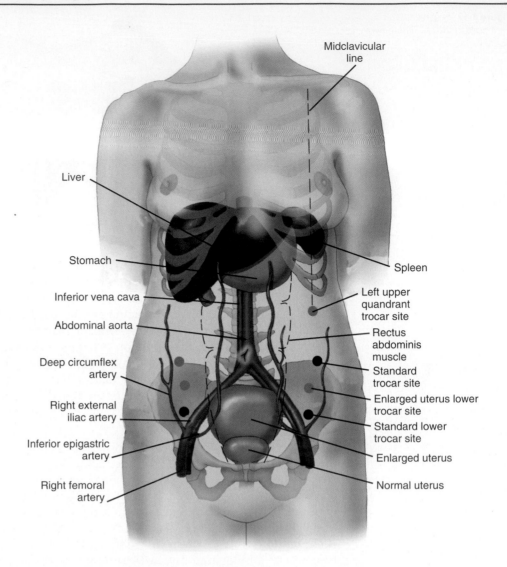

hysterectomy is feasible. If it is not, conversion to laparotomy is appropriate and not considered a complication or failure. The path of the pelvic ureter is traced. In cases where the ureter is not visible transperitoneally, such as with retroperitoneal fibrosis, retroperitoneal dissection may be required to identify the ureter in order to prevent ureteral damage. Lysis of adhesions is performed if necessary. Close examination of the tubes and ovaries is then performed.

There are many options available for ligation of the vascular pedicles using suture or energy sources during laparoscopic hysterectomy. Each has advantages and disadvantages. Though it does incur an additional expense, we prefer a single-use bipolar vessel-sealing device with attached blade. The decision of which instrument or device to use is of personal preference; however, we do not recommend the use of a laparoscopic stapler device for securing the uterine vessels, because lateral firing can damage the ureter.

5. If oophorectomy is planned, the infundibulopelvic ligament is identified. The manipulator may be adjusted to optimize visualization of each side. With the ureter in sight, the infundibulopelvic ligament is ligated and transected bilaterally. If an ovarian-sparing procedure is planned, the utero-ovarian ligament is ligated and transected (Figure 8-3). Safe ligation and trans-ction of these pedicles can be most safely performed from the contralateral side. Although in Figure 8-3 a stapling device is demonstrated, we typically use a bipolar or ultrasonic vibration energy.

6. Attention is turned to the round ligament. The round ligament is transected and ligated approximately 1-3 cm from the cornua (Figure 8-4). This allows the surgical

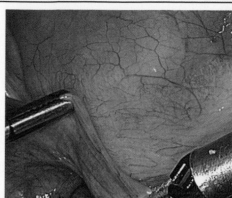

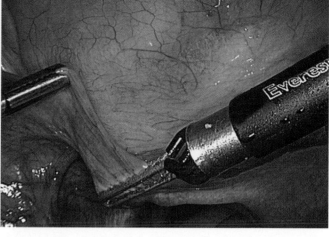

Figure 8-3. The utero-ovarian ligament is transected if an ovarian-sparing procedure is planned.

Figure 8-4. The round ligament is grasped one to three centimeters from the cornua and ligated.

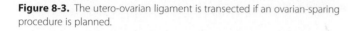

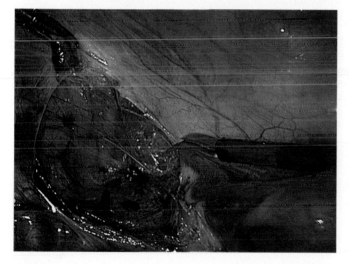

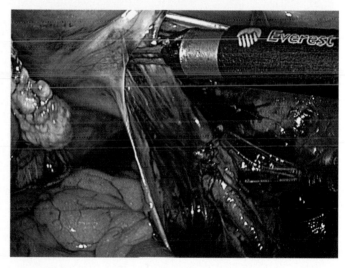

Figure 8-5. The anterior and posterior broad ligament leaves are separated.

Figure 8-6. The posterior leaf of the broad ligament is taken down to the level of the uterosacral ligament.

assistant to use the round ligament remnant for traction. The uterine manipulator and introduction of a laparoscopic tenaculum can optimize visualization. Once the round ligament is completely transected, blunt dissection can be used to separate the anterior and posterior leaves of the broad ligament (Figure 8-5). The posterior leaf should be taken down to the level of the uterosacral ligament (Figure 8-6). This drops the ureter away from the uterine vessels. Certain cases will require that the pelvic sidewall be opened to clearly identify the ureter (Figure 8-7).

7. The anterior leaf should be taken down inferiorly and medially in preparation for bladder flap development. If the vesicouterine peritoneum is difficult to visualize, the bladder can be filled in a retrograde fashion to delineate the border. Once the peritoneum is opened slightly above the bladder border, blunt and sharp dissection can be used to dissect the bladder from the pericervical fascia (Figure 8-8). This is a glistening white layer that can easily be distinguished from the bladder. Judicious use of cautery is necessary, as this is a risk factor for urinary tract injury and subsequent fistula. One should use an instrument to palpate the colpotomizer cup or sponge stick to appreciate the anterior cul-de-sac (Figure 8-9). Once the bladder is 1 cm below this border, there should be sufficient space for adequate cuff closure.

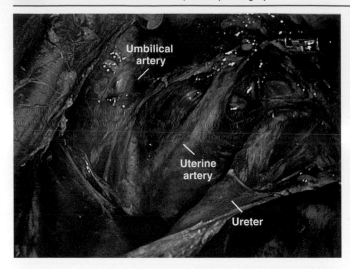

Figure 8-7. Note the proximity of the sidewall vessels and the ureter.

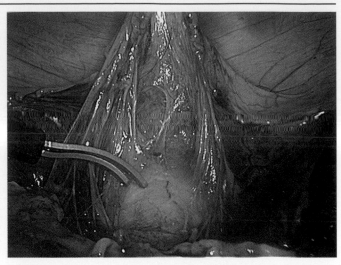

Figure 8-8. The bladder is dissected sharply from the cervix.

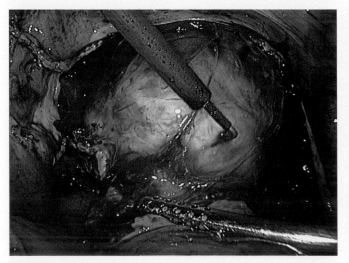

Figure 8-9. The cervico-uterine junction is free of bladder tissue and the colpotomy cup is palpated.

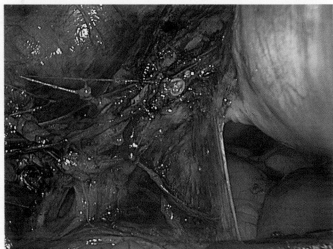

Figure 8-10. The uterine vessels are skeletonized and transected.

8. The uterine vessels are skeletonized, further dropping the ureter, and then ligated (Figure 8-10). If there is any doubt of complete vessel ligation, one may avoid transection until the contralateral side is ligated. At this point in the procedure, the same steps are carried out on the contralateral side after appropriate uterine manipulation and countertraction from the surgical assistant.

9. The colpotomy cup should be palpable circumferentially. The uterine manipulator should be pushed cephalad to facilitate this. Prior to colpotomy, care should be taken to assure that the bladder and rectum are below the colpotomy cup. The vaginal cuff occluder should be filled with saline or water or a laparotomy sponge covered with a sterile glove should be placed in the vagina to maintain pneumo-peritoneum. Amputation of the uterus can be performed with monopolar cautery, sharp dissection, or using ultrasonic vibration energy. Minimal contact with the tissue is preferred as excess cautery can lead to tissue necrosis, which may be a risk factor for cuff dehiscence. Typically, we enter anteriorly or posteriorly (Figure 8-11). Once the colpotomy cup is visualized, one can trace the colpotomy cup. This prevents veering off course, because a two-dimensional view can sometimes be distorting. When performing the colpotomy, keep the uterine vessel pedicles in view and open the vagina above the pedicles laterally.

10. Once the colpotomy is complete, determine if the uterus can be delivered vaginally. If so, remove the occluder and pull the Rumi manipulator and uterus through

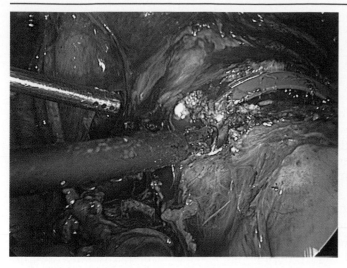

Figure 8-11. An anterior colpotomy is performed with monopolar cautery.

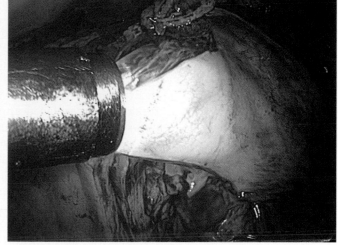

Figure 8-12. The specimen is morcellated.

Figure 8-13. The specimen is removed in strips.

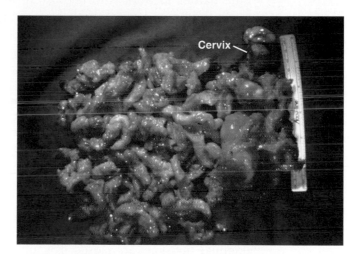

the vagina. The initial suturing of the uterus to the manipulator assists in this step. A single-tooth tenaculum used for traction vaginally can also be helpful during this step. If the uterus is too large, vaginal morcellation can be performed. Otherwise, laparoscopic morcellation will be necessary (Figure 8-12) (see Video 8-2 📹). Replace the vaginal occluder to maintain pneumoperitoneum. As the specimen is morcellated, strips will be removed through the abdominal ports (Figure 8-13). Once the specimen is small enough, it can be removed through the vagina. The abdomen should be carefully surveyed to collect any remaining small uterine pieces.

11. Inspect the vaginal cuff and use judicious bipolar or monopolar cautery to obtain hemostasis. This step can be performed prior to morcellation if necessary. Once hemostasis is achieved, the vaginal cuff is closed. If one does not have adequate laparoscopic suturing abilities or instruments to close the cuff laparoscopically, it can be closed vaginally. There are many possible ways to close the vaginal cuff laparoscopically, including suture placement devices such as the Capio suture device (Boston Scientific, Natick, MA), Endostitch Covidien, Mansfield, MA), Lapra-Ty (Ethicon Endo-surgery, Inc., Somerville, NJ) and free suturing. We prefer free suturing because of its relative simplicity, low cost, and transferable skill set.

When using interrupted sutures, we use 0-polyglactin 910 with extracorporeal knot-tying (see Video 8-5 📹). The vaginal apex corner is identified, the posterior cuff is elevated, and the needle is placed through the posterior vaginal cuff approximately 1 cm medial to the corner and then through the anterior vaginal cuff in the same location. The depth of the tissue bite should be approximately 5 to 10 mm and the vaginal epithelium and pelvic peritoneum should be included on each bite. This ensures that the bite is deep enough and that hemostasis will be achieved. Keep in mind that the laparoscope will provide magnification and the tendency may be to take smaller bites. Anteriorly, care must be taken to avoid incorporating the bladder into the suture line. Continue closing the cuff with interrupted sutures placed approximately 1 cm apart (Figure 8-14). Typically, we will close the contralateral vaginal apex corner prior to completing the remainder of the closure. Closely survey the cuff and place additional sutures if necessary. Alternatively, the cuff can be closed with running suture, using intracorporeal knot-tying (Video 8-3 📹 or see Chapter 5). For this type of closure, we will typically use 0-polydioxanone. Place one suture measuring 6 centimeters in the vaginal apex corner ipsilateral to where the surgeon is standing. Once it is tied intracorporeally, cut the shorter of the free ends. Start at the contralateral corner with another suture measuring 13 centimeters. Place and tie this and then run the suture line towards the surgeon. Once the other corner is reached, tie the two sutures together with intracorporeal knot-tying. Polydioxanone may initially seem a little harder to work with because of its memory, but it can easily be pulled through the tissue after multiple bites are taken.

12. Once the cuff is completely closed, we place a modified McCall culdoplasty to prevent vaginal vault prolapse (see Video 8-4 📹). Using 0-polydioxanone, a stitch is placed through the uterosacral ligament on the right side, then passed through the posterior cuff, and then through the left uterosacral ligament. As this is tied down, the uterosacral ligaments are plicated in the midline.

13. An ampule of indigo carmine is injected intravenously and cystoscopy is performed. This step is absolutely necessary because the incidence of lower urinary tract injury is noteworthy and recognition and repair of any injury is critical. Cystoscopy should include a general survey of the bladder to check for cystotomy and sutures as well as identification of the ureteral orifices with efflux of blue dye bilaterally. Once this is complete, the Foley is replaced and a speculum exam is performed checking for bleeding, uterine fragments, and instruments. All operative pedicles are observed under diminished intra-abdominal pressure and the abdominal incisions are closed. For any port greater than or equal to 10 mm in size, the fascia is closed using a Carter-Thomason endofascial closure device (Inlet Medical, Inc., Eden Prairie, MN).

Figure 8-14. The vaginal cuff is closed using free suturing techniques.

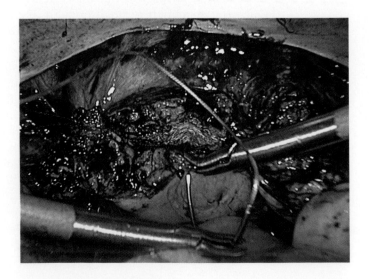

Case 2: Laparoscopic Subtotal Hysterectomy

 View DVD: Video 8-6

This is a 49-year-old woman, gravida 4 para 3, with a 6-year history of menorrhagia. Symptoms consist of heavy vaginal bleeding every 28 to 30 days. She typically bleeds for 7 days, noting clots on the first 2 days. She also complains of dysmenorrhea and pelvic heaviness. Her work-up included a detailed history and physical examination which revealed an enlarged, irregularly shaped uterus. Pap smear and high-risk HPV DNA testing were negative, an endometrial biopsy demonstrated normal secretory endometrium and an ultrasonogram revealed an enlarged uterus measuring 14 × 9 cm with multiple intramural fibroids. The patient elected uterine artery embolization which was performed without incident. Symptoms improved initially, although approximately 4 months after embolization, the patient presented to the emergency room with heavy vaginal bleeding and requested definitive treatment. An ultrasonogram at that time revealed that the uterus had enlarged to 16 × 10 × 10 cm with three discrete fibroids.

Surgical Techniques: Subtotal Laparoscopic Hysterectomy

1. Techniques for subtotal laparoscopic hysterectomy are similar to those described above. Deviations occur during the bladder dissection and amputation of the uterus as described below. If subtotal hysterectomy is planned, a colpotomy cup is not necessary, though a Rumi manipulator can help significantly with an enlarged uterus.

2. Subtotal hysterectomy only deviates from the total laparoscopic hysterectomy description at the point of bladder dissection. If subtotal hysterectomy is planned, minimal bladder dissection is necessary because amputation will occur at the level of the internal os.

3. Once the uterine vessels are coagulated and the level of the internal os is identified, the uterine fundus is amputated from the cervix. This can be performed with monopolar cautery or ultrasonic vibration energy. Ideally, this is performed while angling the device towards the os, creating a reverse cone, which theoretically removes more of the endocervix, potentially decreasing cyclic bleeding (Figure 8-15). Cautery is

Figure 8-15. A reverse cone is performed to prevent cyclic bleeding.

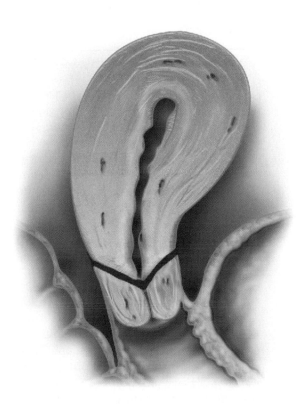

then applied to the endocervix and the anterior and posterior peritoneum are reapproximated over the stump using several interrupted sutures. The entire specimen is then morcellated (see Video 8-2). As with total laparoscopic hysterectomy, cystoscopy and vaginal exam are performed. A prophylactic McCall culdoplasty can be considered (see Video 8-4 📷).

New Technology

In the last five years, variations of the approach to minimally invasive hysterectomy have emerged with the goal of improving patient outcomes and satisfaction. These changes have included the application of robotic surgery and single-port laparoscopy to hysterectomy. For detailed information on robotic surgery, please see chapter X.

Recent technologic advances in endoscopic instrumentation and optics have allowed the development of a less invasive alternative to conventional laparoscopy. Single-port laparoscopy reduces the number of ports required to perform a hysterectomy. This may translate to decreased post-operative pain, fewer port-related complications, and improved cosmetics. Several single port entry systems are currently available and typically consist of an operative sleeve that is introduced into the abdomen through a 3-5 cm incision in the umbilicus. Through this sleeve, two to three operative channels and one camera channel are used to complete the procedure. To facilitate using this new technology, we recommend using a flexible camera and introducing it laterally in the sleeve to prevent collision with the operative instruments. Whether the approach to hysterectomy is using conventional laparoscopy, robotics, or single port, it is important to remember that the steps to hysterectomy are the same.

Postoperative Management

At our institution, patients are admitted for observation and most often are discharged the next morning. However, many physicians perform laparoscopic hysterectomy as an outpatient procedure. Aggressive prophylactic treatment of postoperative nausea and pain is imperative in patients interested in same-day discharge. Furthermore, careful patient selection, appropriate patient expectation, and availability of immediate emergency care are essential when considering outpatient hysterectomy.

Avoiding and Managing Complications

Complications related to the performance of hysterectomy are equally inherent in the laparoscopic and abdominal approach to hysterectomy. However, lower urinary tract injury and vaginal cuff evisceration seem to be increased with laparoscopic hysterectomy. The rates of conversion to laparotomy (3.3%) and vaginal approach (2.0%) are relatively low. A large randomized controlled trial comparing laparoscopic hysterectomy to open and vaginal hysterectomy found that approximately 7% of patients undergoing laparoscopic hysterectomy had at least one complication (including conversion to laparotomy) with the most common complications being major hemorrhage requiring transfusion (4.6%-5.1%), bowel injury (0.2%), ureter injury (0.3%-0.9%), and bladder injury (0.9%-2.1%) (Table 8-2). The complication rate for laparoscopic hysterectomy was noted to be significantly higher than for vaginal and abdominal hysterectomy; however, if conversion to laparotomy had not been considered a major complication, then the complication rates were not different among groups. Single-institution, large case series note similar complication rates.

Avoidance of complications can usually be achieved with careful dissection, identification of anatomic landmarks, and judicious use of cautery. One of the most important considerations in laparoscopic hysterectomy is that this procedure is essentially the same as open hysterectomy, although performed through smaller incisions and with longer instruments. All steps of the open hysterectomy must be performed laparoscopically, using similar techniques in order to avoid complications.

Table 8-2 Complications of Hysterectomy from the eVALuate Trial

	Abdominal Trial		Vaginal Trial	
	Abdominal Hysterectomy (%)	Laparoscopic Hysterectomy (%)	Vaginal Hysterectomy (%)	Laparoscopic Hysterectomy (%)
At least one complication	6.2	7.2	5.4	6.7
Conversion to laparotomy		3.9	4.2	2.7
Major hemorrhage requiring transfusion	2.4	4.6	2.9	5.1
Bowel injury	1	0.2	0	0
Ureter injury	0	0.9	0	0.3
Bladder injury	1	2.1	1.2	0.9
Other*	2.1	2.4	1.8	3.9

*Includes pulmonary complications, anesthesia, return to the operating room, wound dehiscence, and hematoma.

Hemorrhage

Once insufflation is achieved, ligating the infundibulopelvic ligament and the uterine vessels and performing the colpotomy are the most common steps when hemorrhage will be encountered. This can be prevented by dissection, isolation of the pedicle, and ligation. When bleeding is encountered, a surgical assistant must provide visualization using a suction-irrigation device. If an additional port would be of assistance, place one as soon as the need is recognized. Conversion to laparotomy should always be an option and in our minds, is not considered a complication or failure, but rather sound surgical judgment.

Lower Urinary Tract Injury

Lower urinary tract injury including bladder and ureter injury is more common in laparoscopic hysterectomy when compared to other approaches to hysterectomy. Bladder injury can be avoided by identification of the vesicouterine peritoneal plane and careful creation of the bladder flap. Sharp dissection with very minimal use of heat may help avoid thermal injury or fistula creation. Ureteral injury can be avoided by identifying the ureter and ureterolysis, if necessary. Skeletonizing the uterine vessels prior to ligation further allows the ureter to fall from the area of ligation. Furthermore, ligation of the infundibulopelvic ligaments and uterine vessels should be performed with the ureter in sight. Additionally, the ureter can become entrapped or kinked with vaginal cuff closure. Care should be taken to avoid wide, lateral bites at the vaginal apex corners. Equally important as avoidance of lower urinary tract injury is recognition. One single-institution study noted that only 40% of lower urinary tract injuries were noted at the time of laparoscopy with the remainder noted during routine cystoscopy. The great majority of bladder and ureter injuries can be remedied intraoperatively, leading to lower long-term morbidity. For this reason, we consider routine cystoscopy with intravenous administration of indigo carmine an essential step of laparoscopic hysterectomy.

Vaginal Cuff Dehiscence

In one large single-institution study, the vaginal cuff dehiscence rate after laparoscopic hysterectomy was close to 5%, which was significantly higher when compared to abdominal and vaginal hysterectomies. This finding has been supported by other studies and clinical experience, though many surgeons believe that the rate is not as high as this study reports. The majority of these patients reported bowel evisceration during or after the first postoperative episode of intercourse. Study authors hypothesize that electrosurgical thermal energy and techniques unique to laparoscopic hysterectomy are responsible. Though the exact causes of dehiscence are unknown, judicious use of cautery on the vaginal cuff and placing suture at least 1 cm from the vaginal cuff edges may help prevent this complication.

Cyclic Vaginal Bleeding after Subtotal Hysterectomy

Cyclic bleeding posthysterectomy is a complication exclusively seen in supracervical hysterectomy. This problem equally affects open and laparoscopic hysterectomy. Cyclic vaginal bleeding is seen in 11% to 17% of patients after supracervical hysterectomy. Approximately 23% of these patients have trachelectomy at a mean postoperative time of 14 months due to persistent symptoms. This risk can be eliminated by performing total laparoscopic hysterectomy. However, amputation of the fundus using a reverse cone pattern (see Figure 8-15) and cauterization of the endocervix may help decrease the likelihood of this complication.

Outcomes

Laparoscopy is a safe approach to hysterectomy in the appropriate patient. A Cochrane review evaluated 27 randomized controlled trials with a total of 3643 participants to determine the most appropriate approach to hysterectomy (Table 8-3). All trials included in this review compared one approach of hysterectomy to another, but excluded supracervical hysterectomy. There were no significant differences between any route in the incidence of pelvic hematoma, vaginal cuff infection, urinary tract infection, chest infection, or thromboembolic events. Furthermore, there were no differences encountered in fistula formation, urinary dysfunction, sexual dysfunction, or patient satisfaction. Total laparoscopic hysterectomy had the longest operative time and the highest incidence of lower urinary tract injuries but was associated with less wound infections and less blood loss when compared to abdominal hysterectomy. When compared to vaginal hysterectomy, there were no differences between vaginal and laparoscopic hysterectomy in regards to return to normal activities, intraoperative visceral injury, intraoperative bleeding, conversion to laparotomy rates, and duration of hospital stay.

These findings are supported by the single largest randomized controlled trial comparing hysterectomy route, the eVALuate study. In the original analysis, major surgical complications (major hemorrhage, visceral injury, pulmonary embolus, wound dehiscence, anesthetic complications, unintended conversion to laparotomy) occurred more frequently in the laparoscopic group when compared to the abdominal group. However,

---

Table 8-3 Comparison of Laparoscopic To Vaginal and Abdominal Approaches To Hysterectomy For Benign Gynecologic Disease

Laparoscopic Hysterectomy Compared to Vaginal Hysterectomy

Similar outcomes except longer operative time (mean difference 41.5 minutes, 95% CI 33.7–49.4)

Laparoscopic Hysterectomy Compared to Abdominal Hysterectomy

Less blood loss (mean difference 45.3 mL, 95% CI 17.9–72.7)
Shorter hospital stay (mean difference 2 days, 95% CI 1.9–2.2)
Quicker return to normal activities (mean difference 13.6 days, 95% CI 11.8–15.4)
Fewer wound infections or fevers (OR 0.32, 95% CI 0.12–0.85)
Longer operating time (mean difference 10.6 minutes, 95% CI 7.4–13.8)
More urinary tract injuries (OR 2.61, 95% CI 1.22–5.6)

Data from Johnson N, Barlow D, Lehaby A, et al: *Cochrane Database Syst Rev* 2006; 2:CD003677

we strongly believe that conversion to laparotomy should not be considered a major surgical complication. Decision to convert is an important part of surgical judgment. If only unintended conversions to laparotomy due to a major complication were included in the laparoscopic hysterectomy group, then the rate of major complications would have been equivalent in both groups. Furthermore, laparoscopic hysterectomy was associated with less postoperative pain, shorter length of hospitalization, quicker recovery, and a better quality of life at 6 weeks postoperatively when compared to abdominal hysterectomy.

Additional data from this study demonstrate that the complication rate, conversion to laparotomy, and operative time decrease significantly with surgeon experience. Laparoscopic hysterectomy is cost-effective when compared to abdominal hysterectomy, but not when compared to vaginal hysterectomy. Additional observational studies have demonstrated the cost effectiveness of laparoscopic hysterectomy compared to abdominal hysterectomy based on decreased duration of hospitalization and quicker return to work, assuming minimal use of disposable equipment. All data indicate that vaginal hysterectomy, when feasible, is the safest, fastest, and most cost-effective route. However, when vaginal hysterectomy is contraindicated or predicted to be difficult, the laparoscopic approach should be considered.

SUMMARY: Laparoscopic hysterectomy, including total laparoscopic hysterectomy and subtotal hysterectomy, is gaining popularity as surgeons become more familiar with operative laparoscopy. The indications for laparoscopic hysterectomy are the same for hysterectomy in general, and the technique used for hysterectomy should be dictated by the indications for surgery, patient characteristics, and patient preference. Despite the lack of data supporting superior outcomes for subtotal hysterectomy, the decision between total and subtotal hysterectomy is often highly personal. Both total and subtotal laparoscopic hysterectomy are performed using the same steps as a hysterectomy performed through a laparotomy and careful dissection, identification of anatomic landmarks, and judicious use of cautery are necessary to avoid complications. Outcomes for laparoscopic hysterectomy are favorable and this approach should be considered when vaginal hysterectomy is contraindicated or predicted to be difficult.

Suggested Reading

ACOG Committee Opinion #311: Appropriate use of laparoscopically assisted vaginal hysterectomy, *Obstet Gynecol* 105:929-930, 2005.

ACOG Committee Opinion #388: Supracervical hysterectomy, *Obstet Gynecol* 110:1215, 2007.

ACOG Practice Bulletin #84: Prevention of Deep Venous Thrombosis and Pulmonary Embolism, *Obstet Gynecol* 110:429-440, 2007.

ACOG Practice Bulletin #104: Antibiotic Prophylaxis for Gynecologic Procedures, *Obstet Gynecol* 113:1180-1189, 2005.

Altgassen C, Michels W, Schneider A: Learning laparoscopic-assisted hysterectomy, *Obstet Gynecol* 104:308, 2004.

Canis MJ, Wattiez A, Mage G, Bruhat MA: Results of eVALuate study of hysterectomy techniques: laparoscopic hysterectomy may yet have a bright future, *BMJ* 328:642, 2004.

Canis M, Botchorishvili R, Ang C, et al: When is laparotomy needed in hysterectomy for benign uterine disease? *J Minim Invasive Gynecol* 15:38, 2008.

Carter JE: Laparoscopic gynecology procedures: avoid the risks, *Diagn Ther Endosc* 2(3):157, 1996.

Chang WC, Li TC, Lin CC: The effect of physician experience on costs and clinical outcomes of laparoscopic-assisted vaginal hysterectomy: a multivariate analysis, *J Am Assoc Gynecol Laparosc* 10:356, 2003.

Elkington NM, Chou D: A review of total laparoscopic hysterectomy: role, techniques and complications, *Curr Opin Obstet Gynecol* 18:380, 2006.

Falcone T, Paraiso MF, Mascha E: Prospective randomized clinical trial of laparoscopic-assisted vaginal hysterectomy versus total abdominal hysterectomy, *Am J Obstet Gynecol* 180:955-962, 1999.

Falcone T, Walters MD: Hysterectomy for benign disease, *Obstet Gynecol* 111(3):753, 2008.

Garry R: A consensus document concerning laparoscopic entry techniques, *Gynecol Endosc* 8:403, 1999.

Garry R, Fountain J, Mason S, et al: The eVALuate study: two parallel randomised trials, one comparing laparoscopic with abdominal hysterectomy, the other comparing laparoscopic with vaginal hysterectomy, *BMJ* 328:129, 2004.

Hur HC, Guido RS, Mansuria SM, et al: Incidence and patient characteristics of vaginal cuff dehiscence after different modes of hysterectomies, *J Minim Invasive Gynecol* 14(3):311, 2007.

Jelovsek JE, Chiung C, Chen G, Roberts S, Paraiso MFR, Falcone T. Incidence of lower urinary tract injury at the time of total laparoscopic hysterectomy, *JSLS* 11:422, 2007.

Jenkins TR: Laparoscopic supracervical hysterectomy, *Am J Obstet Gynecol* 191:1875, 2004.

Johnson N, Barlow D, Lethaby A, et al: Methods of hysterectomy: systematic review and meta-analysis of randomized controlled trials, *BMJ* 330:1478, 2005.

Johnson, N, Barlow, D, Lethaby A, et al: Surgical approach to hysterectomy for benign gynaecological disease, *Cochrane Database Syst Rev* (2).CD003677, 2006.

Lethaby A, Ivanova V, Johnson NP: Total versus subtotal hysterectomy for benign gynaecological conditions, *Cochrane Database Syst Rev* (2):CD004993, 2006.

McPherson, K, Metcalfe, MA, Herbert A, et al: Severe complications of hysterectomy: the VALUE study, *BJOG* 111:688, 2004.

Parker, WH: Total laparoscopic hysterectomy and laparoscopic supracervical hysterectomy, *Obstet Gynecol Clin North Am* 31:523, 2004.

Ribeiro SC, Ribeiro RM, Santos NC, Pinotti JA: A randomized study of total abdominal, vaginal and laparoscopic hysterectomy, *Int J Gynaecol Obstet* 83:37, 2003.

Sculpher M, Manca A, Abbott J, et al: Cost effectiveness analysis of laparoscopic hysterectomy compared with standard hysterectomy: results from a randomised trial, *BMJ* 328:134, 2004.

Shen CC, Wu MP, Kung FT, et al: Major complications associated with laparoscopic-assisted vaginal hysterectomy: ten-year experience, *J Am Assoc Gynecol Laparosc* 10:147, 2003.

Wattiez A, Soriano D, Cohen SB, et al: The learning curve of total laparoscopic hysterectomy: comparative analysis of 1647 cases, *J Am Assoc Gynecol Laparosc* 9:339, 2002.

Laparoscopic Tubal Surgery

Jeffrey M. Goldberg M.D.

 Video Clips on DVD

9-1 Laparoscopic Neosalpingostomy for a Hydrosalpinx (7 minutes/43 seconds)

9-2 Laparoscopic Salpingectomy for Pyosalpinx (3 minutes/34 seconds)

9-3 Laparoscopic Tubal Ligation (0 minutes/37 seconds)

9-4 Laparoscopic Management of a Tubal Pregnancy (3 minutes/36 seconds)

Introduction

Tubal disease contributes to female infertility in 25% to 35% of cases with over half of these due to salpingitis. While chromotubation at laparoscopy is the gold standard for documenting tubal patency, hysterosalpingography (HSG) is still the standard initial technique for diagnosing fallopian tube disease. Preliminary studies have demonstrated that tubal patency can be assessed with transvaginal ultrasonography and saline and air or sonicated albumen. However, this method is not as informative as HSG. In addition to documenting patency, HSG reveals the tubal caliber, the presence of mucosal folds, and can diagnose salpingitis isthmica nodosa (SIN) and post-spill loculation from peritubal adhesions. This information is very useful in deciding between corrective tubal surgery and in vitro fertilization. HSG may also have a therapeutic effect, as several studies have noted the fecundity rates to be higher following the procedure.

IVF for Tubal Disease

Great advances have been made with both in vitro fertilization (IVF) and the surgical treatment of tubal disease. IVF success rates have been steadily increasing and surgery has been becoming less invasive. Many variables need to be considered in advising tubal infertility patients to undergo corrective surgery or IVF. The age of the patient, presence of other infertility factors, extent of the tubal disease, experience of the surgeon, and success rates of the IVF program are the most important. Patient preference and insurance reimbursement also figure into the equation.

The Society for Assisted Reproductive Technologies (SART) national IVF registry publishes the success rates of each IVF program as well as summary statistics annually. Figure 9-1 shows the national mean clinical pregnancy rates (PRs) and the mean live birth rates (LBRs) in 2005. Unfortunately, meaningful success rates for the various surgical procedures are largely lacking, making comparing options more difficult. Most of the data on tubal surgery is from the 1980s when laparoscopic skills and instrumentation were very much less refined than they are now. Also, surgery and IVF are not directly comparable since surgical success is reported as the pregnancy rate per patient whereas IVF success rates are per cycle.

The advantages of IVF include good success rates and the fact that it is nonsurgical. The disadvantages include cost (especially if more than one cycle is required), the need for one to four daily injections for several weeks, the frequent monitoring required, and the risks of multiple pregnancy and ovarian hyperstimulation syndrome.

Tubal Cannulation

Proximal tubal block on HSG or chromotubation accounts for 10% to 25% of tubal disease. The block may be due to obstruction, caused by spasm of the uterotubal ostium or mucus plugs; or occlusion, which is a true anatomic block from SIN or fibrosis. Obstruction may be relieved by selective salpingography or tubal cannulation. If the obstruction is not overcome with gentle pressure, a true anatomic occlusion is assumed and the procedure terminated. Occasionally the tube may be perforated with the guide-wire; this is of no clinical significance. Tubal occlusion requires resection and micro-surgical anastomosis. Tubal implantation is of historic interest only because it is associated with lower success rates and the risk of cornual rupture in pregnancy.

Unless the proximal block on HSG is clearly due to SIN, tubal cannulation can be attempted. Tubal patency is achieved about 80% of the time and approximately half of those patients subsequently conceive. Although tubal patency rates are similar when tubal cannulation is performed under fluoroscopic guidance, ongoing pregnancy rates are higher with hysteroscopic cannulation, as reported in a meta-analysis (Table 9-1). This may be due to the opportunity to diagnose and treat other pathology during lapa-roscopy or it may be that cannulation under direct vision is less traumatic. Because tubal cannulation is a minor procedure with comparable results to microsurgical resec-tion and anastomosis, it should be the treatment of choice. If unsuccessful, or if the block is due to SIN, IVF is preferred to microsurgical correction. Other cases in which IVF would be the preferred treatment include older women and when a significant male factor is present.

Figure 9-1. 2005 national IVF data showing pregnancy and live birth rates per IVF cycle based on the woman's age.

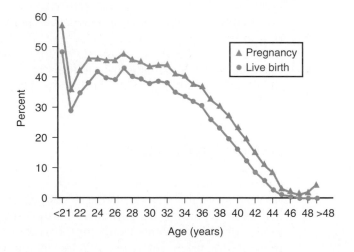

Table 9-1 Ongoing Pregnancy Rates Based on Tubal Cannulation Method		
Studies	**Patients**	**Ongoing PR**
Microsurgery n = 5	175	47.4
Hysteroscopy n = 4	133	48.9
Fluoroscopy n = 9	482	15.6
PR, pregnancy rate. Honore et al: *Fertil Steril* 71:785-795, 1999.		

Case 1: Proximal tubal cannulation

DT is a 32-year-old nulligravida with 3 years of primary infertility. She had regular menstrual cycles with progressive dysmenorrhea. Her husband had a normal semen analysis. An HSG showed a normal uterine cavity and bilateral cornual occlusion which was confirmed at laparoscopy. Superficial endometriosis over the bladder flap, cul-de-sac, left pelvic side wall, and ovary were also noted. Both fallopian tubes were easily cannulated hysteroscopically and patency confirmed. All of the peritoneal lesions were excised and the ovarian lesion was coagulated with bipolar cautery. Her dysmenorrhea improved and a follow-up HSG 6 months postoperatively showed the tubes remained patent. She conceived spontaneously 2 months later and has an ongoing intrauterine pregnancy.

Surgical Techniques

1. Laparoscopy with transcervical chromotubation with dilute indigo carmine is performed to document proximal tubal occlusion.

2. Tubal cannulation is then attempted with the Novy coaxial catheter system (Figures 9-2 and 9-3). The outer catheter is placed through the operating channel of the operative hysteroscope. The catheter is introduced to the tubal ostium. The flexible guidewire within the inner catheter is passed through the outer catheter into the proximal fallopian tube while an assistant observes laparoscopically. The assistant can also facilitate the procedure by straightening the proximal tube. An alternative technique is to place the inner catheter with the guidewire through the operating channel of a 5-mm flexible hysteroscope (Figures 9-4 and 9-5).

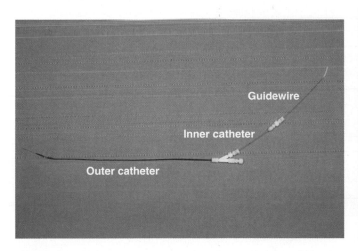

Figure 9-2. The Novy coaxial catheter system includes an outer catheter, an inner catheter, and a flexible guidewire. The outer catheter is placed through the operative channel of the rigid hysteroscope.

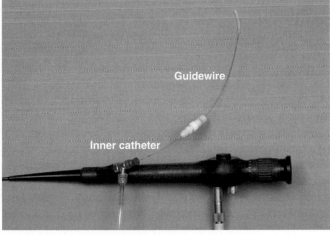

Figure 9-3. The Novy inner catheter with flexible guidewire may also be placed through the operating/fluid instillation channel of the flexible hysteroscope. Normal saline or lactated Ringer's solution is injected to distend the uterus.

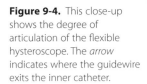

Figure 9-4. This close-up shows the degree of articulation of the flexible hysteroscope. The *arrow* indicates where the guidewire exits the inner catheter.

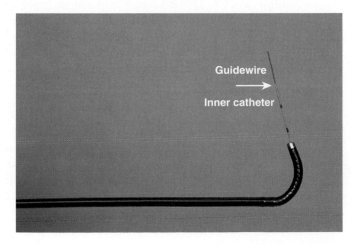

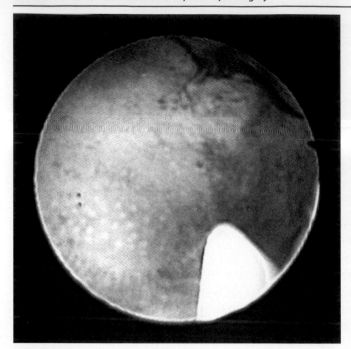

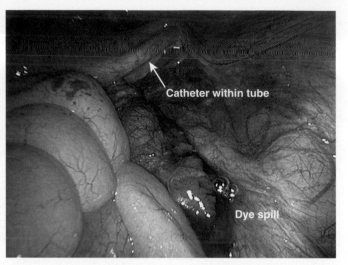

Figure 9-5. The catheter and guidewire are directed through the utero-tubal ostium then advanced into the tube. The laparoscopic surgeon assists by straightening the proximal tube.

Figure 9-6. The catheter and guide wire can be seen negotiating the tube by laparoscopy. The guide wire is then withdrawn and dilute indigo carmine dye injected through the inner catheter. Free spill of indigo carmine is confirmed laparoscopically.

3. There is usually minimal resistance to negotiating the intramural segment and proximal isthmus. Great resistance indicates salpingitis isthmic nodosa or luminal fibrosis, which are not treatable with tubal cannulation. Using excessive force increases the risk for tubal perforation (which is innocuous). Once the cannula is in the lumen of the isthmic segment, the guidewire is removed and indigo carmine is injected through the inner catheter to demonstrate that the remainder of the tube is patent (Figure 9-6).

Microsurgical Tubal Anastomosis

In young women with no other infertility factors, the intrauterine pregnancy rate is about 70% to 90% after sterilization reversal. Age was the most important prognostic factor. Term pregnancy rates of 33% to 51% have been reported in women 40 years of age or older. Isthmic–isthmic repairs and longer final tubal lengths yield higher success rates. The ectopic rate after the procedure is approximately 2% to 5%, comparable to IVF. The decision to perform tubal anastomosis versus. IVF is left up to the patient after reviewing the pros and cons of each.

The procedure can be performed through a minilaparotomy as an outpatient. There have been a few published reports of laparoscopic tubal anastomosis. In general, the procedure times are prolonged and the pregnancy rates are lower, though comparative studies are lacking. We performed a small series of laparoscopic tubal anastomoses with robotic assistance and found no advantage to the robot. In fact, it increased operative time by 1 to 2 hours compared with minilaparotomy as well as laparoscopic tubal anastomosis without robotic assistance.

The laparoscopic procedure is identical to an open microsurgical tubal anastomosis. The tubes are repaired in two layers using interrupted 8-0 delayed absorbable suture. Each tube requires a total of approximately 8 to 10 sutures. The use of a one-stitch technique, titanium clips, and fibrin glue have been suggested to avoid the extensive suturing involved. Again, the goal of laparoscopic surgery should be to duplicate the standard open procedure, and such shortcuts may compromise the clinical results.

Whereas the initial pilot study success rates with laparoscopic tubal anastomosis were discouraging, a recent larger series reported rates comparable to open microsurgery.

The subsequent pregnancy rates depend upon several variables including the age of the woman and the presence of other infertility factors such as ovulatory dysfunction, endometriosis, or an abnormal semen analysis. Contraindications to tubal anastomosis include a final tubal length of less than 4 cm, significant tubo-ovarian adhesions, stage 3 or 4 endometriosis, and/or more than a mild male factor. The site of the anastomosis also influences success rates, with isthmic-isthmic repairs typically giving the best results and cornual-ampullary yielding the worst. Only surgeons who are very facile with intracorporeal knot-tying and extensively trained in conventional tubal microsurgery should attempt this procedure.

Case: See Tubal Anastomosis in Robotics Chapter

Surgical Techniques

1. The procedure begins by inserting a uterine manipulator for manipulation and chromotubation.

2. A 10-mm laparoscope is placed through an umbilical port, as it affords better visualization than a 5-mm laparoscope. This is crucial when working with 8-0 sutures.

3. A 3-mm port is inserted in the right and left lower quadrant for the laparoscopic microsurgical instruments.

4. A 5-mm port is placed suprapubically in the midline for manipulation, inserting/retrieving needles, and suction/irrigation.

5. After assuring adequate tubal length and the absence of significant pelvic disease, dilute Pitressin (vasopressin) (20 units in 100 mL of injectable saline) is infiltrated into the mesosalpinx beneath the occluded ends (Figure 9-7).

6. The ends are then mobilized with the unipolar needle with 20 watts of cutting current, then opened with scissors (Figures 9-8 through 9-11).

7. Patency of the proximal and distal segments is confirmed with transcervical and retrograde chromotubation, respectively, using dilute indigo carmine (Figures 9-12 and 9-13).

8. The tubal ends are brought together with a 6-0 delayed absorbable suture through the mesosalpinx (Figure 9-14).

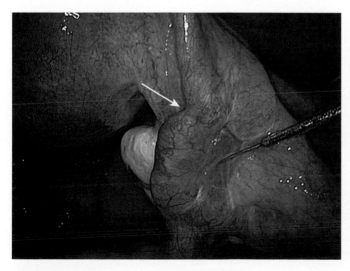

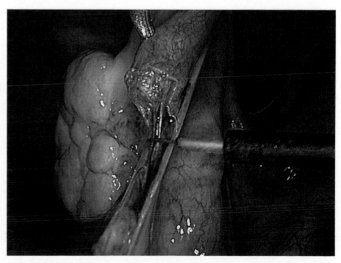

Figure 9-7. The *arrow* indicates the site of occlusion by bipolar cautery. There is adequate tubal length. Dilute Pitressin is injected in the mesosalpinx beneath the occluded segments

Figure 9-8. The serosa is incised with the unipolar micro-needle (on 20 watts cutting current) to separate and mobilize the tubal ends.

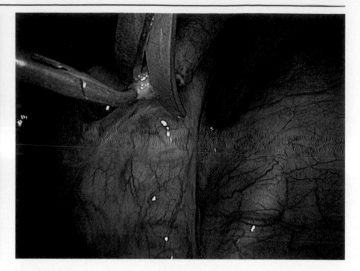

Figure 9-9. The occluded ends have been completely mobilized.

Figure 9-10. The occluded end of the proximal tube is excised with scissors.

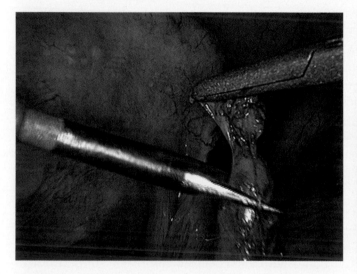

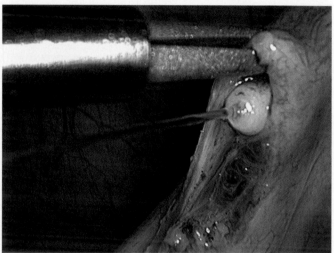

Figure 9-11. The distal segment is also opened with scissors.

Figure 9-12. Transcervical chromotubation with dilute indigo carmine through the uterine manipulator demonstrates patency of the proximal segment.

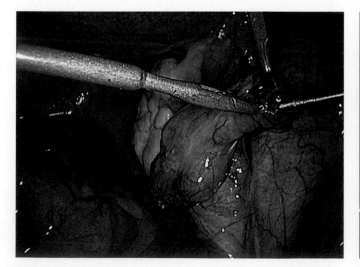

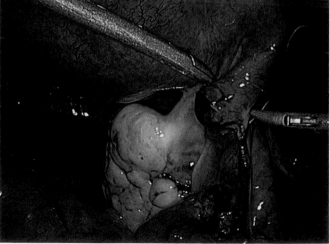

Figure 9-13. Patency of the distal segment can be tested with indigo carmine injected through a cannula placed in antegrade or retrograde fashion.

Figure 9-14. An interrupted 6-0 delayed absorbable suture is placed in the mesosalpinx just beneath the tubal segments to align them and eliminate tension on the anastomosis.

9. The actual anastomosis is performed using interrupted 8-0 delayed absorbable suture (though some surgeons prefer Prolene). The sutures are placed at the 3-, 6-, 9-, and 12-o'clock positions with the 6 o'clock suture placed first. The needle is placed from out to in through one segment and in to out on the other so that the knots are tied extraluminally (Figures 9-15 and 9-16). The first layer is through the muscularis and may include the endosalpinx.

10. The knots are tied intracorporeally with the surgeon and assistant working together with 3-mm needle holders (Figure 9-17). The second layer is the serosa, which is also closed with interrupted 8-0 delayed absorbable suture (Figure 9-18).

11. Transcervical chromotubation is performed to document bilateral tubal patency (Figure 9-19).

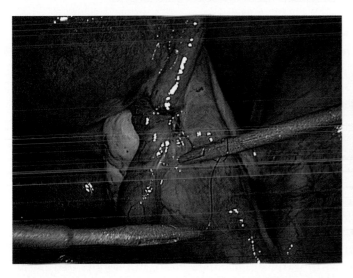

Figure 9-15. All sutures are tied intracorporeally. The tubal segments are ready to be anastomosed

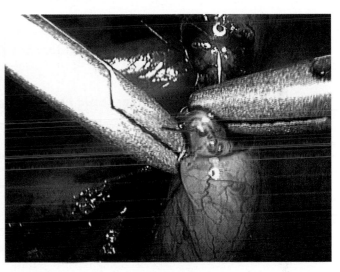

Figure 9-16. Four interrupted 8-0 delayed absorbable sutures are placed incorporating the mucosa and muscularis layers.

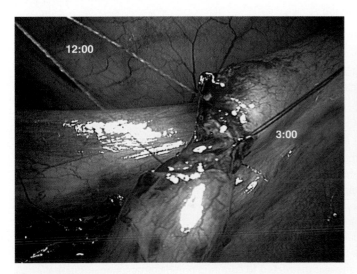

Figure 9-17. The 3-, 6-, 9-, and 12-o'clock sutures are placed from out-to-in on one segment and in-to-out on the other segment such that the knots are tied outside the tubal lumen. The 6-o'clock stitch is placed first.

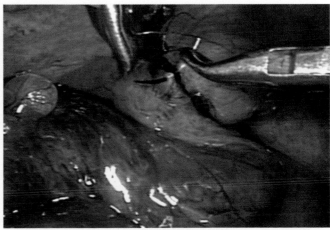

Figure 9-18. The serosa is also reapproximated with several interrupted 8-0 delayed absorbable sutures. Closure of this layer is probably nonessential.

Figure 9-19. The completed repair. Chromotubation demonstrates tubal patency with no anastomotic leak.

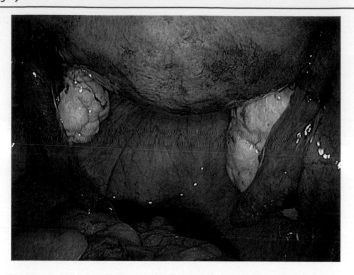

Video Demonstration: See Chapter on Robotic Surgery

Laparoscopic Fimbrioplasty / Neosalpingostomy

Success rates following laparoscopic fimbrioplasty or neosalpingostomy depend on the extent of adnexal adhesions, tubal dilation and wall thickness, and the preservation of the endosalpinx. Intrauterine and ectopic pregnancy rates for patients with mild disease range from 58% to 77% and 2% to 10%, respectively. For severe disease these values were 0% to 22% and 4% to 17%. Irreversible damage to the endosalpinx from the preceding infection is responsible for the discrepancy between the patency rates and pregnancy rates following neosalpingostomy.

A hysterosalpingogram is performed if the patient does not conceive within the first three to six cycles. If patent, in vitro fertilization is offered to all patients that fail to conceive within the first postoperative year, with all other infertility factors corrected. Fimbrial phimosis is a constriction of the distal tube. Often a tuft of fimbria may be extruding from the lumen. On HSG, the tubes are patent and usually demonstrate mild distal dilation. The fimbrioplasty procedure to open the tube wider is virtually identical to neosalpingostomy. Neosalpingostomy and fimbrioplasty should only be performed by laparoscopy; laparotomy for distal tubal disease is obsolete. Tuboplasty is not appropriate for those with severe disease.

Case 2: Neosalpingostomy

   View DVD: Video 9-1

TG is a 30-year-old nulligravida with a 7-year history of primary infertility. She had regular monthly menstrual cycles and her husband had a normal semen analysis. An HSG demonstrated a normal uterine cavity and bilateral hydrosalpinges, greater on the left. She denied any history of sexually transmitted infections. At laparoscopy, the upper abdomen and pelvis were free of adhesions. The left hydrosalpinx was dilated over 4 cm and a salpingectomy was performed. The right was minimally dilated and good mucosal folds were noted when the distal tube was opened. The cut edges were everted and sutured to the tubal serosa to maintain patency. A follow-up HSG 6 months later confirmed tubal patency and she was instructed to continue timed coitus for an additional 6 months and to call immediately when pregnant to follow serial hCG levels and perform an early ultrasonogram to determine the location of the gestation.

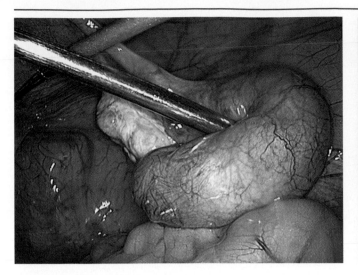

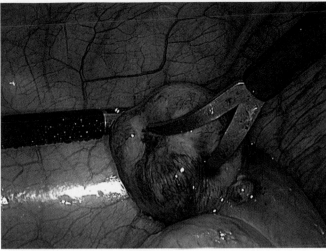

Figure 9-20. Chromotubation confirms that this hydrosalpinx is thin-walled, mildly dilated and free of adhesions. This is the ideal candidate for neosalpingostomy.

Figure 9-21. Following the injection of dilute vasopressin into the mesosalpinx at the distal tube, the tube is opened with scissors or a micro-unipolar needle with cutting current. A linear or cruciate incision is performed, taking care to avoid the mesenteric vessels.

Surgical Techniques

1. A uterine manipulator is inserted for manipulation and chromotubation.
2. A 10-mm port is placed through the umbilicus, both for the better visualization obtained with a 10 mm laparoscope and to remove the hydrosalpinx if a neosalpingostomy is not feasible.
3. Ancillary 5-mm ports are placed in the right and left lower quadrants.
4. If the hydrosalpinx meets the criteria for neosalpingostomy, the procedure begins by lysing any adhesions to fully mobilize the tube (Figure 9-20).
5. Dilute Pitressin (vasopressin) is infiltrated into the distal mesosalpinx.
6. The tube is then opened using scissors or a unipolar needle with cutting current (Figure 9-21).
7. The endosalpinx is inspected and if fairly normal, the edges of the opened tube are everted and sutured to the tubal serosa. Two to three interrupted 4-0 delayed absorbable sutures are placed. The suture end of an SH needle may be straightened to form a "ski needle" to aid suture placement.
8. The knots are tied intracorporeally with the surgeon and assistant working together (Figures 9-22 to 9-24).
9. Chromotubation is then performed to confirm tubal patency (Figure 9-25).
10. The fimbrioplasty procedure for fimbial phimosis is virtually identical (Figure 9-26). The phimotic tubal ostium is incised to create a larger opening and the tubal edges are everted and sutured to the tubal serosa.

Laparoscopic Salpingectomy

Salpingectomy is indicated for ectopic pregnancies when hemostasis cannot be achieved, when the patient is no longer interested in fertility, or with a prior ectopic or tubal reconstructive surgery in the ipsilateral tube. Salpingectomy is performed when the fallopian tube is damaged beyond repair by infection, endometriosis, or ectopic pregnancy. Numerous studies have shown that hydrosalpinges have a detrimental effect on IVF success. Two meta-analyses of these studies noted that the pregnancy, implantation, and delivery rates were significantly lower and the spontaneous abortion rates were higher in the presence of hydrosalpinges. This may be due to mechanical

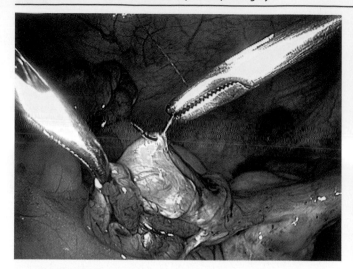

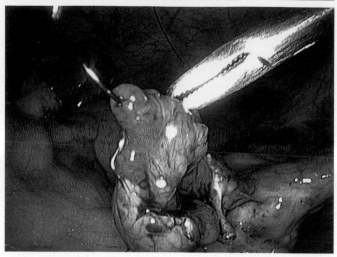

Figure 9-22. The tubal epithelium appears healthy with good mucosal folds. If necessary, bleeding may be controlled with fine-tipped bipolar forceps. A 4-0 delayed absorbable suture is placed superficially through the tubal serosa. The suture end of the SH needle has been straightened because the "ski" needle may facilitate suturing in these cases.

Figure 9-23. The needle is then placed through the mucosal edge from outside to inside.

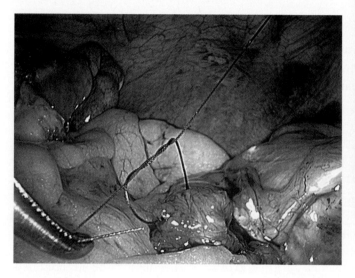

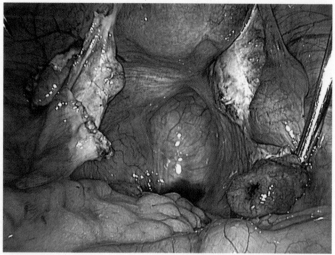

Figure 9-24. The suture is tied intracorporeally to evert the fimbria.

Figure 9-25. Additional sutures are placed in the same fashion to complete the cuff salpingostomy. The fimbriated end has been completely everted. The mucosa appears healthy and transcervical chromotubation demonstrates free spill. The contralateral tube was not reparable, so a left salpingectomy had been performed. The excised left hydrosalpinx is seen lateral to the ovary prior to removal from the peritoneal cavity. Interceed or Adept may be used to reduce the risk of postoperative adhesion formation.

Figure 9-26. This tube, while patent, is phimotic with a distal constriction ring around a small tuft of fimbria. Dilute Pitressin is injected in the distal mesosalpinx and the fimbrioplasty is performed using the same steps as in neosalpingostomy.

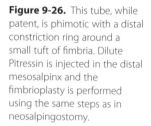

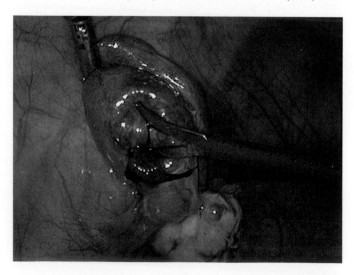

flushing of the embryos from the uterine cavity, decreased endometrial receptivity, or a direct embryotoxic effect.

Patients with bilateral hydrosalpinges, as well as hydrosalpinges visible on ultrasonography, were more significantly affected. Laparoscopic salpingectomy prior to initiating an IVF cycle restores the rates back to normal. Whether proximal tubal ligation, laparoscopic neosalpingostomy, or ultrasound-guided aspiration just prior to IVF are as effective as salpingectomy is as yet unknown. Although laparoscopic salpingectomy is a simple procedure, it is critical to avoid any compromise of the ovarian blood supply because that may result in diminished ovarian reserve and reduced IVF success rates.

(See Video 9-1 📹)

Cases 3 and 4: Salpingectomy

MH is a 41-year-old woman, para 2012. Her last delivery was 20 years ago. She presented with infertility with her new husband. A hysterosalpingogram demonstrated a right hydrosalpinx with evidence of salpingitis isthmica nodosa. The uterine cavity was normal and the left tube was normal and patent. Her husband had a normal semen analysis. Her day 3 FSH was 15. Laparoscopic right salpingectomy was recommended. Laparoscopy confirmed a right hydrosalpinx. It was attached to the right pelvic sidewall by filmy adhesions. Perihepatic adhesions were also noted. The appendix and the remainder of the pelvis were normal. A right salpingectomy was performed. Her photos are shown below. The plan was to initiate treatment with in vitro fertilization due to her age, elevated FSH, and tubal disease but she conceived spontaneously 3 months postoperatively. She had an uneventful pregnancy and vaginal delivery at term.

The patient in the video is a 29-year-old para 1011. She underwent a laparoscopic left distal salpingectomy for an ectopic pregnancy with concurrent right neosalpingostomy for a hydrosalpinx 3 years earlier. There were perihepatic and adnexal adhesions consistent with a prior episode of pelvic inflammatory disease. She conceived spontaneously and had a cesarean delivery 1 year later. She presented with acute severe right lower quadrant pain with guarding and rebound tenderness as well as nausea and vomiting. Her evaluation included a negative hCG, normal CBC with a left shift, and pelvic ultrasonogram and CT were normal with a small amount of fluid in the cul-de-sac. Laparoscopy revealed a right pyosalpinx and purulent fluid in the cul-de-sac (many polymorphonuclear leukocytes were present but cultures were negative). A right salpingectomy was performed.

Surgical Techniques

1. The setup is the same as for a salpingostomy with the insertion of a uterine manipulator and placement of a 10-mm umbilical and 5-mm lower quadrant ports.

2. Adnexal adhesions, which are usually present, are lysed to fully mobilize the tube and ovary (Figure 9-27).

3. The proximal tube is coagulated and transected just lateral to the uterine cornua. A harmonic scalpel, tripolar device, or bipolar forceps with scissors may be used to accomplish this (Figures 9-28 and 9-29).

4. The mesosalpinx is then serially coagulated and cut (Figure 9-30). It is very important to stay as close to the fallopian tube as possible so as not to compromise the vascular supply to the ovary.

5. The tube is then grasped and withdrawn through the 10-mm umbilical port while observing with a 5-mm laparoscope through one of the lower quadrant ports (Figure 9-31).

(See Video 9-2 📹)

Tubal Ligation

Tubal ligation was the original operative laparoscopic procedure, and is still one of the most common. The three basic methods are cauterization and the application of bands or clips. The tube can be cauterized by bipolar forceps, then divided. Monopolar cautery should not be used because it destroys an excessive amount of the tube. The banding

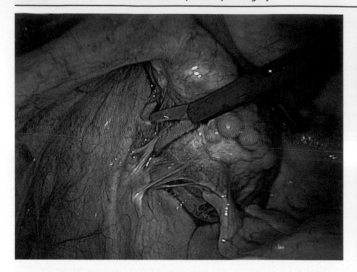

Figure 9-27. Lysis of peritubal adhesions may be required prior to performing the salpingectomy.

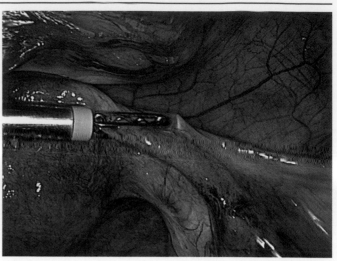

Figure 9-28. The proximal tube is coagulated with bipolar cautery.

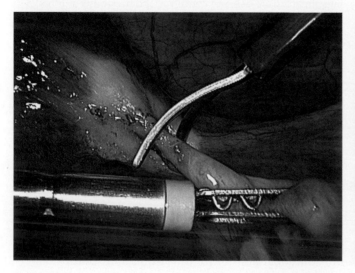

Figure 9-29. The proximal tube is divided with scissors. The bipolar forceps are used to hold the tube in the event that any bleeding occurs after the tube is cut.

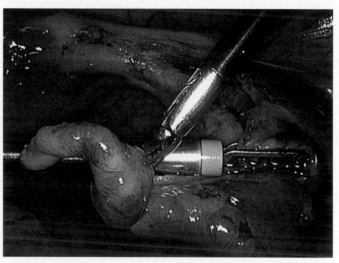

Figure 9-30. The mesosalpinx is serially coagulated and cut, staying close to the tube to avoid compromising the blood supply to the ovary.

Figure 9-31. The tube has been excised. It is then removed through a 10-mm trocar. Observe for hemostasis and evidence of devascularization of the ovary.

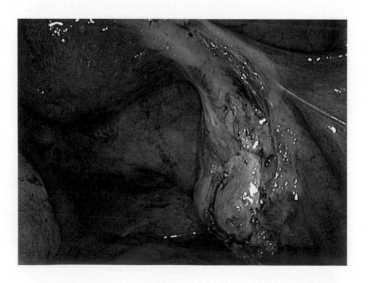

technique is accomplished by placing a silastic Falope ring over a knuckle of tube. A classic Pomeroy tubal ligation can be also performed in a similar fashion by placing a 0-chromic endoloop around a knuckle of tube and then excising it. Filshie or Hulka clips are placed across the tube with dedicated appliers.

While the goal is to permanently sterilize the patient, it must be kept in mind that she may someday regret her decision and desire further fertility, usually due to remarriage or loss of a child. For this reason the procedure should provide a low failure rate yet not compromise the patient's chance for success if she ultimately pursues tubal anastomosis. The ligation should be performed at the mid-isthmic segment and should sacrifice as little tubal length as possible. In the interest of restoring fertility by tubal anastomosis, clips are preferred because they damage only a minimal amount of the tube, providing the best chance for success after repair. The Filshie clip is the device of choice because it has a lower failure rate than the Hulka clip.

Case 5: Tubal ligation with Filshie clips

 View DVD: Video 9-3

JW is 37-year-old woman, para 2032, who had term vaginal deliveries 9 and 5 years ago. She also had three spontaneous abortions believed to be due to antiphospholipid antibody syndrome. She presented with severe pelvic pain before and during menses. She underwent laparoscopic treatment of endometriosis 7 years previously for similar pain which resolved. She is no longer interested in fertility and desires sterilization. Hormonal contraception was not advised in this 37-year-old with a predilection for thromboembolism related to the antiphospholipid antibody syndrome. She was not interested in an IUD or barrier methods and her husband refused a vasectomy. Tubal ligation was planned during her laparoscopy for dysmenorrhea which revealed a left ovarian endometrioma, dense adhesions between the ovary and pelvic sidewall, and deep endometriosis of the sidewall with fibrosis around the ureter. The ovary was mobilized, an ovarian cystectomy performed, and the pelvic peritoneum was excised from the left pelvic sidewall after fully mobilizing the ureter. Bilateral tubal ligation was then performed using Filshie clips.

Surgical Techniques

1. Tubal ligation is usually accomplished with a 5-mm laparoscope through the umbilicus and a midline suprapubic port. The fallopian tubes must be traced throughout their length, because there have been reports of the round ligaments being ligated by mistake. Three methods for performing tubal ligation are shown here.

2. The Filshie clip is loaded in the clip applier and the mid-isthmic segment of the tube is grasped perpendicular to the tube (Figure 9-32). The clip is carefully placed so the tube is completely occluded (Figure 9-33).

3. The mid-isthmus may also be coagulated with bipolar cautery (monopolar cautery should never be used) (Figure 9-34).

4. The tube is then completely divided with scissors (Figure 9-35).

5. The Falope ring is a small silastic band which is loaded on an applicator. The mid-isthmic segment is grasped with the applicator to elevate a knuckle of tube (Figure 9-36). The Falope ring is then slid over the loop of tube (Figure 9-37). Be careful not to pull up on the tube because it may be transected. Once the ring is placed the knuckle of tube is seen to blanch.

(See Video 9-3)

Ectopic Pregnancy

Linear salpingostomy for ectopic pregnancy was one of the first procedures to compare the results of laparoscopy with laparotomy in a prospective randomized fashion, and demonstrated the advantages of laparoscopy over laparotomy. However, laparoscopy may carry a higher incidence of persistent ectopic. All patients must continue to be

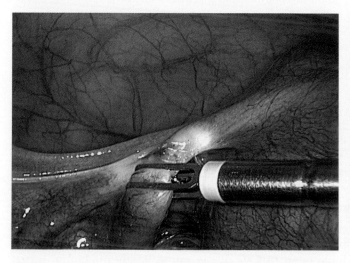

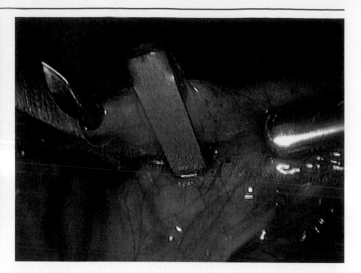

Figure 9-32. The entire tubal length must be identified to be certain that it is in fact the fallopian tube which is being ligated. Here the Filshie clip applier is being placed on the mid-isthmic segment of the tube.

Figure 9-33. The clip is securely in place across the tube. Minimal tissue has been damaged.

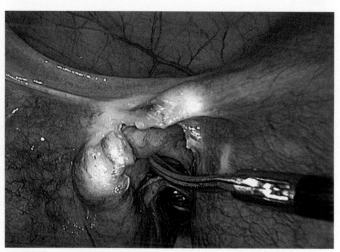

Figure 9-34. The tube is grasped with the bipolar forceps and coagulated with 40 watts of current. An adjacent area is then coagulated as shown here.

Figure 9-35. The tube is transected with scissors to assure that the burn was transmural. This may not be required if the electrosurgical generator is equipped with an ammeter to indicate the tube has been completely coagulated based on the cessation of current flow through the tubal tissue.

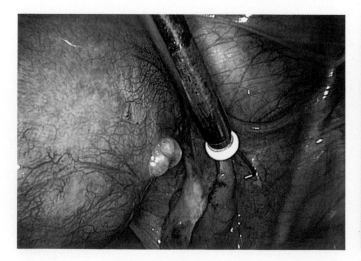

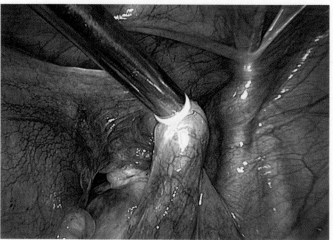

Figure 9-36. The mid-isthmic segment is grasped with the Falope ring applicator.

Figure 9-37. A knuckle of tube is elevated into the Falope ring application device and the Falope ring is slid over it.

followed with serial quantitative serum hCG levels. Any rise or plateau is an indication for treatment. Methotrexate has been shown to be effective for treating these patients. Also, do not forget to administer RhoGAM in Rh-negative patients.

The use of dilute vasopressin and coagulation of the serosal vessels greatly reduces the need for electrocautery with the risk of thermal injury to the tubal muscularis and endosalpinx. Total or partial salpingectomy is performed when the tube is beyond repair, the patient has had prior tubal surgery or a previous ectopic pregnancy within the ipsilateral tube, or fertility is no longer desired. The technique for performing salpingectomy is described earlier. Milking the ectopic out of the tube is discouraged because it results in greater tubal damage and a poorer prognosis for future reproduction.

Cases 6 and 7: Ectopic pregnancy

 View DVD: Video 9-4

NG is a 22-year-old woman, para 0020. She has had two elective pregnancy terminations and was treated for *Chlamydia* as an outpatient. She presented with acute right lower quadrant pain and was uncertain when her last menstrual period was. A quantitative hCG was 4896 IU/mL. An ultrasonogram revealed a normal uterus with an empty cavity, and the endometrium measured 14 mm. Both ovaries were normal but there was a 2-cm elongated cystic structure adjacent to the right ovary. There was a small amount of fluid in the cul-de-sac consistent with blood.

Because she presented with pain and her compliance with follow-up hCG levels after methotrexate treatment was uncertain, a decision was made to proceed to laparoscopy. She consented to salpingostomy or salpingectomy depending on the condition of the tube. Laparoscopy demonstrated perihepatic adhesions as well as filmy adnexal adhesions bilaterally. The pelvis was otherwise normal except for a fusiform swelling of the right ampullary segment and some blood in the cul-de-sac. A linear salpingostomy was performed. She was discharged home 2 hours later and was instructed to return for weekly hCG levels until negative to rule out persistent trophoblast growth. She was also counseled to call as soon as she is pregnant for close follow-up due to the increased risk for another ectopic.

The patient in the video is a 32 year old para 0010 who underwent a laparoscopic right distal salpingectomy for an ectopic pregnancy. A left hydrosalpinx was noted at the time. She was referred for secondary infertility. A laparoscopic left salpingostomy was performed as the tube met all of the criteria for repair as discussed in the salpingostomy section above. She conceived spontaneously a few months later. Despite appropriately rising quantitative hCG levels, no intrauterine gestation was seen on ultrasonography. No adnexal masses were noted either. Laparoscopy revealed that the pelvis was free of adhesions and the fimbriated end looked normal. An ectopic pregnancy was located in distal ampullary segment. Laparoscopic salpingectomy was performed due to the risk of a subsequent ectopic pregnancy.

Surgical Techniques

1. If there is any question as to whether the patient may have an intrauterine pregnancy, no uterine manipulator is placed.

2. A 10 mm umbilical port is placed to allow for later tissue removal. A 5-mm port is inserted in each lower quadrant. The hemoperitoneum is aspirated and the pelvis carefully inspected (Figure 9-38). Any adhesions are lysed. If the tube is not to be conserved, a salpingectomy is performed as described earlier. If tubal preservation is appropriate, the linear salpingostomy is performed as follows.

3. Dilute vasopressin is injected into the mesosalpinx beneath the ectopic (Figure 9-39).

4. The serosal vessels over the tubal bulge may be coagulated in an effort to further reduce bleeding (Figure 9-40).

5. The tube is incised on the antimesenteric side with scissors or unipolar needle (Figure 9-41).

6. The tube is gently compressed beneath the ectopic to facilitate expression of the products of conception (POC) (Figure 9-42). Resist the urge to manually remove the tissue with graspers because this tends to cause more damage to the tubal epithelium and increases bleeding, resulting in more cautery injury.

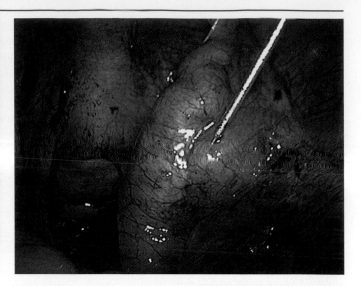

Figure 9-38. This is an unruptured ectopic in the ampullary segment of the right tube.

Figure 9-39. Five to 10 mL of vasopressin (10 IU in 50 mL of injectable saline solution) is injected subserosally into the mesosalpinx beneath the ectopic. Delayed bleeding with the use of vasopressin is a theoretical concern but has not been a problem in actual clinical practice.

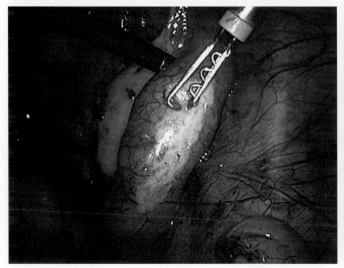

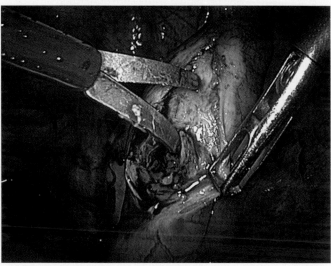

Figure 9-40. The serosa of the antimesenteric aspect of the ectopic is superficially coagulated with bipolar cautery.

Figure 9-41. The tubal wall is incised with scissors. The unipolar needle or harmonic scalpel can also be used for this step, taking care to limit thermal injury to the endosalpinx.

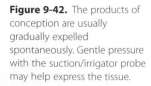

Figure 9-42. The products of conception are usually gradually expelled spontaneously. Gentle pressure with the suction/irrigator probe may help express the tissue.

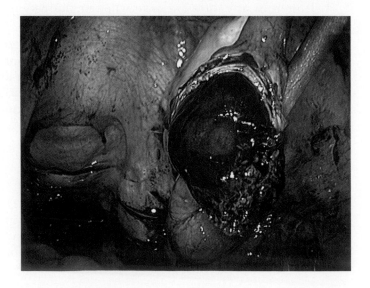

7. Irrigation is then used to ensure that all the POC are out and to identify any bleeders for coagulation with bipolar cautery (Figure 9-43). Increased bleeding may be managed by suture ligating the mesosalpingeal vessels below the ectopic with 4-0 delayed absorbable suture.

8. The tube is left open to heal without sutures (Figure 9-44).

9. The POC are removed through the 10-mm umbilical port using a 10-mm spoon forceps or endopouch while watching with a 5-mm laparoscope from one of the lower ports (Figure 9-45). It is important to confirm that no POC have been left in the peritoneal cavity because they may continue to proliferate, leading to an abdominal pregnancy.

(See Video 9-4 📹)

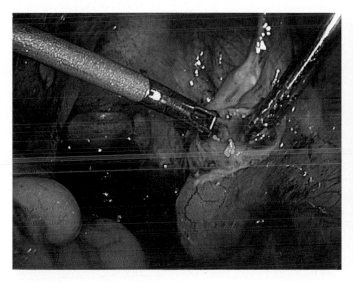

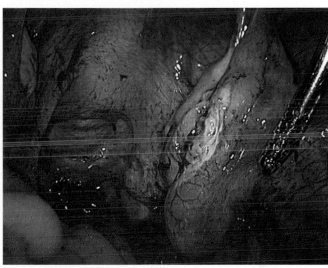

Figure 9-43. The implantation site is irrigated to flush out any remaining blood clots and/or products of conception. Evacuating the ectopic with gentle pressure and irrigation results in less bleeding and subsequent cautery injury than attempting to remove the tissue with grasping forceps.

Figure 9-44. The tubal defect is left open. It is observed for hemostasis. Any bleeding sites are controlled with bipolar cautery.

Figure 9-45. The products of conception are placed in an endopouch for removal through the 10-mm umbilical port. The tissue can also be removed with the 10-mm spoon forceps, but care must be used to avoid leaving any tissue behind which may implant and continue to grow.

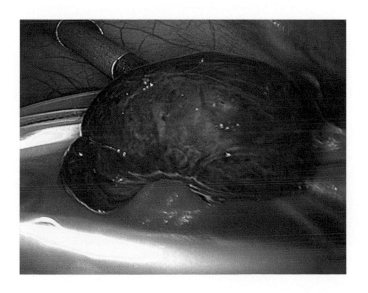

SUMMARY: In general, fertility-enhancing surgery for tubal disease is recommended in the following situations: hysteroscopic tubal cannulation under laparoscopic guidance for proximal tubal occlusion, tubal anastomosis for sterilization reversal by laparoscopy or minilaparotomy, laparoscopic neosalpingostomy for mild hydrosalpinges, and salpingectomy for selected ectopic pregnancies as well as for moderate to severe hydrosalpinges prior to IVF. IVF is indicated for patients who fail to conceive within a year following tubal cannulation, anastomosis, or salpingostomy; or instead of those procedures in older women and those with additional infertility factors, as well as following salpingectomy for moderate to severe hydrosalpinges.

Tubal ligation remains one of the most commonly performed gynecologic laparoscopic procedures. All of the methods are easy to perform and have low failure rates. If properly performed, good pregnancy rates can be achieved with tubal anastomosis. While methotrexate treatment has replaced surgery for many ectopic pregnancies, laparoscopic linear salpingostomy or salpingectomy still have a role in managing this condition.

Suggested Reading

Bissonnette F, Lapensee L, Bouzayen R: Outpatient laparoscopic tubal anastomosis and subsequent fertility, *Fertil Steril* 72:549-552, 1999.

Camus E, Poncelet C, Goffinet F, Wainer B, Meriet F, Nisand I, Philippe HJ: Pregnancy rates after in-vitro fertilization in cases of tubal infertility with and without hydrosalpinx: a meta-analysis of published comparative studies, *Hum Reprod* 14:1243-1249, 1999.

Centers for Disease Control: 2005 Assisted Reproductive Technology Success Rates. *National Summary and Fertility Clinic Reports.* Published 2007. Available online at http://www.cdc.gov/nccdphp/drh/art.htm.

Dubuisson JB, Chapron CL, Nos C, et al: Sterilization reversal: fertility results, *Hum Reprod* 10:1145-1151, 1995.

Filshe GM, Casey D, Pogmore JR, et al: The titanium/silicone rubber clip for female sterilization, *Br J Obstet Gynaecol* 88:655-662,1981.

Goldberg J, Falcone T, Attaran M: Contrast-enhanced sonography (letter), *Hum Reprod* 13:3282, 1998.

Goldberg J, Falcone T: Laparoscopic microsurgical tubal anastomosis with and without robotic assistance, *Hum Reprod* 18:145-147, 2003.

Honore GM, Holden AEC, Schenken RS: Pathophysiology and management of proximal tubal blockage, *Fertil Steril* 71:785-795, 1999.

Hoppe DE, Bekkar BE, Nager CW: Single-dose systemic methotrexate for the treatment of persistent ectopic pregnancy after conservative surgery, *Obstet Gynecol* 83:51-54, 1994.

Jeanty P, Besnard S, Arnold A, Turner C, Crum P: Air-contrast sonohysterography as a first step assessment of tubal patency, *J Ultrasound Med* 19:519-527, 2000.

Kim JD, Kim KS, Doo JK, et al: A report on 387 cases of microsurgical tubal reversals, *Fertil Steril* 68:875-880, 1997.

Lipscomb GH, Stovall TG, Tamanathan JA, Ling FW: Comparison of silastic rings and electrocoagulation for laparoscopic tubal ligation under local anaesthesia, *Obstet Gynecol* 80:645-649, 1992.

Lundorff P, Thorburn J, Hahlin M, Kallfelt B, Lindblom B: Laparoscopic surgery in ectopic pregnancy: a randomized trial versus laparotomy, *Acta Obstet Gynecol Scand* 70:343-348, 1991.

Lundorff P, Thorburn J, Lindblom B: Fertility outcome after conservative surgical treatment of ectopic pregnancy evaluated in a prospective randomized trial, *Fertil Steril* 57:998-1002, 1992.

Milingos SD, Kallipolitis GK, Loutradis DC, Liapi AG, Hassan EA, Mavrommatis CG, Miaris SG, Michalas SP: Laparoscopic treatment of hydrosalpinx: factors affecting pregnancy rates, *J Am Assoc Gynecol Laparosc* 7:355-361, 2000.

Murphy AA, Nager CW, Wujek JJ, Kettel LM, Torp VA, Chin HG: Operative laparoscopy versus laparotomy for the management of ectopic pregnancy: a prospective trial, *Fertil Steril* 57:1180-1185, 1992.

Murray DL, Sagoskin AW, Widra EA, Levy MJ: The adverse effect of hydrosalpinges on in vitro fertilization pregnancy rates and the benefit of surgical correction, *Fertil Steril* 69:41-45, 1998.

Nackley AC, Muasher SJ: The significance of hydrosalpinx in in vitro fertilization, *Fertil Steril* 69:373-384, 1998.

Peterson HB, Xia Z, Hughes JM, et al: The risk of pregnancy after tubal sterilization: findings from the US Collaborative Review of Sterilization, *Am J Obstet Gynecol* 174:1161-1179, 1996.

Rioiux JE, Cloutier D: Bipolar cautery for sterilisation by laparoscopy, *J Reprod Med* 13:6, 1974.

Rodgers AK, Goldberg JM, Hammel JP, Falcone T: Tubal anastomosis by robotic compared with outpatient minilaparotomy, *Obstet Gynecol* 109:1375-1380, 2007.

Seifer D, Gutmann JN, Grant WD, Kamps CA, DeCherney AH: Comparison of persistent ectopic pregnancy after laparoscopic salpingostomy versus salpingostomy at laparotomy for ectopic pregnancy, *Obstet Gynecol* 81:378-382, 1993.

Stadtmauer LA, Riehl RM, Toma SK, Talbert LM: Cauterization of hydrosalpinges before in vitro fertilization is an effective surgical treatment associated with improved pregnancy rates, *Am J Obstet Gynecol* 183:367-371, 2000.

Strandell A, Lindhard A, Waldenstrom U, Thorburn J, Janson PO, Hamberger L: Hydrosalpinx and IVF outcome: a prospective, randomized multicentre trial in Scandinavia on salpingectomy prior to IVF, *Hum Reprod* 14:2762-2769, 1999.

Trimbos-Kemper TCM: Reversal of sterilization in women over 40 years of age: a multicenter survery in the Netherlands, *Fertil Steril* 53:575-577, 1990.

Vermesh M, Silva PD, Rosen GF, Stein AL, Fossum GT, Sauer MV: Management of unruptured ectopic gestation by linear salpingostomy: a prospective, randomised clinical trial of laparoscopy versus laparotomy, *Obstet Gynecol* 73:400-404, 1989.

Vermesh M, Presser SC: Reproductive outcome after linear salpingostomy: a prospective 3-year follow-up, *Fertil Steril* 57:682-684, 1992.

Van Voorhis BJ, Sparks AE, Syrop CH, Stovall DW: Ultrasound-guided aspiration of hydrosalpinges is associated with improved pregnancy and implantation rates after in-vitro fertilization cycles, *Hum Reprod* 13:736-739, 1998.

Watson A, Vandekerckhove P, Lilford R, Vail A, Brosens I, Hughes E: A meta-analysis of the therapeutic role of oil soluble contrast media at hysterosalpingography: a surprising result? *Fertil Steril* 61:470-477, 1994.

Yoon TK, Sung HR, Kang HG, et al: Laparoscopic tubal anastomosis: fertility outcome in 202 cases, *Fertil Steril* 72:1121-1126, 1999.

Zeyneloglu HB, Arici A, Olive D: Adverse effects of hydrosalpinx on pregnancy rates after in vitro fertilization – embryo transfer, *Fertil Steril* 70:492-499, 1998.

Laparoscopic Surgery for Müllerian Anomalies, Incompetent Cervix, and Ovarian Transposition

Marjan Attaran M.D.
Mohamed A. Bedaiwy M.D.
Tommaso Falcone M.D.

 Video Clips on DVD

10-1 Anatomic Implications and Treatment of Rudimentary Uterine Horn (8 minutes/5 seconds)

10-2 Laparoscopic Transabdominal Cerclage in a Patient with a

Bicornuate Uterus (6 minutes/23 seconds)

10-3 Laparoscopic Lateral Ovarian Transposition (7 minutes/50 seconds)

Introduction

Fertility preservation must be the ultimate goal of every gynecologic procedure performed on children, adolescents, and women of childbearing age. Management of congenital anomalies of the müllerian system remains challenging to the clinician due to its rarity, the variable anatomy, and the degree of surgical skill required. Surgical management of cervical incompetency is also an uncommon event, with indications that are somewhat controversial. This chapter will also review the techniques of ovarian transposition that may be used in patients who will undergo potentially-sterilizing chemotherapy and/or radiation treatment.

Müllerian Malformations

Normal differentiation and development of the müllerian ducts lead to formation of the uterus, fallopian tubes, cervix, and upper vagina. The type of abnormality will determine whether this anomaly is appreciated or not. Some patients will present at the time of puberty with the obstructive symptomatology of primary amenorrhea and cyclic pelvic pain, while others go unrecognized until faced with an obstetric problem. Indeed, many patients' anomalies are never realized until surgery or imaging is performed for an unrelated problem. Thus, the true incidence of müllerian anomalies is difficult to calculate accurately. Given these limitations, the prevalence of these anomalies has been reported to range from 0.16% to 10%. As may be expected, the incidence of müllerian anomalies is greater in the infertility population than in the general unselected population.

Müllerian anomalies have been classified both to help with diagnosis and to compare the various modes of management and outcomes. But there is no single classification that has encompassed all anomalies. When a patient presents with a müllerian anomaly, great thought and time must be given to determine the correct diagnosis and best subsequent treatment. One must maintain the ability to think "outside the box" and recognize the great anatomic variability of these anomalies. The first step is to manage the immediate symptom, which is usually pain. After the pain is under control, a thorough investigation is necessary to clarify the anomaly. This investigation may include various imaging studies, examination under anesthesia, diagnostic laparoscopy and hysteroscopy, and evaluation of the urinary system.

Noncommunicating and Communicating Uterine Horns

Preoperative Evaluation

A unicornuate uterus may be associated with a communicating or noncommunicating rudimentary horn. Such patients have monthly regular periods, which may or may not be associated with pain. If the noncommunicating horn is not functioning, that is there is no endometrial cavity, the patient is pain-free and the diagnosis is not usually made until the time of investigation for infertility, obstetric problems, or recurrent pregnancy loss. However, if the noncommunicating rudimentary horn is functional, severe dysmenorrhea unresponsive to medical therapy will bring the patient in for an evaluation (Figure 10-1). A patent connection between a functional uterine horn and unicornuate uterus does not usually lead to any symptoms. However, these patients are at risk of developing a pregnancy in the rudimentary horn with subsequent rupture due to failure of diagnosis.

Physical examination may reveal a deviated uterus or an adnexal mass. Ultrasound imaging may show an adnexal mass believed to be an endometrioma or a pedunculated fibroid. An MRI, which is more likely to elucidate this diagnosis, is recommended in younger patients with a suspicion of an obstructive müllerian anomaly. Because the embryologic development of the müllerian and metanephric ducts is closely linked, patients with müllerian anomalies may also have urologic anomalies such as horseshoe and pelvic kidneys and renal agenesis on the side of the absent or obstructed uterine horn. Imaging studies must also be performed to uncover malformations of the urinary system to avoid inadvertent damage to these structures.

Figure 10-1. Laparoscopic image of noncommunicating right rudimentary horn.

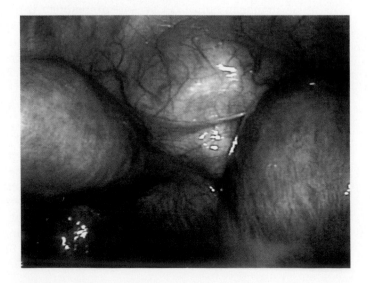

Case 1: Rudimentary Horn

 View DVD: Video 10-1

LS is a 16-year-old female who presented to her pediatrician with progressively worsening dysmenorrhea. Her periods began at age 13 and were not regular until the past 2 years. Each month she had associated nausea and vomiting. She was placed on a trial of NSAIDs without success. Multiple days of school had been skipped and she had been seen in the emergency department at least twice. During her second visit she had a pelvic ultrasound that revealed a 4-cm left ovarian cyst and a possible 5-cm right adnexal mass. Gynecology was consulted and due to the severity of her pain, she underwent diagnostic laparoscopy and a diagnostic hysteroscopy. The findings were consistent with a left unicornuate uterus and a right rudimentary uterine horn. A simple left ovarian cyst was also noted. Stage II endometriosis was detected with most of the lesions present on the ovaries and in the cul-de-sac. Because the findings were unexpected, a decision was made not to proceed with surgery at this time and instead the patient was placed on suppressive therapy. She did well on continuous oral contraceptive pills and eventually presented

for a second opinion to a referral center. An MRI was performed to determine the extent of myometrial attachment of the rudimentary horn to the unicornuate uterus, whether there was endometrium present in the rudimentary horn, and if there were any urologic abnormalities (Figure 10-2). She was scheduled for an operative laparoscopy with resection of the rudimentary horn.

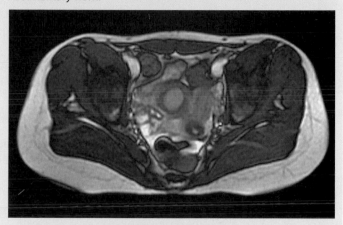

Figure 10-2. MRI showing obstructed rudimentary horn.

Surgical Techniques

A nonfunctioning uterine horn does not need to be removed. However, a noncommunicating functioning uterine horn should be removed upon diagnosis. The rudimentary horn may share myometrial tissue with the unicornuate uterus or be attached by a band of fibrous tissue. In the former case, significant variations are seen from patient to patient.

1. A 5-mm port is placed in the umbilicus. After gaining visualization of the pelvis, the abdominal wall anatomy and the pelvis are examined carefully. A 10-mm port is placed on the side of the obstructed rudimentary horn, lateral to the inferior epigastic vessels, under direct visualization. It is absolutely crucial to determine without doubt the side that is indeed the rudimentary horn. Because it is obstructed, in many instances it is larger than the unicornuate uterus. Two other 5-mm ports are placed under direct visualization, one in the lower abdomen on the contralateral side to the rudimentary horn and the other higher in the abdomen at the level of the umbilicus.

2. Once the round ligament of the uterine horn is identified, it is coagulated or ligated, then cut. Access is gained into the retroperitoneal space, the ureter (if present) is identified, and the bladder is dissected off the lower border of the rudimentary horn. The fallopian tube attached to the rudimentary horn must be removed to forestall a future ectopic pregnancy via sperm transmigration. After disconnecting the tube from the mesosalpinx, the utero-ovarian ligament is transected.

3. The uterine artery supplies the rudimentary horn. In cases where the uterine horn is attached to the uterus via fibrous tissue, the blood supply is found within this plane between the uterus and rudimentary horn. In cases where the rudimentary horn is attached to the uterus via shared myometrium, the blood supply cannot be easily identified and thus the uterine artery ascending beneath the rudimentary horn should be identified and ligated. On occasion, aberrant vessels may be noted arising directly from the internal iliac artery to the rudimentary horn. It may be difficult to find a plane of dissection between the horn and the uterus so care must be taken to avoid entry into the cavity of the unicornuate uterus. In some instances, placing a hysteroscope into the unicornuate uterus will help identify the myometrial

border to avoid cutting into it. After this dissection, myometrial stitches are frequently necessary to reapproximate the tissue.

(See Video 10-1 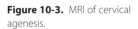)

Cervical Agenesis

Cervical agenesis is a rare müllerian anomaly whose true incidence remains unknown despite several case reports in the literature. One review of the literature cited an incidence of 1:80,000 to 100,000 births. Cervical agenesis/dysgenesis is typically classified as a Ib müllerian anomaly according to the ASRM guidelines. As with all müllerian anomalies, a range of cervical defects may be seen. In some instances there is complete agenesis of the cervix, but in the majority, the cervical region is described as lacking normal anatomical landmarks. In these cases, the cervical region may just have fibrous tissue or have disconnected and fragmented portions of the cervix. In addition, the vagina may or may not be present in patients with cervical agenesis. In a series of 58 patients with cervical atresia, 48% had isolated congenital cervical atresia with a normal vagina. The rest of the patients had either a vaginal dimple or complete atresia.

Preoperative Evaluation and Patient Selection

Unlike some of the other müllerian anomalies, patients with cervical agenesis present very early during adolescence. The typical age of presentation is between the ages of 12 to 16, and the primary complaint is pelvic/abdominal pain. The pain is secondary to obstruction of flow from the uterus. Initially the patient has cyclic pain, which may evolve with time to continuous pain. It is not uncommon for such patients to have been evaluated by their pediatricians for other causes of abdominal pain. Although these girls have amenorrhea, this symptom fails to raise a red flag because the patients are so young at presentation that lack of a period is not worrisome.

Continuing menstruation in an obstructed uterus forms a hematometra, and possibly hematosalpinges, endometriosis, and pelvic adhesions. Imaging of such a pelvis can easily lead to a misdiagnosis. While ultrasound may be helpful in looking for a cervix, one's clinical suspicion must be communicated directly to the radiologist performing the procedure. Magnetic resonance imaging is very helpful in visualizing the cervix but is certainly not definitive (Figure 10-3).

Patients with cervical agenesis who lack a vagina must be differentiated from those with a high obstructing transverse vaginal septum. MRI is very helpful in making this differentiation by showing accumulation of blood in the upper vagina and a cervix in patients with a high transverse septum. However, the cervix may also be dilated with blood in these cases making it difficult to see. Lack of a hematocolpos helps make the

Figure 10-3. MRI of cervical agenesis.

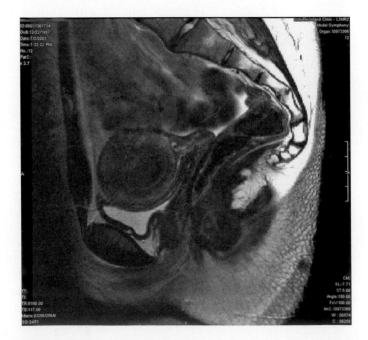

diagnosis of cervical agenesis/dysgenesis. Theoretically, an MRI should detect absence of the cervix, but it is unable to clearly differentiate among the various degrees of cervical dysgenesis.

Pain control should be the first goal of treatment. Although analgesia may be required, severe pain will resolve within several days. Until definitive surgery can be performed, suppressive therapy is used to prevent further endometrial shedding. Agents that are commonly used to achieve this suppression are: continuous oral contraceptive pills, norethindrone acetate, depo-medroxyprogesterone acetate, and GnRH agonists or antagonists.

Most adolescents are neither emotionally ready nor equipped to decide on a surgical course of action, which may be as radical as hysterectomy. Thus, if suppressive therapy has provided pain relief, many may choose to hold off on definitive surgical therapy until they can fully understand the possible consequences. In addition, this alleviates the burden placed upon parents to make a decision regarding their daughter's reproductive future.

There are no specific guidelines in the literature to determine the correct surgical procedure. It is clear however that each patient should be assessed individually. The classic and definitive treatment of cervical agenesis remains total abdominal hysterectomy. Certainly a hysterectomy would diminish continued physical pain and discomfort. In addition, an early hysterectomy would potentially preserve more ovarian tissue which may be used to achieve a pregnancy via in vitro fertilization with a gestational carrier. On the other hand, it is a daunting decision to have a hysterectomy at a young age.

The other surgical options for management of cervical dysgenesis are cervical canalization and uterovaginal anastomosis. There are many reports in the literature of cervical canalization and stent placement. Although success has been reported with menses established, many patients have required reoperation secondary to refibrosis of the cervical tract and obstruction. The primary concern when performing this surgery is subsequent upper genital tract infection and peritonitis. Indeed fulminant sepsis and death has been reported. In addition, pregnancy rates are very low. In Fujimoto's review of patients with cervical agenesis, 59% of those who underwent cervical canalization achieved normal menstruation. Four of the 23 who achieved cervical patency required multiple surgeries.

In more recent years, there have been episodic reports of uterovaginal anastomosis. Deffarges and colleagues have published the results of this procedure on 18 patients via laparotomy in 2001. Ten of these patients attempted pregnancy and only four achieved it spontaneously. Several years later, Creighton and colleagues reported the first laparoscopic surgical uterovaginal anastomosis for cervical agenesis. Given the complexity of these procedures and the lower pregnancy rates, it seems prudent to attempt such procedures on individuals whose pelvic organs are fairly free of any disease and those patients with cervical agenesis who have a normal caliber vagina.

Case 2: Cervical Agenesis

TR presented at 16 years of age to the gynecology department for primary amenorrhea. She had been investigated thoroughly for many years for constipation and abdominal pain. She could not clearly recall cyclic abdominal pain. She currently felt abdominal pelvic pain continually. Thelarche occurred at age 10 and abdominal pain began 2 years later. She had attempted intercourse once unsuccessfully.

On examination, the patient was noted to have complete development of her secondary sexual characteristics. Breasts were Tanner stage 5. Her abdominal examination was normal. Evaluation of her external genitalia revealed only a vaginal dimple. Rectal examination failed to show any evidence of a hematocolpos. An MRI of the pelvis was performed and revealed a uterus with some blood in the endometrial cavity. In addition, a collection of blood was noted in the upper vagina.

The patient was placed on Depo-Provera and her symptoms promptly dissipated. She began using vaginal dilators with the purpose of extending the distal vagina. She was able to increase the vaginal length by 4 cm. At this time she was scheduled for surgery to excise the "presumed" transverse vaginal septum. At the time of the surgery, intraoperative ultrasound guidance was used to facilitate access to the presumed hematocolpos. However, the collection of blood was very anterior and when it was drained it was felt that it was not an upper vagina but rather a fistulous tract from the uterus to the uterovesical region. A repeat MRI in fact confirmed the lack of cervical tissue. The patient did well on her suppressive therapy and continued with the vaginal dilation. When she turned 18 she decided to proceed with total laparoscopic hysterectomy with preservation of the ovaries.

Surgical Technique

1. Patient positioning: The patient is first placed in lithotomy position with the arms tucked by her sides. A Foley catheter is placed inside the bladder, and if a vagina is present, a sponge stick is placed inside the vagina.

2. Trocar placement: Initially a 5-mm umbilical port is placed. A 10-mm Step port is then introduced in the right lower quadrant lateral to the inferior epigastic vessels under direct visualization. Cephalad to this port, a 5-mm port is placed at the level of the umbilicus. Two additional 5-mm ports are introduced on the left side.

3. A 10-mm single tooth laparoscopic tenaculum is positioned through the 10-mm port and the uterus is grasped. Graspers and harmonic scalpel are placed through the other 5-mm ports to transect the fallopian tubes from the ovary and divide the utero-ovarian ligaments.

4. The harmonic scalpel is then used to transect the round ligament and access is gained into the retroperitoneal area. Blunt dissection is carried out to identify the course of the ureter. Anteriorly, the bladder flap is created. As the bladder is dissected away and pushed caudad, the sponge stick in the vagina helps delineate the border of the vagina and the lower uterine segment. Once the uterine arteries are coagulated and cut, blanching of the uterus is noted. Staying close to the lower border of the uterus, the cardinal ligaments are sequentially coagulated and cut until the uterus is free.

5. The 10-mm port is then extended to accommodate a 12-mm morcellator. The uterus is morcellated and removed in strips.

Case 3: Cervical Agenesis

SB presented at age 15 to a gynecologist, complaining of monthly abdominal and pelvic pain associated with nausea and vomiting for the past 6 months. She had not yet experienced menarche. Breast development began at age 12. On examination she is reported to have Tanner 3 breasts and Tanner 4 pubic hair development. Evaluation of the external genitalia revealed "imperforate hymen" on review of the examiner's notes. Rectal examination only revealed a uterus to palpation. A pelvic ultrasound was performed, which showed a uterus that was 9.0 × 3.0 × 5.9 cm with a 1.3 cm thick endometrium. There was no mention of a hematocolpos.

The patient underwent a hymenectomy which failed to reveal a vagina. A tract was made from the perineum in the cephalad direction until access was inadvertently gained into the posterior cul-de-sac. At this point the procedure was terminated and the patient with placed on Depo-Provera to stop her periods.

She underwent an MRI of the pelvis which revealed cervical agenesis. On subsequent consultation with a specialist, the patient and her family felt very strongly about keeping the uterus in the hopes that she would be able to conceive in future. She experienced breakthrough pain periodically (presumably from cryptomenorrhea), and would occasionally be admitted for pain management. Eventually, she was placed on Depo-Lupron with add-back therapy using Prem-Pro. Subsequent evaluation of the vagina revealed that it was scarred; thus she was started on vaginal dilators which she has used inconsistently.

Discussion of Case

From the initial encounter, this patient expressed an extreme interest in the preservation of the uterus at all cost. Indeed, despite continued pain and lack of control of breakthrough bleeding she has continued to persevere in the hopes that surgical advancements in this field may provide her an opportunity to conceive. Since reports on uterovaginal anastomosis have been published, she has expressed an interest in proceeding with this surgery. If her pelvis is free of adhesions and the fallopian tubes are normal, she may be a candidate for this surgery. Creighton and colleagues have described the laparoscopic technique they employed for this procedure. After introduction of the laparoscope and the auxiliary ports, retention sutures were placed through the uterus to help elevate it away from the vagina. The bladder was then dissected off the lower uterine segment, a hysterotomy was performed at the fundus of the uterus, and a blunt probe was placed in it to help identify the lower border of the uterus. The lower border of the uterus and the upper portion of the vagina were transected, and a Foley catheter was placed via the vagina through this opening into the lower uterine segment. The created vaginal cuff and lower uterine segment were then reapproximated and the Foley balloon was kept in the uterus for several weeks. Unfortunately, our patient has scarring in her vagina, which may pose a problem for this surgery. If she can successfully dilate the vagina with dilators, this option may be viable.

Laparoscopic Cervicoisthmic Cerclage

The incidence of cervical insufficiency varies from 0.5 to 5 per 1000 deliveries, which reflects the variation in the definition and diagnostic criteria used. The definition of cervical insufficiency is either based on the history of repeated second-trimester pregnancy loss or on the presence of short cervix. Regardless of the definition, women with cervical insufficiency have a 50% probability of preterm labor, and a 10% probability of perinatal mortality. Over the past 50 years, cervical stitch "cerclage" has been the most utilized therapy for cervical insufficiency. Despite its wide utilization, the benefit of conventional cervical cerclage (CCC) in women with repeated second-trimester miscarriage has not been established when compared to no treatment in large randomized clinical trials. In a recent systematic review of randomized clinical trials, it has been concluded that CCC will not be a cure for all women with cervical insufficiency and other interventions should be explored.

Cervicoisthmic cerclage was first described by Benson and Raphael in 1965 to provide an alternative surgical approach for CCC by placing the cerclage stitch at the level of the uterine isthmus instead of the cervix in those patients with very short or deformed cervices who do not benefit from CCC. Extremely short or deformed cervices can be caused by congenital hypoplasia, obstetric laceration, scarred cervices, extensive cone biopsy, or associated with in utero exposure to diethylstilbestrol (DES). These women have a higher risk of unfavorable obstetric outcomes and usually fail CCC. In this high-risk cohort, transabdominal cervicoisthmic cerclage has been reported to significantly increase the duration of gestation and to reduce the incidence of preterm labor compared to CCC. Despite the reported favorable pregnancy outcomes after the originally described "open" cervicoisthmic cerclage, the morbidity of the procedure prevented wide-scale utilization. Since 1965, several modifications of the procedure have been proposed to minimize morbidity and to improve obstetrical outcomes. To date, two other approaches besides the original laparotomy route have been utilized: laparoscopic and transvaginal. In addition, two timing options of the procedure have been reported: "interval" before pregnancy and "prophylactic" during pregnancy. In addition, robotic assistance has been recently implemented in cervicoisthmic cerclage to overcome the limitations of the traditional laparoscopic surgery. Case reports are accumulating on the use of the da Vinci robotic technology for such indications. It is considered to be less invasive, is associated with quicker recovery and shorter duration of hospital stay, and is effective for both interval and prophylactic procedures.

Preoperative Work-up

The exact risk of recurrent fetal loss without cerclage in women at high risk for cervical incompetency is unknown. Consequently, in women with a history suggestive of cervical insufficiency, prophylactic cerclage is strongly justifiable. Careful counseling is mandatory, particularly if the diagnosis of cervical insufficiency is made after a single fetal loss. In this scenario, the advantages and disadvantages of cerclage should be weighed against the other options, including expectant management. In addition to the routine work-up for recurrent pregnancy loss, ultrasound should be performed during pregnancy to measure cervical length for assessment of cervical shortening or dilatation, with or without bulging of the membranes. Preoperative evaluation of patients selected for laparoscopic cerclage should include a thorough history and physical and possibly assessment for fetal anatomical and chromosomal integrity. Patients should be made aware of the risks of fetal loss during or after the procedure.

Case 1: Cervical insufficiency

A 34-year-old white female, gravida 5, para 1131, presented with a history of four consecutive pregnancy losses after a term pregnancy. The patient was thought to have an cervical insufficiency based on pregnancy losses at 19, 23, 8, and 15 weeks, respectively. In the last pregnancy, an unsuccessful McDonald cerclage operation was performed. Following this loss, examination revealed a very short cervix that was flush with the vaginal wall. The patient was informed that she is not

Continued

Case 1: Cervical insufficiency—cont'd

a candidate for a transvaginal cerclage and that the abdominal cerclage was the best option.

At the time of the procedure, the uterus, fallopian tubes, and ovaries appeared normal. There was minimal superficial endometriosis on the left pelvic sidewall lateral to the uterosacral ligament. The liver and bowel appeared to be within normal limits. There was no evidence of adhesions. After the procedure, an 8-mm dilator could be passed through the cervix without any problems (Figure 10-4).

Five months later, she conceived spontaneously. An ultrasonogram at 7 weeks of gestation demonstrated a normal ongoing singleton pregnancy. The pregnancy progressed uneventfully. An uncomplicated elective low transverse cesarean section was conducted at 38 weeks with the delivery of a healthy 3050 g male infant. At the time of the cesarean section, the Mersilene band used for the cerclage was palpable circumferentially in the lower uterine segment through the hysterotomy incision, forming a ring approximately 1.5 cm in diameter.

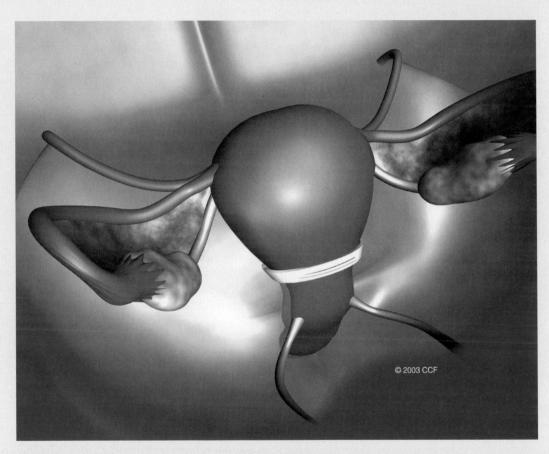

© 2003 CCF

Figure 10-4. Mersilene mesh around the cervico isthmic area. Reprinted with the permission of the Cleveland Clinic Center for Medical Art & Photography © 2003. All rights reserved.

Technique of Interval Laparoscopic Cerclage

1. For the interval laparoscopic approach, as shown in the video, the laparoscope was introduced through a 5-mm intraumbilical port and pneumoperitoneum was obtained. Two ancillary ports were placed under direct visualization.

2. The uterus was manipulated using a Hulka tenaculum. The vesicouterine fold was incised and the bladder was dissected downward as necessary.

3. Windows were made in the broad ligament medial to the uterine vessels at the level where the uterosacral ligaments inserted into the cervix.

4. The ends of the 5-mm Mersilene tape (RS-21; Ethicon, Inc., Somerville, NJ) were sutured with a 2-0 Surgitek to facilitate placement of the tape. The Mersilene tape was then brought circumferentially around the cervix at the level of the internal os medial to the uterine vessels.

5. The Hulka tenaculum was removed and an 8-mm Hegar dilator was placed into the cervix. The Surgitek was cut from each end of the 12-inch Mersilene tape. The tape was tied tightly with six square knots with the dilator in place. The tape was then trimmed so that the ends were approximately 2-cm long bilaterally.

6. Finally, the bladder peritoneum was closed over the Mersilene tape.

Case 2: Cervical insufficiency

 View DVD: Video 10-2

A healthy 31-year-old white female, gravida 2, para 1001, was referred for cervical insufficiency. This patient had a uterine didelphys, and had previously undergone removal of a longitudinal vaginal septum (Figure 10-5). She had had a previous McDonald cerclage that tore through her cervix and she was on bed rest from weeks 25 to 34 of gestation. Her first pregnancy was delivered by elective classical cesarean section at 36 weeks of gestation after confirmation of fetal lung maturity.

The procedure described in this report was performed at 10 weeks of gestation after ultrasonographic confirmation of fetal viability. Before the procedure, cervical examination revealed a markedly short, distorted exocervix with the cervical opening nearly flush with the vaginal apex. A transvaginal cerclage was not feasible. It was discussed with the patient that transabdominal cerclage would be her best option and this could be done either abdominally or laparoscopically. Accordingly, a decision was made to proceed with laparoscopic placement as a prophylactic procedure as described later.

At the time of the procedure, uterus didelphys bicollis with a pregnancy in the right horn was documented. The left uterine horn appeared soft, but within normal limits. There were bilateral functional ovarian cysts and normal fallopian tubes. There were adhesions from the sigmoid colon to the bladder flap and a well-healed uterine incision on the right uterine horn. She had an accessory spleen; otherwise, the bowel, liver, and appendix appeared to be within normal limits. An ultrasonogram at the end of the procedure demonstrated fetal cardiac activity. The pregnancy progressed uneventfully. An uncomplicated elective repeat cesarean section was conducted at 36 weeks after confirmation of fetal lung maturity with the delivery of a healthy female infant.

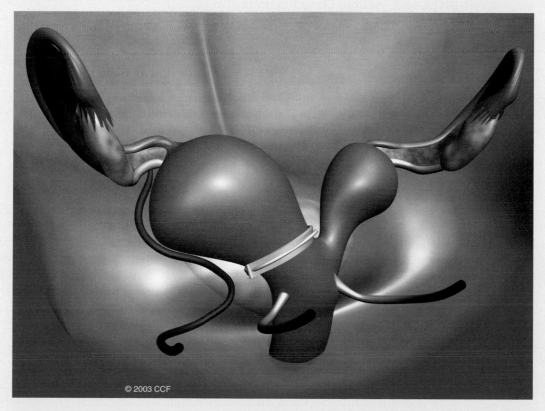

© 2003 CCF

Figure 10-5. Mersilene mesh around the cervico isthmic junction of a patient with a unicornuate uterus with a non-functional rudimentary horn. Reprinted with the permission of the Cleveland Clinic Center for Medical Art & Photography © 2003. All rights reserved.

Technique of Prophylactic Laparoscopic Cerclage

1. The prophylactic cervicoisthmic cerclage was initiated by a direct left upper quadrant entry approach with a 5-mm trocar, as shown in Video 10-2. Ancillary ports were placed in the right and left lower quadrants under direct visualization. The umbilical port was also placed under direct visualization.

2. The 10-mm laparoscope was then introduced. The uterus was manipulated as little as possible. The bladder was dissected downward to the lower cervix after delineating it by retrograde filling through the Foley catheter with 200 mL of irrigation fluid.

3. In cases where manipulation of the uterus is not satisfactory (e.g., in case of congenitally malformed uteri), the round ligament may be cauterized and transected to provided an atraumatic approach to manipulate the uterus.

4. The right retroperitoneal space was dissected at the level of the uterine vessels where the descending cervical branch meets the uterine artery.

5. A window was made in the peritoneum medial to the vessels. The Mersilene tape, which had been stitched to Ethibond suture, was introduced into the abdominal cavity. This was then brought in through the left side, taking care not to injure the uterus, then brought around the right side and introduced through the right broad ligament.

6. Again, the Mersilene band was medial to the blood vessels in order to decrease any devascularization of the lower uterine segment. After confirmation of fetal cardiac activity, intracorporeal knot-tying was then performed, first with a surgical knot and then throwing six more half-hitches for a total of seven knots.

7. The procedure was completed as in the interval procedure. The surgical technique used is depicted in the video.

   (See Video 10-2)

Risks and Possible Complications

There is potential to injure the uterine vessels. Bowel injury, which could result in a pelvic abscess, has also been reported. Moreover, bladder and ureteric injuries could be inflicted, causing a need for further procedures. There are no actual figures on the precise incidence of these maternal complications. The procedure could cause problems with the pregnancy such as injury to the uterus, hemorrhage, intrauterine fetal death, preterm birth and intra-amniotic infection. Stitching the cervix could cause certain surgical difficulties in delivering the baby if it dies in utero or at the time of cesarean section.

Outcomes

To date, several cases with favorable outcomes have been performed laparoscopically, with and without robotic assistance. The majority of these cases were performed on an anatomically normal uterus as a prophylactic procedure during pregnancy, while fewer cases were performed as an interval procedure. Any surgical team with a combination of good operative laparoscopic and intracorporeal knot-tying skills could use the afore mentioned technique. The laparoscopic approach has the advantage of obviating the need for sequential laparotomies to perform cerclage. Abdominal cerclage via laparotomy may be associated with pelvic adhesions, which might be a cause of subsequent infertility if performed as an interval procedure. On the other hand, if an abdominal cerclage is to be delayed until viability is ascertained, the consequences of laparotomy on pregnant women should be considered.

Careful laparoscopic dissection and hemostasis along the cervicoisthmic junction help avoid jeopardizing the uterine vessels and/or the ureter. This clearly alleviates the doubts raised by some earlier reports that a laparoscopic approach during pregnancy might be associated with a higher risk of bleeding because of a diminished ability to distinguish between the isthmus and adjacent vessels by tactile feedback. Most of the reports on laparoscopic cerclage are limited by the absence of a control group from the same population at the same time period.

SUMMARY: Laparoscopic abdominal cerclage, with or without robotic assistance, is becoming an increasingly popular approach for the management of cervical insufficiency where a vaginal approach is technically impossible or deemed to fail. It could be performed during pregnancy or as an interval procedure. It is less invasive and is associated with less bleeding, quicker recovery, and shorter duration of hospital stay compared to an open abdominal cerclage. As for the majority of laparoscopic procedures, the outcome of laparoscopic cerclage was never assessed by prospective randomized controlled trials. Until enough satisfactory evidence is available, the laparocopic approach for surgical management of cervical insufficiency should be offered to patients after adequate counseling.

Ovarian Transposition

Introduction

Pelvic radiotherapy damages both the ovaries and the uterus. Ovarian damage from radiotherapy results in impaired fertility and premature ovarian failure. Irradiation-induced uterine damage manifests as impaired growth and blood flow. The effects on subsequent pregnancies can be substantial. The ovarian follicles are remarkably vulnerable to DNA damage from ionizing radiation. Irradiation results in ovarian atrophy and reduced follicle stores. As a result, serum FSH and LH levels progressively rise and estradiol levels decline within 4 to 8 weeks following radiation exposure.

On the cellular level, irradiation of oocytes results in rapid onset of pyknosis, chromosome condensation, disruption of the nuclear envelope, and cytoplasmic vacuolization. The irreversibility of this damage has been attributed to the lack of germline stem cells in the ovary. However, a recent study suggested the presence of germline stem cells in the adult ovary. If these findings are confirmed by others, they leave open the possibility that new oocytes might be able to be regenerated after depletion by chemotherapy or radiotherapy.

Patient Selection

Cancer patients are at high risk for premature ovarian failure after treatment with pelvic or total body irradiation. The degree of ovarian damage is related to the patient's age, the radiation field, the total dose of radiation to the ovaries, and the number of treatments that are required to deliver the dose. For example, it may take 18 to 20 Gray (Gy; 1 rad = 1 cGY) to induce permanent ovarian failure in prepubertal girls and only 14 Gray to achieve the same result in women 30 years of age. A dose-dependent reduction in the primordial follicle pool occurs when exposing ovaries to radiotherapy. It is estimated that as little as 2 Gy is enough to destroy 50% of the oocyte population in young reproductive-age women (LD_{50}). Ovarian failure will occur in virtually all patients exposed to pelvic radiation at doses necessary to treat a cervical cancer (85 Gy), rectal cancer (45 Gy), or total body radiation for bone marrow transplantation (8 to 12 Gy to the ovaries). The addition of chemotherapy to radiotherapy further decreases the dose required to induce premature ovarian failure.

Even if the ovaries are not directly in the radiation field, radiation scatter can reduce ovarian function. Periaortic lymph node irradiation for treatment of Hodgkin disease exposes the ovaries to approximately 1.5 Gy and the short-term functioning of the ovaries is not affected. The effect of this dose on long-term function remains uncertain. It is very important to discuss with the radiotherapist the expected dose that will be delivered to the ovaries either directly or through scatter.

Transposing the ovaries out of the field of irradiation appears to help to maintain ovarian function in patients scheduled to undergo gonadotoxic radiotherapy. Transposing the ovaries reduced the radiation dose to each ovary by approximately 5% to 10%

compared to ovaries left in their original location. Transposed ovaries receive a dose of 126 cGy during intracavitary radiation, 135 to 190 cGy during external radiation therapy with a total dose of 4500 cGy, and 230 to 310 cGy during para-aortic node irradiation with a dose of 4500 cGy. The ovary should be at least 3 cm from the upper border of the radiation field.

Case 1: Transposition Prior to Radiotherapy

 View DVD: Video 10-3

A 23-year-old woman with recently diagnosed rectal cancer consults to discuss her options to preserve her fertility. She will receive radiotherapy to the pelvis as well as chemotherapy. Her chemotherapy will consist of 5-fluorouracil (5-FU). This drug has a low incidence of gonadotoxicity. For this reason this patient does not need ovarian tissue removal for cryopreservation. The patient is offered ovarian transposition. The radiotherapist calculates the scatter radiation dose outside the field and determines that the ovaries should be placed 2 to 3 cm above the anterior superior iliac spine.

Ovarian Transposition

Lateral transposition of the ovary out of the pelvis and into the colic gutters appears to be more effective than medial transposition. In pediatric patients who are receiving spinal irradiation for a brain tumor, medial transposition into the lowest point in the pelvis, typically to the utero-ovarian ligaments, is best. However, in patients receiving pelvic radiation, such as with a rectal or gynecologic tumor, lateral transposition is best.

Ovarian transposition can be performed by either laparotomy or laparoscopy. When laparotomy is required for the treatment of cervical cancer with radical hysterectomy or during staging of Hodgkin disease, lateral ovarian transposition can be performed simultaneously. However, staging laparotomy and splenectomy are no longer required for stage I and II Hodgkin disease. In cases where laparotomy is not required or transposition was not done during initial laparotomy, transposition can be performed laparoscopically.

There are several advantages to laparoscopic transposition, and as a result, this approach has become the most common. Laparoscopic transposition can be performed as an outpatient procedure with little disruption of the planned therapeutic schedule. The ability to do this easily will eliminate unnecessary transposition in the majority of cervical cancer cases where radiation therapy is not required. An important advantage of laparoscopic ovarian transposition is that radiation therapy can be initiated immediately postoperatively, preventing failure due to the ovaries migrating back to the irradiation field. In cases of vaginal or cervical cancers being treated by brachytherapy, laparoscopic ovarian transposition can be performed under the same anesthetic used for inserting the brachytherapy device.

Before surgery, it should be discussed with the radiotherapist how far the ovaries need to be moved out of the field. For example, in patients with rectal cancer, the field usually goes up to the sacral promontory. Radiotherapists often request that the ovaries be moved above the anterior superior iliac spines. The deep inguinal ring where the round ligament inserts to course through the inguinal canal is midway between the pubic tubercle and the anterior superior iliac spine and can easily be seen at laparoscopy. The ovaries usually need to be moved above this location. Postoperatively, the ovarian dose can be calculated.

Surgical Technique for Lateral Ovarian Transposition

There are different techniques depending on how much mobilization of the ovary is required and whether the surgeon is willing to transect the fallopian tube. Transecting the tube allows the entire adnexa to be moved as a unit and has the advantage of not dissecting the mesovarium where there is the anastomosis of the blood supply to the tube and ovary.

The surgery starts with transection of the utero-ovarian ligament and proximal fallopian tube. The adnexae are mobilized with the ovarian vessels to the paracolic gutters (Figure 10-6). It is important to dissect the ureter away from the ovarian vessels (Figure 10-1). Ideally, the vascular pedicles are kept retroperitoneal to avoid tension, torsion or trauma, and bowel herniation while the ovaries remain intraperitoneal to reduce cyst formation (Figure 10-7). The ovary is then sutured with nonabsorbable suture to the posterior abdominal peritoneum. Clips are placed so that the radiotherapist can assess where the ovaries are located.

A different technique for ovarian transposition has been reported that requires less mobilization of the ovary. The utero-ovarian ligament and mesovarium, but not the fallopian tube, are divided and the ovarian vessels are not mobilized. The ovary is not separated from the fimbriated end of the fallopian tube. Although this approach has been described in a case report to have resulted in a spontaneous pregnancy, this technique may not allow sufficient movement of the ovaries out of the radiation field in most cases of malignancies requiring pelvic radiation. It is unlikely that most fallopian tubes would stretch as far as the anterior superior iliac spine.

High mobilization of the ovaries without the tube has been described by Morice and colleagues. In this technique, the tube is not detached from the uterus but is separated from the ovary. The ovary is detached and the ovarian vessels dissected to the aortic bifurcation. The pedicle is then rotated and attached to the paracolic gutters.

(See Video 10-3 📹)

Outcomes and Complications

Most ovaries will maintain function if they are transposed at least 3 cm from the upper edge of the field. The dose of radiation that the ovaries receive after transposition has been calculated. It has been shown that when cervical cancer is treated with a radiation dose of 4000 cGy, ovaries 3 cm from the radiation field edge receive 280 cGy and those 4 cm from the field edge receive 200 cGy, due to scatter. One study found that the ovaries will maintain function when transposed above the iliac crest. It has been shown that approximately 80% of women undergoing laparoscopic ovarian transposition will maintain ovarian function after radiation therapy for various indications. The majority of women with stage I or II Hodgkin disease treated with radiation alone or

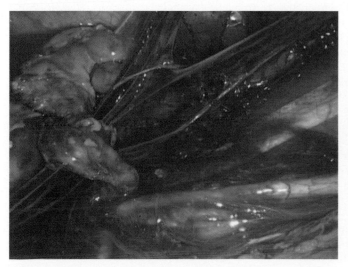

Figure 10-6. The figure shows a dissection for a left ovary transposition. The radiation field was such that the ovarian vessels had to be mobilized high. The ureter was dissected free of the ovarian vessels to allow better mobilization of the pedicle. The tendon of the psoas muscle is seen, along with the ureter, the ovarian vessels, and ovary

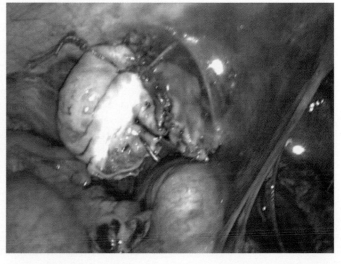

Figure 10-7. Final position of transposed ovary on the abdominal wall. The suture is nonabsorbable.

with minimal chemotherapy following laparoscopic ovarian transposition will retain their ovarian function and fertility.

Causes of Failure

Ovarian failure following transposition can be on the basis of several different mechanisms: the ovaries are not moved far enough out of the radiation field, the ovaries migrate back to their original position (this may occur if absorbable suture is used), and the ovarian blood flow may be compromised from surgical technique or radiation injury to the vascular pedicle. Another concern with ovarian transposition is the development of symptomatic ovarian cysts. The mechanism causing the cysts is unknown, but they can be suppressed with oral contraceptives.

Fertility after Radiotherapy

In a study of 37 women who underwent preradiation ovarian transposition, 15% became pregnant after brachytherapy, with or without external radiation, for vaginal or cervical clear cell carcinoma, and 80% became pregnant after external radiation for dysgerminomas and pelvic sarcomas. Interestingly, 75% of these pregnancies occurred without repositioning of the ovaries.

Several papers have addressed pregnancy outcomes after pelvic irradiation. In a study of 31,150 atomic bomb survivors, there was no increase in stillborns, major congenital malformations, chromosomal abnormalities, or mutations. Likewise, in women treated with radiotherapy for Hodgkin disease addition, there was no increase in stillbirths, low birth weight, congenital malformations, abnormal karyotypes, or cancer. However, one study found an increase in low birth weight and spontaneous abortions if conception occurred less than a year after radiation exposure. On this basis, it seems reasonable to advise delaying pregnancy for a year after completing radiation therapy.

Suggested Readings

Müllerian Anomalies

Aittomaki K, Eroila H, Kajanoja P: A population based study of the incidence of mullerian aplasia in Finland, *Fertil Steril* 76:624-625, 2001.

The American Fertility Society: Classifications of adnexal adhesions, distal tubal occlusion, mullerian anomalies and intrauterine adhesions, *Fertil Steril* 49:944-955, 1988.

Creighton SM, Davies MC, Cutner A: Laparoscopic management of cervical agenesis, *Fertil Steril* 85:1510 e.13-15, 2006.

Deffarges JV, Haddad B, Musset R, Paniel BJ: Utero-vaginal anastomosis in women with uterine cervix atresia: long-term follow-up and reproductive performance. A study of 18 cases, *Human Reprod* 16:1722-1725, 2001.

Falcone T, Gidwani G, Paraiso M, et al: Anatomic variations in the rudimentary horns of a unicornuate uterus: implications for laparoscopic surgery, *Hum Reprod* 12:263-265, 1997.

Fujimoto VY, Miller JH, Klein NA, Soules MR: Congenital cervical atresia: report of seven cases and review of the literature, *Am J Obstet Gynecol* 177:1419-1425,1997.

Rock J, Breech L: Surgery for anomalies of the mullerian ducts. In Rock JA, Jones HW 3rd, editors: *Te Linde's Operative Gynecology*, ed 9, Philadelphia, 2003, Lippincott Williams & Wilkins.

Suganuma N, Furuhashi M, Moriwaki T, Tsukahara S, Ando T, Ishihara Y: Management of missed abortion in a patient with congenital cervical atresia, *Fertil Steril* 77:1071-1073, 2002.

Laparoscopic Cervicoisthmic Cerclage

Al-Fadhli R, Tulandi T: Laparoscopic abdominal cerclage, *Obstet Gynecol Clin North Am* 31:497-504, 2004.

Davis G, Berghella V, Talucci M, Wapner RJ: Patients with a prior failed transvaginal cerclage: a comparison of obstetric outcomes with either transabdominal or transvaginal cerclage, *Am J Obstet Gynecol* 183:836-839, 2000.

Karaman Y, Bingol B, Günenc Z: Laparoscopic transabdominal isthmic cerclage in a case of cervical agenesis and a successful pregnancy with ICSI, *Gynecol Surg* 4:45-48, 2007.

Laparoscopic Ovarian Transposition

Bedaiwy MA, Falcone T, Attaran M, Goldberg JM, Agarwal A: Preservation of fertility in the cancer patient. In Falcone T, Hurd W: *Clinical Reproductive Medicine and Surgery*, Mosby Elsevier Philadelphia, PA, 2007.

Wallace WH, Anderson RA, Irvine DS: Fertility preservation for young patients with cancer: who is at risk and what can be offered? *Lancet Oncol* 6(4):209-218, 2005.

Indications and Techniques for the Laparoscopic Management of Endometriosis

11

Amy J. Park M.D.
Jeffrey M. Goldberg M.D.
Tommaso Falcone M.D.

 Video Clips on DVD

Introduction

Endometriosis is a condition characterized by the presence of functional endometrial glands and stroma outside the endometrial cavity, which induces a chronic inflammatory reaction. These implants can be located throughout the pelvis, including the ovaries, uterosacral ligaments, rectovaginal septum, peritoneum, appendix, intestinal tract, and urinary tract; although less commonly, they have also been reported in the umbilicus, in cesarean section or episiotomy scars, in the cervix, in hernia sacs, and in the pleural and pericardial cavities.

The pathogenesis and classification of endometriosis remains elusive, despite awareness of this clinical entity for over a century. The diagnosis must be made by direct visualization, although typical symptoms and preoperative imaging, in addition to a response to medical management, may be suggestive of endometriosis. Nevertheless, patients with endometriosis may be asymptomatic, have a completely negative preoperative work-up, or not respond to medical therapy. Although suppression of endometriosis-related symptoms can be achieved in some cases with medical therapies, definitive treatment remains surgical, especially in the setting of more advanced disease.

In performing laparoscopic surgery, the surgeon should follow the same surgical principles used in performing the procedure by laparotomy. Laparoscopy offers the advantages of improved visualization, decreased postoperative pain, shorter postoperative recovery time, and decreased trauma, which results in reduced de novo adhesion formation.

The exact prevalence of endometriosis is unknown, due to its variable presentation and the necessity of surgery to make a definitive diagnosis. It is estimated to be approximately 10% in reproductive-aged women. However, the prevalence varies according to the specific subpopulation. In women with dysmenorrhea, the prevalence ranges from 40% to 60%, while in infertile women, it is approximately 40%, and it has been estimated to be as high as 80% in those women with both infertility and pain. Endometriosis has been identified in 70% of teenagers undergoing diagnostic laparoscopy for chronic pelvic pain. A polygenic, multifactorial inheritance pattern has been suggested for endometriosis, with an occurrence rate of 7% in first-degree female relatives compared to unrelated females.

The costs of endometriosis are not insignificant. Endometriosis is one of the main gynecologic conditions leading to hospitalization and surgery, with an estimated annual cost of $579 million in 1992 dollars in the United States.

When extensive pelvic adhesions or large endometriomas are present, infertility can be attributed to anatomic distortion. However, the cause of infertility in patients with mild disease is likely due to an aberrant local inflammatory response, as evidenced by the altered cytokine levels in the follicular and peritoneal fluid of patients with endometriosis. Other contributing etiologies may include altered folliculogenesis or ovulation, and an adverse effect on tubal function, fertilization and implantation.

Pathophysiology

The mechanism by which endometriosis develops remains unknown, although there are four main theories as to its pathogenesis.

Retrograde Menstruation

This theory posits that endometriotic lesions result from the reflux of endometrial tissue through the fallopian tubes from the endometrial cavity during menstruation. The anatomic distribution of endometriotic lesions supports this theory, because the most common sites are the ovary, uterosacral ligaments, posterior uterus, posterior cul-de-sac, and posterior broad ligament. Endometrial tissue has been shown to be capable of developing into endometriotic lesions in the peritoneal cavity in animal studies where the uterus has been manipulated to cause retrograde menstruation. Endometriosis has been reported in laparotomy, cesarean section, and episiotomy scars after procedures where the endometrial tissue directly seeded the incision. Additionally, patients who have anomalies of the müllerian tract or cervical stenosis with outlet flow obstruction have a higher incidence of endometriosis.

Nevertheless, 90% of women with patent fallopian tubes who undergo laparoscopy during the perimenstrual period have demonstrated bloody peritoneal fluid, which is a much higher percentage than the prevalence of endometriosis, suggesting that other factors must contribute to the development of endometriosis.

Coelomic Metaplasia

The ovary, endometrium, and peritoneum all develop from totipotential coelomic epithelium. This theory postulates that certain hormonal or infectious stimuli trigger these cells to transform into endometrial implants. This hypothesis would explain the presence of endometriotic lesions in premenarchal girls and women with primary amenorrhea who lack a functional endometrium. It may also account for ovarian endometriomas, because they may result from the invagination of the mesothelial layer of the ovarian cortex.

Vascular Dissemination

Endometrial cells may travel to extrauterine sites via the lymphatic or vascular systems. Lymphovascular spread of endometriosis may account for retroperitoneal endometriosis and the spread of endometriosis to the lung or pericardial cavity. Vascular spread can explain the findings of endometriosis lesions in remote locations such as the nasal cavity and the brain.

Autoimmune Disease

Altered immune function may result in endometrial cells' successful implantation. This theory proposes that a decreased cytotoxic response to endometrial cells may be from a defect in natural killer cell activity, allowing the development of ectopic endometrial tissue implants. There also may be an increased resistance of endometrium to natural killer cytotoxicity in patients with endometriosis. Alterations in both humoral and cell-mediated immunity have been shown in the peritoneal fluid of endometriosis patients. Patients with endometriosis also have an increased percentage of B lymphocytes, natural killer cells, and monocyte-macrophages in their follicular fluid, indicating a possible altered immunologic function. Increased concentrations of interleukins IL-6, IL-1β, IL-10, tumor necrosis factor-α (TNF-α), and decreased concentrations of vascular endothelial growth factor (VEGF) have been documented in the follicular fluid of endometriosis patients.

Diagnosis and Clinical Presentation

Endometriosis must be diagnosed via direct visual inspection at surgery or pathologic confirmation of a biopsy specimen. Ultrasound or magnetic resonance imaging (MRI) may be helpful in diagnosing endometriomas preoperatively, but negative findings on preoperative imaging or examination do not exclude the presence of disease. Given the costs of MRI, its routine use as a diagnostic tool should be limited when surgical diagnosis and treatment are indicated.

The classic symptoms of endometriosis are dysmenorrhea, dyspareunia, and infertility. However, patients with extensive endometriosis may be asymptomatic, while others with mild disease may have severe pelvic pain. Conversely, women with dysmenorrhea and pelvic pain may have no identifiable endometriosis lesions. If the endometriosis has invaded the rectovaginal septum or uterosacral ligaments, the patient may complain of rectal or lower back pain, or dyspareunia. Other symptoms may include dyschezia and constipation. If there is rectosigmoid involvement, the patient may suffer from cyclic hematochezia. Urinary tract involvement can entail hematuria, urinary urgency, or ureteral obstruction. Patients may also present with low back pain or adnexal masses. In general, the extent or location of disease does not correlate with the severity of symptoms.

These symptoms typically wax and wane according to the hormonal milieu of the menstrual cycle, as the endometriotic lesions respond to the estrogen and progesterone-mediated effects in a similar fashion to the normal endometrium.

Physical examination may reveal pelvic tenderness, cul-de-sac nodularity, a fixed retroverted uterus, an indurated rectovaginal septum, or adnexal masses. However, the absence of these physical findings does not exclude disease. In order to increase the sensitivity of detecting deeply infiltrating nodules, the clinician should consider performing the physical examination during menstruation.

Classification

In 1996, the American Society for Reproductive Medicine published its recommendations for the classification of endometriosis in order to systematically document the severity, extent, and location of disease ranging from stage I to IV (Figure 11-1). This classification schema assigns higher severity according to depth of invasion into the peritoneum and ovary, presence of adhesions, and partial or complete obliteration of the cul-de-sac. Although this system attempts to provide a reproducible framework by which clinicians can communicate, several studies have demonstrated that there is

AMERICAN SOCIETY FOR REPRODUCTIVE MEDICINE
REVISED CLASSIFICATION OF ENDOMETRIOSIS

Patients' Name_____ Date_____

Stage I   (Minimal)   - 1–5   Laparoscopy_____ Laparotomy _____ Photography_____
Stage II   (Mild)   - 6–15
Stage III   (Moderate) - 16–40   Recommended treatment _____
Stage IV   (Severe)   - >40   _____
Total _____ Prognosis _____

	ENDOMETRIOSIS	<1 cm	1–3 cm	<3 cm
Peritoneum	Superficial	1	2	4
Peritoneum	Deep	2	4	6
Ovary	R Superficial	1	2	4
Ovary	Deep	4	16	20
Ovary	L Superficial	1	2	4
Ovary	Deep	4	16	20
	POSTERIOR CULDESAC OBLITERATION	Partial		Complete
		4		40
	ADHESIONS	<1/3 enclosure	1/3–2/3 encolsure	>2/3 enclosure
Ovary	R Filmy	1	2	4
Ovary	Dense	4	8	16
Ovary	L Filmy	1	2	4
Ovary	Dense	4	8	16
Tube	R Filmy	1	2	4
Tube	Dense	4*	8*	16
Tube	L Filmy	1	2	4
Tube	Dense	4*	8*	16

*If the fimbirated end of the fallopian tube is complete closed, change the point assignment to 16.
Denote appearance of superficial implant types as red [(R), red, red-pink, flamelike, vesicular blobs, clear vesicles], white [(W), opacifications, peritoneal defects, yellow-brown], or black [(B) black, hemosiderin deposits, blue]. Denote percent of total described as R ___%, W ___% and B ___%. Total should equal 100%.

Denote appearance of superficial implant types as red [(R), red, red-pink, flamelike, vesicular vesic

Additional endometriosis: _____ | Associated pathology:_____
_____ | _____
_____ | _____
_____ | _____

To be used with normal
tubes and ovaries | To be used with abnormal
                                      | tubes and/or ovaries
L   R   L   R

A

Figure 11-1. The American Society for Reproductive Medicine classification of endometriosis.

STAGE I (MINIMAL)

PERITONEUM
    Superficial endo – 1–3 cm –2
R OVARY
    Superficial endo – <1 cm –1
    Filmy adhesions – <1/3 –1
        TOTAL POINTS 4

STAGE II (MILD)

PERITONEUM
    Deep endo – >3 cm –6
R OVARY
    Superficial endo – <1 cm –1
    Filmy adhesions – <1/3 –1
L OVARY
    Superficial endo – <1 cm –1
        TOTAL POINTS 9

STAGE III (MODERATE)

PERITONEUM
    Deep endo – >3 cm –6
CULDESAC
    Partial obliteration –4
L OVARY
    Deep endo – 1–3 cm –16
        TOTAL POINTS 26

STAGE III (MODERATE)

PERITONEUM
    Superficial endo – >3 cm –4
R TUBE
    Filmy adhesions – <1/3 –1
R OVARY
    Filmy adhesions – <1/3 –1
L TUBE
    Dense adhesions – <1/3 –16*
L OVARY
    Deep endo – <1 cm –4
    Dense adhesions – <1/3 –4
B   TOTAL POINTS 30

STAGE IV (SEVERE)

PERITONEUM
    Superficial endo – >3 cm –4
L OVARY
    Deep endo – 1–3 cm –32**
    Dense adhesions – <1/3 –8**
L TUBE
    Dense adhesions – <1/3 –8**
        TOTAL POINTS 52

*Point assignment changed to 16
**Point assignment doubled

STAGE IV (SEVERE)

PERITONEUM
    Deep endo – >3 cm –6
CULDESAC
    Complete obliteration –40
R OVARY
    Deep endo – 1–3 cm –16
    Dense adhesions – <1/3 –4
L TUBE
    Dense adhesions – >2/3 –16
L OVARY
    Deep endo – 1–3 cm –16
    Dense adhesions – >2/3 –16
        TOTAL POINTS 114

Figure 11-1, cont'd.

poor correlation between symptom severity and stage of disease. It may provide some value in the prognosis and management of infertility.

General Surgical Principles

The goals of surgery are to restore normal anatomy, alleviate pain symptoms and enhance fertility. The surgical procedures can be divided into conservative management, with excision or ablation of endometriotic lesions, or radical treatment, which entails the addition of hysterectomy with or without oophorectomy. If possible, excision of endometriotic lesions should be performed in order to obtain pathologic diagnosis, exclude malignancy, and decrease recurrence rates. The main disadvantage is the potential for bleeding due to sharp dissection. Ablative surgery, using monopolar or bipolar cautery or laser, carries a decreased risk of bleeding, but at the expense of increased peripheral damage to surrounding structures and undertreatment of lesions, which increases the risk of recurrent disease. The most commonly used lasers are CO_2, KTP532, and NdYAG. Excision should be performed for all deeply infiltrating lesions as well as superficial lesions in patients with pain symptoms. There is no data to show that excision is superior to ablation for superficial lesions in women with infertility.

If urinary or gastrointestinal involvement is suspected, an appropriate work-up with preoperative imaging or studies should be obtained. The surgeon should address the extent of surgery the patient desires, for example, partial bladder or bowel resection, and enlist the assistance of a urologic or colorectal surgeon if the patient chooses extirpative surgery. Treatment must be individualized, and the patient and physician should establish the primary goals of the surgery preoperatively. For example, the infertile patient who is undergoing an initial diagnostic laparoscopy may desire excision of endometriosis with preservation of her tubes, ovaries, and uterus. In contrast, a patient who has undergone multiple laparoscopies and remains infertile and has an endometrioma and hydrosalpinx may opt for a salpingectomy and ovarian cystectomy to prepare for in vitro fertilization. The patient with chronic pelvic pain may desire a bilateral salpingo-oophorectomy with or without a hysterectomy, in addition to excision or ablation of her endometriotic lesions. Nevertheless, in spite of adequate medical or surgical treatment, patients may still suffer from pain or infertility, and a multidisciplinary approach with counseling, consultation with pain specialists, or assisted reproduction may still be required.

The surgeon should approach the patient in a systematic fashion in order to restore normal anatomy. A Foley catheter and uterine manipulator should be placed prior to the initiation of the case in order to decompress the bladder and allow intraoperative manipulation of the uterus. The initial step of the operation often entails adhesiolysis in order to obtain adequate visualization of the pelvic organs, because endometriosis can often cause an inflammatory response that results in distorted anatomy due to adhesions involving the adnexae, pelvic sidewalls, uterus, and bowel.

The surgeon should redundant have an awareness of the location of the ureters at all times. Because retroperitoneal fibrosis is also common, the ureters may follow an aberrant course. Thus, the surgeon should have a low threshold to perform a retroperitoneal dissection and ureterolysis. Often, the localization and identification of the ureters is the key to the surgery. Once the ureters are identified and followed throughout the course of the pelvis, the surgeon can safely remove endometriotic implants of the pelvic sidewall peritoneum or uterosacral ligaments, identify the uterine arteries if performing a hysterectomy, secure the ovarian blood supply, or perform a pararectal dissection in order to mobilize the rectum.

Specific Indications for Surgery

Pelvic Pain

It is reasonable to consider an empiric trial of medical management for endometriosis when there is no indication for immediate surgery. However, symptoms often recur after the patient discontinues the medical therapy.

Conservative surgical management of endometriosis results in relief in symptoms in two thirds of patients. Concomitant oophorectomy may also provide additional pain relief, due to the removal of the hormonal effects on the endometriotic implants. Hysterectomy alone should not be considered as a primary treatment option for pelvic pain due to endometriosis. The decision to perform a hysterectomy with or without oophorectomy should be tailored to the individual needs and desires of the patient and after extensive counseling regarding the options.

Infertility

Surgery to remove endometriosis may result in improved fertility rates, whereas medical treatments have not been shown to improve fertility and only delay pregnancy. Although the benefit of performing laparoscopy in those patients with mild disease is controversial, those patients with moderate or severe endometriosis do have improved fertility rates with laparoscopic excision or ablation. The choice as to perform a repeat laparoscopic surgery for recurrent endometriosis versus proceeding to in vitro fertilization depends on such factors as the severity of previous endometriosis, concomitant pain symptoms, and the patient's age.

Adnexal Mass/Ovarian Endometrioma

Patients with an adnexal mass suggestive of an endometrioma often present with similar symptoms to other patients with endometriosis: pain and infertility. In addition, malignant transformation can occur, albeit less than 1% of the time. Drainage or ablation alone is associated with a high recurrence rate. Therefore, surgical excision is of paramount importance in order to pathologically confirm the diagnosis and to prevent recurrence.

Urinary Tract Endometriosis

Endometriosis is estimated to affect the urinary tract in 0.3% to 6% of cases. Urinary tract endometriosis most commonly affects the bladder (84%), followed by the ureter (15%), the kidney (4%), and then the urethra (2%). The symptoms and signs of urinary tract endometriosis include cyclic or noncyclic hematuria; urinary frequency; urgency; vesical, suprapubic, or back pain and the presence of a tender anterior vaginal wall mass. Ureteral obstruction may also occur which can result in renal failure. Hormonal therapy is only a palliative measure, and surgery remains the definitive treatment with excellent relief of symptoms.

Bowel Endometriosis

Rectovaginal and colorectal endometriosis is estimated to affect 5% of patients with endometriosis. In this patient population, the vast majority have endometriosis involving other pelvic organs, and 76% of these patients have rectal involvement. Deep dyspareunia, dyschezia, tenesmus, or rectal pain (which may be associated with menstruation) may all be indicative of rectovaginal endometriosis. Signs of rectovaginal endometriosis include hematochezia (which may be associated with menses), change in bowel habits, and rectovaginal septum nodularity.

Similar to urinary tract endometriosis, medical management is associated with almost 100% recurrence. Definitive treatment consists of surgical excision of all endometriotic lesions with or without hysterectomy and/or oophorectomy.

Case 1: Endometriosis of the Peritoneum

 View DVD: Videos 11-1 and 11-2

Ms. H is a 27-year-old with debilitating dysmenorrhea, with abdominal pain that radiates to her lower back and legs during her menses. She also complains of mid-cycle dyspareunia and infertility. She has previously been on oral contraceptive pills which diminished the pain. Ibuprofen also helps with the pain. She has associated nausea and vomiting with the pelvic pain. Her sister has had three laparoscopies for endometriosis. Physical examination revealed a normal-sized uterus and no adnexal masses or tenderness. An ultrasonogram was also normal.

Intraoperative findings include a normal-sized anteverted uterus, adhesions of the tubes to the ovaries, adhesions between the ovaries and bilateral pelvic sidewalls, bilateral uterosacral ligament and pelvic sidewall endometriotic implants, bilateral retroperitoneal fibrosis with the ureters following an aberrant course close to the uterine arteries, and normal anterior cul-de-sac, appendix, and upper abdomen.

Preoperative Preparation

This patient has pelvic pain due to endometriosis that involves the pelvic sidewalls and uterosacral ligaments. Her symptoms are classic for endometriosis; however, it is important to remember that some patients may not have these symptoms and still have endometriotic lesions and vise versa. Pelvic ultrasound did not reveal any abnormalities, which is also often the case with endometriosis. Further work-up with MRI or other preoperative testing or imaging besides a complete blood count or pregnancy test is not indicated. The patient should be consented for a diagnostic laparoscopy and excision of endometriosis.

Surgical Techniques

1. The surgeon initially surveys the pelvis, appendix, and upper abdomen thoroughly for any relevant pathology. Endometriotic lesions may be pigmented or nonpigmented. Pigmented lesions can range in color from black (Figure 11-2), blue, brown, or red. Nonpigmented lesions can be clear, yellow, or white (Figure 11-3), or have areas of hypervascularization (Figure 11-4). Their appearance may range from a puckering of the peritoneum to glandular excrescences to petechial patches, or peritoneal defects.

2. One of the primary goals of surgery is to restore normal anatomy. Endometriosis often causes retroperitoneal fibrosis and pelvic adhesions. Adhesiolysis of bowel, peritubal, or periovarian adhesions frequently must be undertaken first in order to correct the resultant anatomic distortion. In this patient, the adhesions are taken down sharply using scissors between the tubes and ovaries. Blunt dissection is used to peel the ovaries off the pelvic sidewalls.

3. In order to perform an excision of pelvic sidewall peritoneal endometriosis, the ureter is identified and followed throughout its course in the pelvis. If endometriosis extensively involves the retroperitoneal space, the pelvic ureter may be difficult to locate. One of the cardinal principles of endometriosis surgery is to start the dissection in normal tissue where structures can be identified and travel towards the abnormal tissue. Even with anatomic distortion due to endometriosis, the ureter can usually be identified at or just below the pelvic brim where it crosses over the bifurcation of the common iliac artery into the external and internal iliac vessels, and followed caudally into the pelvis (Figure 11-5).

4. The initial incision into the pelvic sidewall peritoneum is made while tenting the peritoneum medially, away from the pelvic sidewall, in order to avoid injury to the underlying structures. This incision, ideally, should be located superior to the ureter, in normal-appearing tissue (Figure 11-6).

5. After the initial incision is made, blunt dissection is performed to skeletonize the pelvic sidewall peritoneum and identify the ureter. Once the ureter is identified, the surgeon performs the ureterolysis by bluntly dissecting the ureter off the overlying peritoneum and then continuing the pelvic sidewall peritoneal incision in a sequential fashion (Figure 11-7A and B). The surgeon and his or her assistant applies traction and countertraction principles in order to perform the ureterolysis by holding the pelvic sidewall peritoneum close to the surgical plane of dissection and then using the suction irrigator or laparoscopic scissors in order to bluntly sweep

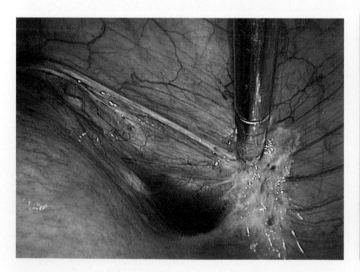

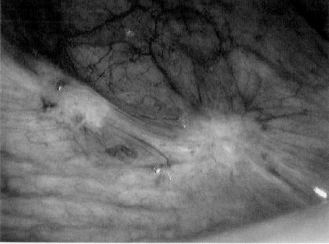

Figure 11-2. A black endometriotic implant on the right bladder peritoneum.

Figure 11-3. A white endometriotic implant on the left pelvic sidewall.

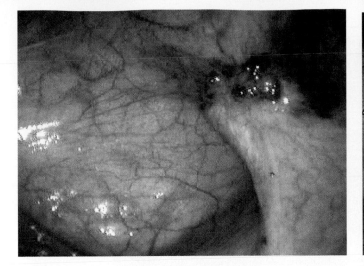

Figure 11-4. A red pigmented endometriotic implant with hypervascularization on the right uterosacral ligament.

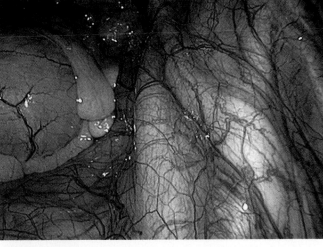

Figure 11-5. The ureter is most easily identified at the pelvic brim, where it crosses over the bifurcation of the common iliac artery into the external and internal iliac vessels. The right ureter crosses the right external iliac artery.

Figure 11-6. A, Entry into the retroperitoneal space should start in the normal tissue where structures can be identified and travel towards the abnormal tissue. **B,** The laparoscopic Allis tents the right pelvic sidewall peritoneum off the pelvic sidewall and a small incision is made in the normal tissue cephalad to the endometriotic lesion.

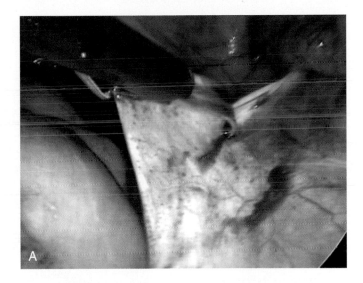

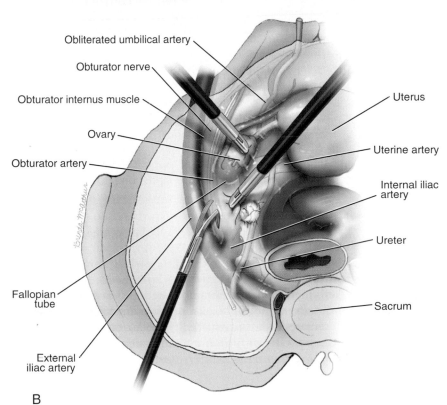

Obliterated umbilical artery

Obturator nerve

Obturator internus muscle

Ovary

Obturator artery

Fallopian tube

External iliac artery

Uterus

Uterine artery

Internal iliac artery

Ureter

Sacrum

B

Figure 11-7. A, The ureterolysis is performed by bluntly dissecting the ureter off the overlying peritoneum. The ureter is typically seen on the medial leaf of the broad ligament after opening the retroperitoneal space—in this case, the right pelvic side wall. **B,** The peritoneal incision is extended caudally, with the ureter visualized at all times. The endometriotic lesion is left on the medial leaf of the pelvic sidewall peritoneum and should be excised with the peritoneum once the ureterolysis is performed.

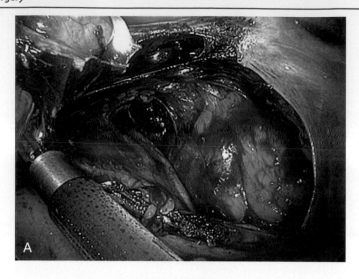

A

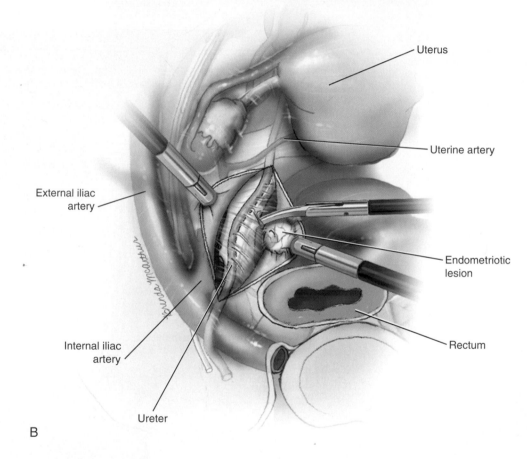

Uterus

Uterine artery

External iliac artery

Endometriotic lesion

Internal iliac artery

Rectum

Ureter

B

the ureter laterally. This incision is made superior to any endometriotic lesions that need to be excised.

6. Once the pelvic sidewall peritoneum with endometriotic lesions is mobilized off the retroperitoneal structures, and the location of the ureter is well visualized away from the peritoneum, medial traction is applied to the peritoneum and monopolar cautery can be used to excise the specimen. As long as the ureter is identified, the portion of the uterosacral ligament with endometriotic involvement can also be safely removed with monopolar cautery which prevents bleeding that can often occur from this area.

7. Prior to excising the diseased portion of the uterosacral ligament, the lesion is circumscribed, in order to avoid unintentional rectal injury, by dissecting the medial border, making a sharp incision into the peritoneum, bluntly dissecting the underlying layers off the peritoneum, and isolating the endometriotic lesion (see Videos 11-1 and 11-2).

Avoiding and Managing Potential Complications

The path of the ureter is often aberrant due to retroperitoneal fibrosis and may travel intimately with the uterine artery (Figure 11-8). Therefore the uterine artery may need to be cauterized proximal to the area of entanglement in order to prevent bleeding; the extensive anastomotic vascular supply to the uterus prevents its compromise.

Endometriosis may also encase the ureter, requiring isolation of the endometriotic nodule from the surrounding structures, such as peripheral involvement of the branches of the internal iliac vessels and possible coagulation of these vessels (Figure 11-9). Once the endometriotic lesion is isolated, the surgeon can apply traction on the endometriotic nodule and sharply dissect around the ureter in order to excise as much of the nodule as possible.

The ureter may be injured by two main mechanisms—transection or thermal injury. If either of these injuries is suspected, a urologic consult should be obtained. If transection has occurred, a ureteral reanastomosis or reimplantation may be performed, with a possible psoas hitch or Boari flap depending on the location of the ureteral injury. A ureteral stent should be placed. A thermal injury may also require the placement of a ureteral stent, and the surgeon may consider placing an omental flap in order to prevent the formation of a ureteral fistula.

The peritoneal attachments between the sigmoid colon and left pelvic sidewall (the white line of Toldt) often need to be taken down in order to visualize the left ureter. This process can endanger the genitofemoral nerve, which runs along the psoas muscle, as well as the external iliac vessels. Sharp dissection should be performed for adhesions that are transparent or filmy and applying traction-countertraction to the pelvic sidewall and sigmoid colon can prevent unnecessary damage to underlying structures.

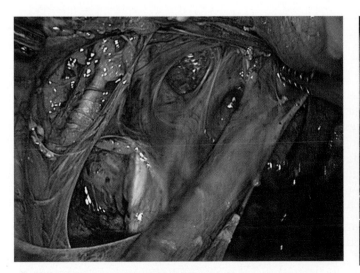

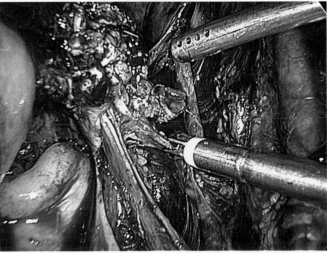

Figure 11-8. A, The left retroperitoneal anatomy is demonstrated here. Endometriosis often implants on the pelvic sidewalls, in close proximity to the ureter. The surgeon should always be aware of the location of the ureter, as well as the other retroperitoneal structures during the pelvic sidewall dissection. **B,** Shown here is the left pelvic sidewall. From left to right of the image we can identify the obturator nerve, the obliterated umbilical artery and uterine artery from a common trunk, and the ureter.

Figure 11-9. This endometriotic lesion encases the right ureter. The bipolar cautery occludes the right uterine artery.

Case 2: Ovarian Endometriosis

 View DVD: Video 11-3

Mrs. A is a 33-year-old gravida 0 with a history of infertility for 3 years. She has had regular ovulatory menstrual cycles with progressive dysmenorrhea, and underwent an appendectomy 12 years ago. Her husband had a normal semen analysis. Physical examination revealed a normal-sized midposition uterus with minimal bilateral adnexal fullness. A pelvic ultrasonogram demonstrated bilateral 4-cm persistent ovarian cysts consistent with endometriomas. Because laparoscopic bilateral ovarian cystectomy was planned, transcervical chromotubation to assess tubal patency and diagnostic hysteroscopy to evaluate the uterine cavity were recommended instead of performing a hysterosalpingogram. Intraoperative findings included a normal-sized uterus, 6-cm ovaries with 4-cm endometriomas bilaterally with spillage of chocolate fluid, dense adhesions between the ovaries and bilateral pelvic sidewalls, bilateral retroperitoneal fibrosis with the ureters traveling more medially, and adhesions between the left pelvic side wall, ovary and sigmoid colon.

Preoperative Preparation

This patient has infertility with endometriosis as a likely etiology. The appropriate infertility work-up should be performed preoperatively to evaluate for male or female causes of infertility. Pelvic ultrasounds can be a useful adjunctive test to detect ovarian endometriomas, although the absence of any findings does not preclude endometriosis.

Surgical management is indicated in this particular patient, because medical management entails a contraceptive effect that is undesired in the setting of her infertility. Removal of endometriomas has been shown to improve subsequent fertility rates, especially in the setting of moderate to severe endometriosis. She also has never had prior surgery for endometriosis. Those patients who have had prior surgeries for endometriosis may choose to have a repeat surgery or proceed to assisted reproductive techniques. If the patient is older than 35 years old, has tubal factor or concomitant male factor infertility, or has a history of more severe (stage III or IV) endometriosis, it may be more cost-effective to bypass surgery in favor of in vitro fertilization (IVF). However, some studies have reported that IVF pregnancy rates are lower in women with endometriosis than in those with tubal infertility. The main risk of performing IVF in patients with endometriomas is infection; several cases of tubo-ovarian abscess have been reported in this setting.

Bilateral laparoscopic ovarian cystectomies, in addition to the excision of the endometriotic lesions and lysis of adhesions, are the treatment of choice in this patient. Laparoscopic cystectomy for ovarian endometriomas greater than 4 cm in diameter has been shown to improve fertility as compared to drainage and coagulation. Drainage, coagulation, or laser vaporization of endometriomas without excision of the pseudocapsule is associated with a significantly increased risk of recurrence, associated pain, and decreased spontaneous conception rates. However, ovarian cystectomy may result in decreased ovarian reserve.

Surgical Techniques

1. The ovary is often adhesed to the pelvic sidewall when an endometrioma is present, and endometriosis usually involves the pelvic sidewall, as is the case in this patient. These adhesions are lysed using blunt dissection, which is the preferred technique. The ureter must be identified prior to performing any sharp dissection of the pelvic sidewall by entering the retroperitoneal space, as described previously. If there are adhesions between the tube and ovary, these should be taken down prior to manipulating the ovary. In this patient, the adhesions between the tubes and ovaries are lysed using sharp dissection.

2. Small endometriotic implants (<1 cm) of the ovary may be ablated by opening the cyst followed by coagulation of the cyst wall using monopolar or bipolar cautery or laser vaporization until no further pigmented fluid or tissue is seen. However, larger endometriomas must be excised in order to avoid recurrence (Figures 11-10 and 11-11).

3. Dilute vasopressin may used for hemostasis and to help develop a plane.

4. The cortex is first incised using monopolar cautery on the antimesenteric surface away from the hilum, in order to avoid excess bleeding (Figure 11-12A and B). The incision is extended until the cyst is easily accessed. The cut and coagulation set-

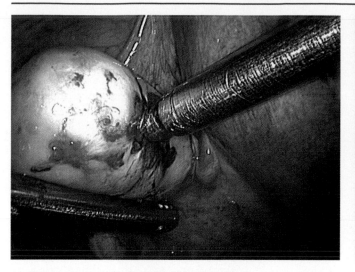

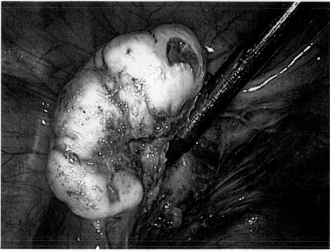

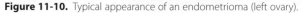

Figure 11-10. Typical appearance of an endometrioma (left ovary).

Figure 11-11. The small endometrioma cavity and superficial endometriotic implants on this ovary have been ablated using bipolar cautery.

tings are lowered to 20 to 25W in order to avoid making too deep an incision, because the goal is to incise the ovarian cortex until the endometrioma is reached, without spilling its contents—the surgical planes between the ovarian cyst and surrounding stroma are more easily identified if the cyst is not ruptured. Also, although the rate of malignancy is low if an endometrioma is suspected from preoperative imaging, spillage of malignant ovarian cyst contents can result in seeding the pelvis with malignant cells. If the endometrioma is breached as in this case, copious irrigation is performed in order to remove the chocolate fluid and clearly visualize the appropriate surgical planes. Suction irrigation is also used to decompress the cyst. The incision is extended once the appropriate level is reached until the cyst is easily accessed.

5. Hydrodissection assists in separating the cyst wall from the ovarian stroma. At times, sharp dissection or monopolar cautery may be necessary in order to separate the planes, because endometriosis can cause dense tethering of the tissue (Figure 11-12C).

6. After arriving at the correct surgical plane between the cyst wall and ovarian stroma, atraumatic yet strong traction-countertraction is applied using two 5-mm Allis forceps in order to peel the cyst wall off the normal ovarian tissue. It is important to apply this traction-countertraction close to the dissection plane to minimize tissue trauma (Figure 11-12D).

7. Once the surgeon approaches the ovarian hilum, bipolar cautery may be used to coagulate the base of the cyst wall as this area tends to bleed because of its proximity to the vascular supply (Figure 11-12E). One must take care to remove the cyst wall in its entirety in order to prevent recurrence.

8. The cyst is then placed in the anterior or posterior cul-de-sac where it can easily be found for later removal.

9. The ovarian bed is irrigated and inspected thoroughly for any bleeding areas; bipolar cautery can then be used in order to achieve hemostasis (Figure 11-13). Cautery should be used sparingly so as not to compromise ovarian reserve. Reducing the CO_2 pressure and reinspecting the ovarian bed is helpful to ensure that there are no other bleeding areas that have been suppressed because of the pneumoperitoneum.

10. Once hemostasis is obtained, the ovarian cyst wall is placed into an Endocatch sac and removed through a 10-mm port. Extension of the incision may be required.

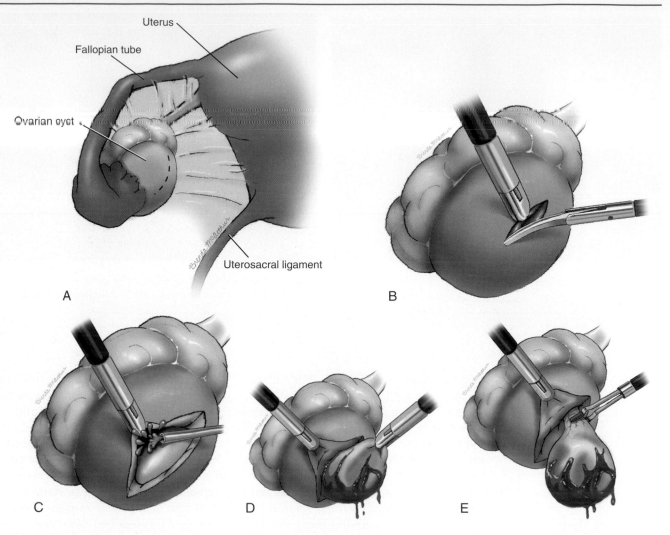

Figure 11-12. A, The ovarian cortex is incised on its antimesenteric side. **B,** Monopolar cautery is used on a low power setting so that the endometriotic cyst is not entered. **C,** Hydrodissection may assist in separating the cyst wall from the ovarian stroma. The instrument can also be used to peel off the cyst from the ovary. **D,** Once the correct surgical plane between the cyst wall and ovarian stroma is reached, traction-countertraction is used to peel the cyst wall off the normal ovarian tissue. **E,** Bipolar cautery is used at the ovarian hilum, because this area tends to bleed due to its proximity to the vascular supply.

Figure 11-13. The bed of the ovary is inspected and any bleeding areas are cauterized in order to achieve hemostasis.

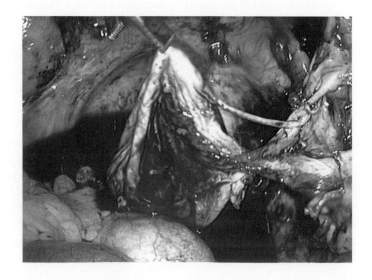

11. The ovarian defect is usually left open though surgeon may choose to close the ovary with a 2-0 or 3-0 Vicryl or polydioxanone suture if the cyst dimensions are large (e.g., >5 cm). The surgeon can also elect to use an anti-adhesion barrier. (See Video 11-3)

Avoiding and Managing Potential Complications

The lysis of dense peri-ovarian adhesions to restore the normal anatomy can put the tube and retroperitoneal structures at risk. If the adhesions between the ovary and pelvic sidewall cannot be lysed using blunt dissection, the ureter must be isolated and identified via a retroperitoneal dissection. Endometriosis involving the pelvic sidewall peritoneum also needs to be removed. While manipulating the ovary and using cautery, the surgeon should have an awareness at all times of the proximity of the ovary to the pelvic sidewall, because thermal injury to the ureter and vasculature can occur through the ovarian stroma, which can be quite thin after performing a cystectomy.

Performing an ovarian cystectomy can lead to removal or thermal damage of normal ovarian tissue and reduce ovarian reserve. Therefore, the surgeon should take care to perform the traction-countertraction close to the plane of dissection in order to remove only the cyst wall. Also, when approaching the hilum, meticulous dissection can prevent the need for extensive coagulation of the ovarian blood supply and subsequent devascularization of the ovary.

Once the specimen is loaded into the Endocatch bag, it is brought to the end of the trocar, and the trocar is then removed in order to deliver the open end of the Endocatch bag through the anterior abdominal wall. After opening the neck of the Endocatch bag, an intact cyst is punctured and its contents suctioned. Puncturing inside the bag, not through the bag, is important, as is having the suction irrigator immediately available, in order to avoid unnecessary spillage into the port site or peritoneal cavity. If the specimen is large, it may require morcellation or extension of the port site in order to extract the ovarian cyst, which should always be done under direct visualization with the camera.

Case 3: Bladder Endometriosis

Ms. L is a 36-year-old gravida 0 with a history of endometriosis for which she had a bowel resection. She presented with dysmenorrhea, bladder pain, and hematuria. An endometriotic lesion of the bladder was diagnosed and resected by cystoscopy. She had relief for a few months but her pain recurred and magnetic resonance imaging revealed evidence of an endometriotic lesion growing into the posterior bladder wall. Repeat cystoscopy preoperatively showed an endometriotic lesion close to the right ureteral orifice. Intraoperative findings included a fixed retroverted uterus, adhesions completely obscuring visualization of both adnexa, and partial obliteration of the posterior cul-de-sac with adhesions to the sigmoid colon. There was extensive endometriosis involving the vesicouterine fold and lower uterine segment with infiltration transmurally through the bladder.

Preoperative Preparation

This patient with severe endometriosis has involvement of the urinary tract. This involvement may be intrinsic, arising within the affected organ, or extrinsic, due to involvement of adjacent structures that has invaded through the bladder wall into the mucosa. Prior surgery where the endometrial cavity has been breached, such as cesarean section, can also introduce endometriotic lesions into the urinary tract.

Endometriosis of the urinary tract is suspected with symptoms of pelvic pain, vesical or suprapubic pain, flank pain, dyspareunia, dysmenorrhea, irritative voiding symptoms, hematuria, or the presence of a tender anterior vaginal wall mass or pelvic mass. If there is ureteral involvement and subsequent obstruction, renal failure may result. An intravenous pyelogram may demonstrate a filling defect in the bladder. However, MRI is the most accurate imaging modality for suspected urinary tract endometriosis and has the added advantage of demonstrating the presence of other endometriotic lesions. Pathologic confirmation should be performed by biopsy via laparoscopy or cystoscopy.

Although hormonal therapy is an option, it is only a palliative measure. Surgery to excise the endometriosis, with or

Continued

Case 3: Bladder Endometriosis—cont'd

without adjunctive oophorectomy, remains the definitive therapy for this condition. Cystoscopic removal may risk bladder perforation because of the propensity of the endometriotic lesion to be transmural, and may also result in incomplete treatment and subsequent recurrence, as in this patient's case.

Preoperative consultation with a urologist should be obtained in order to appropriately plan the surgery and counsel the patient regarding the extent of excision or reconstruction needed. Cystoscopy should be performed to

evaluate the extent and location of bladder involvement (e.g., whether there is mucosal invasion and proximity to the ureteral orifices). Ureteral stents may need to be placed if the endometriotic lesion is close to a ureteral orifice, or if there is evidence of obstruction. If ureteral obstruction is present, the preoperative work-up should also include an evaluation of residual renal function for prognostic purposes. If a ureteral resection is deemed necessary, the urologist may need to perform a ureteroneocystotomy, with or without a psoas hitch or Boari flap, or a uretero-ureterostomy.

Surgical Techniques

Endometriosis of the urinary tract most commonly involves the bladder peritoneum and uncommonly the muscularis and mucosa.

1. If endometriosis affects the bladder peritoneum, the surgeon can grasp the peritoneum and incise it, starting in the normal tissue and circumscribing the entire affected area. The loose areolar tissue and underlying structures are then dissected off the peritoneum, and the lesion is then excised sharply or with monopolar cautery (Figures 11-14 through 11-17).

2. When there is involvement of the bladder muscularis, the overlying peritoneum is grasped and incised, and the underlying tissue is bluntly dissected away (Figure 11-18). Dissection is first performed in the normal area, progressing towards the lesion (Figure 11-19). Pushing the uterus cephalad may assist in identification of the correct plane of dissection.

3. The surgeon should then provide traction on the endometriotic nodule in order to isolate and circumscribe the lesion using sharp and blunt dissection, as well as judicious use of monopolar cautery. Traction-countertraction is of utmost importance, in order to prevent unnecessary damage to surrounding structures. This dissection consists of making an incision, then bluntly dissecting the underlying structures in order to enter the correct surgical plane and to keep the amount of tissue excised to the minimal amount necessary (Figure 11-20). Monopolar cautery

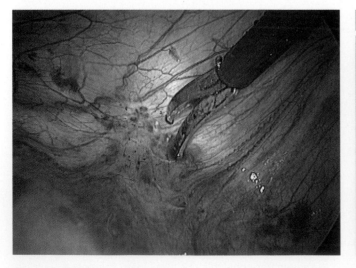

Figure 11-14. This endometriotic lesion is on the right aspect of the bladder peritoneum.

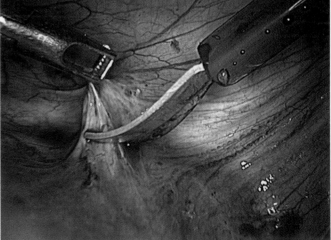

Figure 11-15. The lesion is grasped and incised, starting in the normal tissue. The entire lesion is then circumscribed.

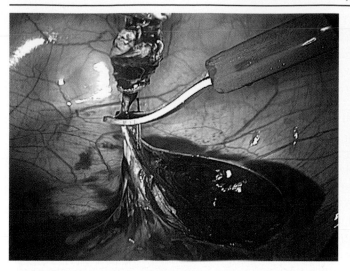

Figure 11-16. The loose areolar tissue is dissected off the peritoneum then the lesion is excised sharply or with monopolar cautery.

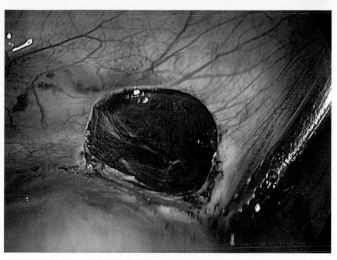

Figure 11-17. The bladder peritoneum has been excised with no compromise of the bladder integrity.

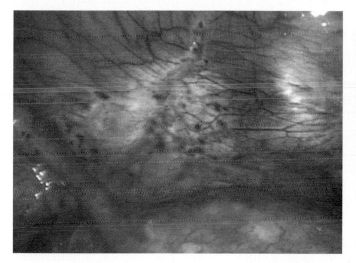

Figure 11-18. This area of endometriotic implants infiltrates into the bladder muscularis (left round ligament), which would not be apparent unless an excision were performed.

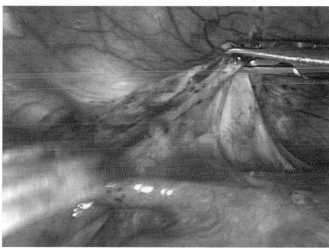

Figure 11-19. The normal peritoneum is grasped and incised and the underlying tissue is bluntly dissected away. Left round ligament seen on the uterus.

Figure 11-20. Dissection is first performed in the normal area, progressing toward the lesion, then bluntly dissecting the underlying structures in order to enter the correct surgical plane and to minimize the amount of tissue excised to the smallest amount necessary.

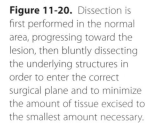

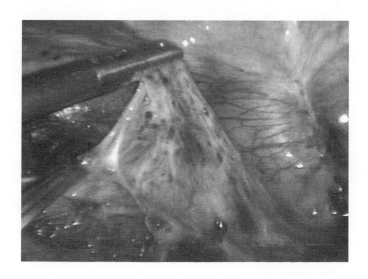

may be used cautiously for hemostasis without compromising the integrity of the bladder.

4. Once the lesion is completely circumscribed, it can be excised using sharp dissection or monopolar cautery (Figure 11-21). The surgeon may elect to retrograde fill the bladder with saline or indigo carmine in order to better define the bladder anatomy. Once the correct plane is identified, the lesion may be excised without compromising bladder wall integrity.

5. If the bladder is entered, it should be reapproximated in a two layer closure using 2-0 or 3-0 Vicryl suture in order to first close the mucosal defect, and then perform an overlying imbricating layer. The bladder should be retrograde filled to check that it is watertight (Figure 11-22), and drained continuously with the Foley catheter for at least 7 to 10 days postoperatively.

6. Endometriosis of the bladder mucosa, as in the patient in the video, entails first performing cystoscopy with bilateral stent placement, which also reconfirms the location of the lesion. Cautery is used to incise the normal peritoneum, and blunt dissection is performed in order to develop the appropriate surgical plane to the vesicouterine fold.

7. The bladder is opened in order to excise the endometriosis lesion and perform a partial cystectomy. Visualization of the Foley catheter and ureteral stents verifies entry into the bladder.

8. A transmural excision of the bladder endometrioma is performed, using both cautery and sharp dissection, taking care to avoid the ureters distally. The same technique as the excision of the bladder muscularis is used—initiating the dissection in normal tissue traveling towards the area of disease, undermining the tissue around the endometriotic nodule, and circumscribing it using traction-countertraction principles.

9. The bladder mucosa is then reapproximated with 3-0 Vicryl running suture. An intracorporeal knot is placed at one angle of the bladder defect in order to perform a running nonlocking closure of the bladder mucosa.

10. A second imbricating layer incorporating the bladder muscularis and serosa is then performed using 2-0 Vicryl.

11. Once reapproximated, the bladder is retrograde filled with dilute indigo carmine solution to check for leakage. Prior to the end of the case, cystoscopy should be performed to confirm bladder integrity, rule out any other lesions, and to check

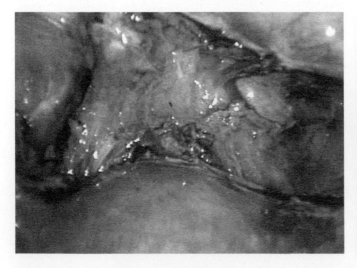

Figure 11-21. Once the lesion is completely circumscribed, it can be excised using sharp dissection or monopolar cautery. The surgeon may elect to retrograde fill the bladder with saline or indigo carmine in order to better define the bladder anatomy. Once the correct plane is identified, the lesion may be excised without compromising bladder wall integrity.

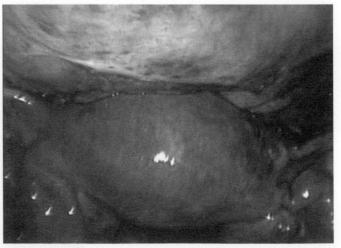

Figure 11-22. The bladder should be retrograde filled to check that it is watertight.

for ureteral efflux by administering intravenous indigo carmine. A Jackson-Pratt drain can be placed through one of the port sites if the surgeon deems it necessary.

Avoiding and Managing Potential Complications

One of the main risks of excising bladder endometriosis is subsequent urine leakage from unrecognized cystotomy. Hence the surgeon should have a low threshold to retrograde fill the bladder with dilute indigo carmine solution and to decompress the bladder with Foley catheter drainage postoperatively to allow for adequate tissue healing. The surgeon should be able to obtain a watertight closure at the end of the procedure.

While excising bladder endometriosis, the surgeon should be aware of the location of the ureters at all times. If the lesion is in close proximity to one of the ureteral orifices, the patient should be counseled about the possibility of needing a ureteral reimplantation in order to completely excise the endometriosis. The surgeon should also try to minimize the amount of surrounding tissue excised, in order to avoid compromising bladder capacity and function. These cases should be undertaken in conjunction with a urologist who is skilled in laparoscopy, although the patient should be counseled about the potential for conversion to laparotomy.

Case 4: Bowel Endometriosis

 View DVD: Videos 11-4 and 11-5

Ms. K. is a 26-year-old gravida 0 with dysmenorrhea, dyspareunia, and chronic lower abdominal pain that is constant and radiates to her back with associated nausea, anorexia, and dysuria. She has associated bowel symptoms consisting of rectal pain, dyschezia, and cyclic hematochezia with her menses. She has had three diagnostic laparoscopies at outside hospitals, which reported severe endometriosis but only minimal excision was performed. She has undergone three cycles of IVF without success. Physical examination reveals a normal-sized uterus, no adnexal masses, and rectovaginal nodularity. Transvaginal ultrasound shows a 2.5-cm right ovarian endometrioma and an otherwise normal pelvis. A colonoscopy is inconclusive for endometriosis—the findings were suggestive of an endometriotic lesion but biopsy was negative.

Intraoperative findings include an obliterated cul-de-sac with adhesions of the uterus to the rectosigmoid, a 3-cm right ovarian endometrioma, bilateral retroperitoneal fibrosis and endometriosis involving the pelvic sidewall, aberrant course of the ureters with tethering to the right uterine artery, adhesions between the right ovary, right tube, right pelvic sidewall, and posterior uterus, adhesions of the left ovary to the left pelvic sidewall and sigmoid colon, and a 3-cm endometriotic nodule invading the rectovaginal septum, uterosacral ligaments, and posterior vagina.

Preoperative Preparation

This patient has severe endometriosis involving her rectovaginal septum with possible invasion into the rectum.

Endometriotic lesions of the bowel may involve the serosa, muscularis (causing hypertrophy of the muscle layer, and/or infiltration of levator muscles), or uncommonly the mucosa. The rectosigmoid is the most common area of involvement, but endometriosis can also affect the appendix or small bowel.

Preoperative consultation with either general or colorectal surgery should be obtained in order to appropriately plan the extent of surgery necessary to excise the disease. The patient must be counseled as to whether she wishes to have a bowel resection at the time of surgery; she may choose to remove as much disease as possible without having a bowel resection, especially if the primary indication for surgery is infertility as opposed to pelvic pain. The extent of surgery may run the gamut from superficial excision of serosal implants to a partial or full thickness disc resection of infiltrating disease to a segmental bowel resection with reanastomosis. The potential risks of a bowel leak or need for colostomy should also be discussed. These patients also usually have endometriomas, pelvic sidewall involvement, and obliteration of the posterior cul-de-sac. Both the surgeon and the patient should be prepared for a lengthy procedure.

Preoperative planning may also entail adjunctive studies and preparation. Pelvic ultrasound may indicate the presence of endometriomas. MRI, barium enema, and/or colonoscopy can assess the extent of endometriosis involving the bowel and aid in preoperative planning. Preoperative mechanical bowel preparation and perioperative intravenous antibiotics may be recommended, especially if the need for a bowel resection is anticipated.

Surgical Techniques

1. The involvement of the rectovaginal septum and/or rectum almost always translates into a partially or completely obliterated cul-de-sac, as is the case in this patient (Figure 11-23 A and B). In addition to the uterine manipulator, a rectal end-to-end anastomosis sizer, and a sponge on a stick in the posterior fornix, are placed in order to aid in the identification of the posterior vagina, rectovaginal septum, and rectum (Figure 11-24).

2. The systematic approach to restoring normal anatomy is crucial to the success of this complex surgery. First, the retroperitoneum is entered in order to identify the ureter, as previously described. A bilateral ureterolysis is performed caudally towards the pelvis (Figure 11-25).

3. The pararectal space is developed with sharp and blunt dissection with good visualization of the ureter at all times (Figure 11-26). In cases of a full-thickness bowel lesion a concomitant rectosigmoid resection and anastamosis is performed.

4. The dissection should be carried down to the levator muscles bilaterally. A sponge on a stick to delineate the posterior fornix and rectal probe to identify the rectum aid in the dissection of the rectovaginal adhesions (Figure 11-27).

5. All of the rectovaginal septum disease should be removed so that the rectum is freed from the posterior vagina and the normal cul-de-sac anatomy restored. Sharp dissection is used when in close proximity to the bowel in order to avoid thermal injury (Figure 11-28A–C).

Figure 11-23. A, The posterior cul-de-sac is obliterated with the rectum adherent to the posterior cervix and uterus. **B,** Another example of an obliterated cul-de-sac from endometriosis.

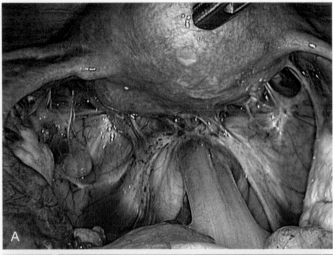

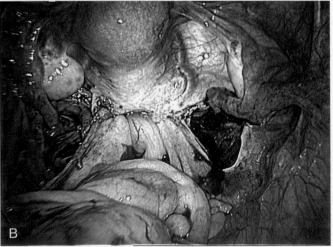

Figure 11-24. In addition to the uterine manipulator, a rectal probe and a sponge on a stick in the posterior fornix are placed in order to aid in the identification of the posterior vagina, rectovaginal septum, and rectum.

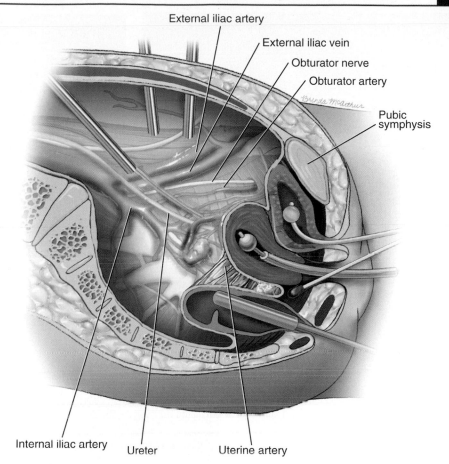

External iliac artery

External iliac vein

Obturator nerve

Obturator artery

Pubic symphysis

Internal iliac artery   Ureter   Uterine artery

Figure 11-25. The peritoneum of the pelvic sidewall is incised and the ureter is identified throughout its course.

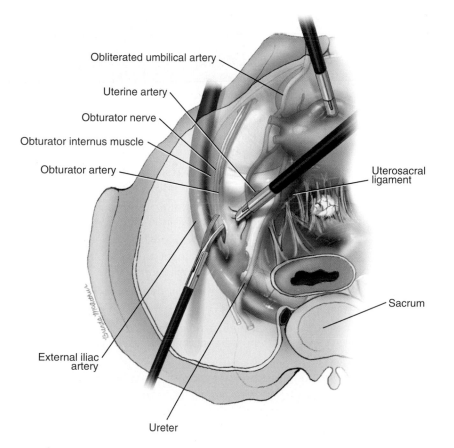

Obliterated umbilical artery

Uterine artery

Obturator nerve

Obturator internus muscle

Obturator artery

Uterosacral ligament

Sacrum

External iliac artery

Ureter

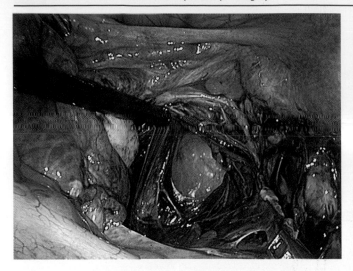

Figure 11-26. The pararectal space is developed with sharp and blunt dissection with good visualization of the ureters at all times.

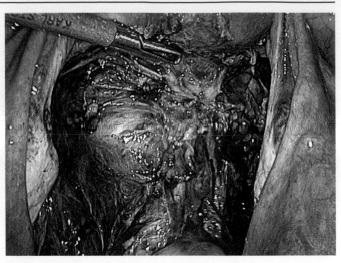

Figure 11-27. The laparoscopic Allis is pointing to the sponge on a stick in the vagina. A rectal probe is in the rectum. These aid in the dissection of the rectovaginal adhesions.

Figure 11-28. A, The bilateral ureterolysis and development of the pararectal space has been performed.

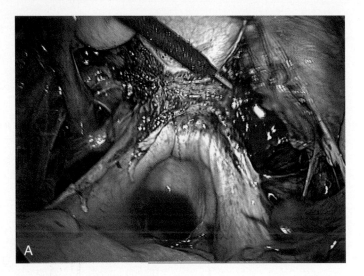

6. Once these steps have been performed, the endometriotic lesion, which is usually an hourglass-or S-shaped lesion on the rectosigmoid, can be shaved off using sharp dissection if the endometriotic lesion is serosal (Figure 11-29).

7. If there is disease infiltrating the bowel and a bowel resection is to be performed, the bowel is transected with a stapling device below the bowel lesion (Figure 11-30).

8. The proximal bowel loop is then exteriorized through a small mini-laparotomy incision, and the specimen can be transected and removed (Figure 11-31). The left sigmoid mesentery contains the blood supply and should be dissected carefully in order to avoid significant devascularization of the remaining rectosigmoid with compromise of the anastomosis.

9. The bowel is then anastomosed (Figures 11-32 and 11-33).

10. In cases of a deeply infiltrating local lesion a disc resection can be performed (Figure 11-34). After excision of the lesion, the defect can be closed with interrupted delayed absorbable sutures (Figures 11-35 and 11-36).

11. At the end of the case, a rigid proctoscopy bubble test can be performed to check for any bowel leakage. The surgeon fills the pelvis with irrigation fluid, uses a bowel grasper across the sigmoid colon above the area of dissection or anastomosis line, then fills the rectosigmoid with air using the rigid proctoscopy. A large Foley

Text to be continued on p. 173

Figure 11-28, cont'd. B, The peritoneal incision is extended across the cul-de-sac adjacent to the rectum. **C,** Blunt dissection is used to dissect the rectum off the peritoneum.

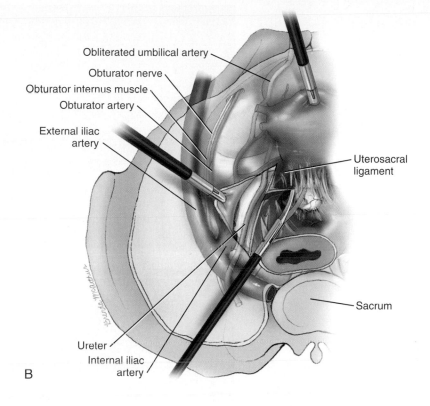

Obliterated umbilical artery

Obturator nerve

Obturator internus muscle

Obturator artery

External iliac artery

Uterosacral ligament

Sacrum

Ureter

Internal iliac artery

B

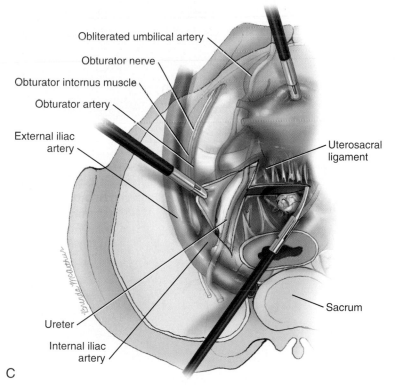

Obliterated umbilical artery

Obturator nerve

Obturator internus muscle

Obturator artery

External iliac artery

Uterosacral ligament

Sacrum

Ureter

Internal iliac artery

C

Figure 11-29. The endometriotic lesion is grasped with an Allis forceps and has been excised from the back of the vagina and anterior rectum.

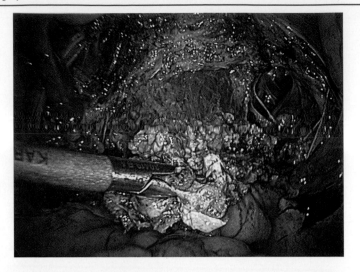

Figure 11-30. The bowel was stapled laparoscopically below the lesion. In order to perform a bowel resection for a transrectal lesion, the bowel is transected with a stapling device below the lesion. In this figure the bowel stump with staples across and the dissected ureters are easily seen.

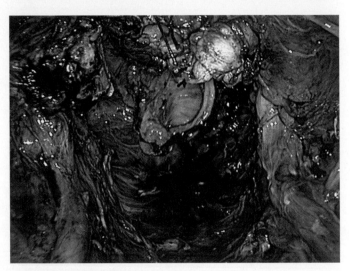

Figure 11-31. A small mini-laparotomy incision is made in order to exteriorize the proximal bowel, and the specimen is then transected and removed.

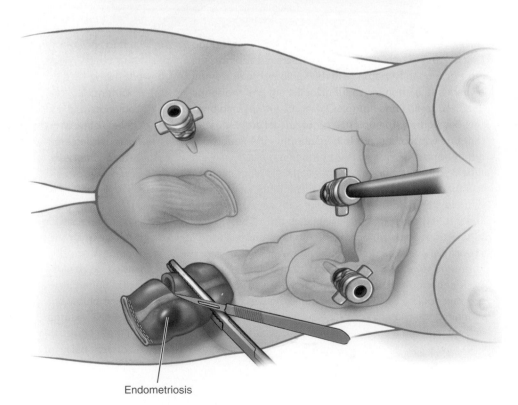

Endometriosis

Figure 11-32. A and **B,** An anvil for the stapling procedure is placed into the proximal colon.

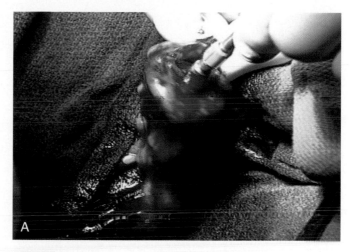

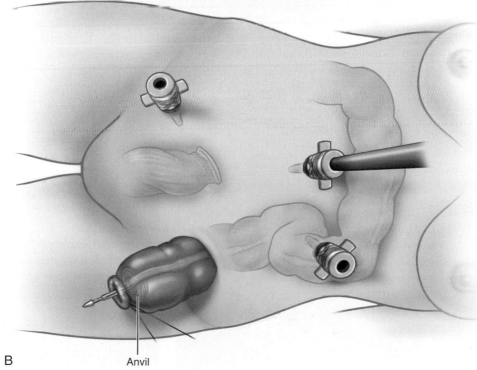

Anvil

Figure 11-33. The bowel anastomosis then proceeds again by laparoscopy.

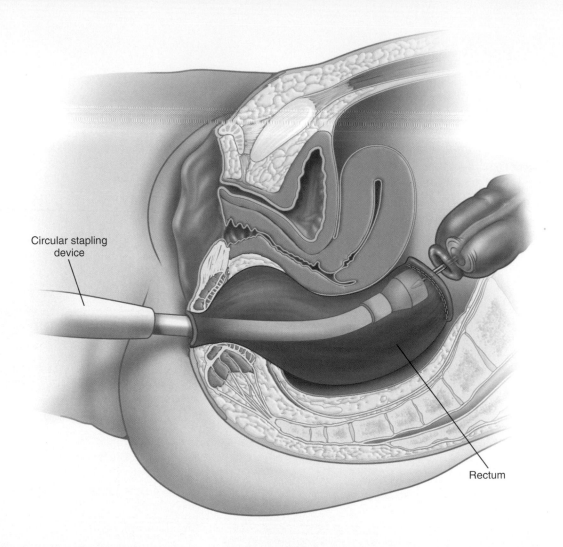

Circular stapling device

Rectum

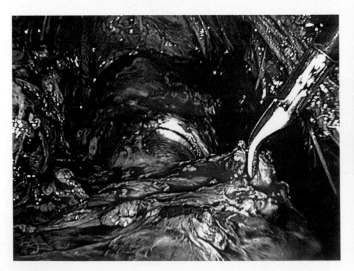

Figure 11-34. Excision of an implant on the rectum. A rigid proctoscope is in the rectum.

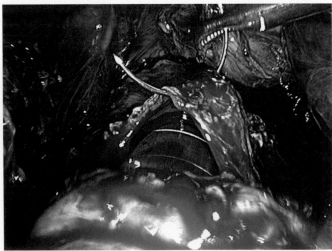

Figure 11-35. The defect is closed with interrupted Vicryl stitches.

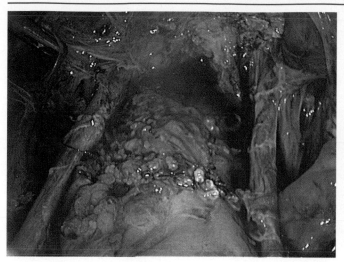

Figure 11-36. Completion of the closure of the defect. The ureters were completed dissected out because of endometriosis.

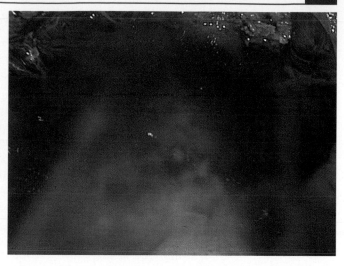

Figure 11-37. The pelvis is filled with fluid and a bowel grasper is used across the sigmoid colon above the anastomosis line. The rectosigmoid is filled with air using the rigid proctoscopy; if air bubbles are seen, the surgeon should search for the area of bowel leakage and repair it.

catheter with a 30 cc balloon can be used instead of a proctoscope. If air bubbles are seen in the fluid, the surgeon should search for the area of bowel leakage and repair it (Figure 11-37).

(See Videos 11-4 and 11-5 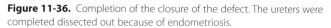)

Avoiding and Managing Potential Complications

These patients usually have retroperitoneal fibrosis from endometriotic involvement of the pelvic sidewall as well as obliteration of the cul-de-sac. This situation often translates to an altered course of the ureters, as well as distortion of the usual paths of the branches of the internal iliac artery. The surgeon should be aware of the location of the ureters at all times. Starting the initial dissection from a normal area and progressing toward the area of disease is one of the major tenets of this surgery. A systematic approach as outlined is also of utmost importance.

Compromise of bowel integrity is a major concern during this surgery. Serosal lesions can often be successfully debulked using the principles of traction and countertraction and careful sharp dissection without causing deeper damage. Deeper lesions into the muscularis or mucosa should be evaluated in conjunction with the general or colorectal surgery consultant.

Other serious complications include rectovaginal fistula and pelvic abscess. The surgeon should have a low threshold for checking for bowel leakage via the rigid proctoscopy bubble test. Intravenous antibiotics should be redosed at the appropriate intervals during the surgery, which often takes several hours.

Surgical Outcomes

Pelvic pain

If endometriosis is the suspected etiology for pelvic pain, an empiric trial of medical management with progestins or combined oral contraceptives is reasonable, rather than proceeding directly to surgery in order to obtain a definitive diagnosis. A GnRH agonist is also an option but is more expensive and is associated with more side effects, for example, postmenopausal symptoms and loss of bone density.

Two randomized trials have demonstrated the efficacy of conservative laparoscopic surgery in the treatment of pelvic pain. Sutton and colleagues conducted a randomized double blind study comparing laparoscopic ablation of endometriosis lesions, lysis of adhesions, and nerve ablation versus a diagnostic laparoscopy only. These patients had stage I to III endometriosis. There was a follow-up of 6 months, at which time they were unblinded to whether they had resection of their disease. Sixty-three percent of patients who had treatment of endometriosis and nerve ablation had significant improvement in their pain, as opposed to 23% in the untreated group. Those patients who had more severe disease had more relief than those who had milder disease. Abbott and colleagues randomized women to a blinded crossover study of laparoscopic excision of endometriosis versus a diagnostic laparoscopy. At 12 months, 80% of women who underwent the excisional surgery had improvement in symptoms and quality of life compared to 32% of those patients who had the sham surgery. Approximately 20% of women reported no improvement after surgery for endometriosis. These studies demonstrate a significant placebo effect of surgery, in the range of 20% to 30%. These same authors also demonstrated in a prospective observational study that patients benefit from conservative laparoscopic excision of endometriosis in terms of pain, quality of life, and sexual function for up to 5 years. Approximately one third of these patients required reoperation, but the return of pain symptoms was not always associated with clinical evidence of recurrence.

Another added advantage of excisional surgery is that it accurately diagnoses the depth of endometriotic lesions; deeply infiltrating endometriosis may have the appearance of superficial disease, resulting in an underestimation of disease.

No randomized trials comparing conservative versus radical surgery have been performed to date. However, some retrospective studies have demonstrated conflicting results. Namnoum and coworkers demonstrated that hysterectomy with oophorectomy can provide good symptom relief, but that ovarian conservation was associated with an increased risk for pain recurrence and reoperation. Falcone et al. retrospectively compared a cohort of women who underwent local excision of endometriosis versus a cohort who underwent hysterectomy with or without oophorectomy. Those women who had a local excision of endometriosis had a higher reoperation rate compared to those who had a hysterectomy. Removal of the ovaries in younger women (aged 30 to 39 years) did not significantly improve the surgery-free time, indicating that ovarian preservation can be a viable option. In any case, if a hysterectomy with or without oophorectomy is performed, all visible endometriotic lesions should be removed concomitantly.

In terms of ovarian endometriomas, there have been two randomized trials of laparoscopic ovarian cyst excision versus ablation of endometriomas greater than 3 cm for the treatment of pelvic pain or infertility. Both excision and ablation techniques result in symptom relief; however, the time to recurrence of pain (e.g., dysmenorrhea, dyspareunia, and nonmenstrual pelvic pain) was significantly shorter in the drainage and ablation group. Spontaneous conception rates were significantly higher in the excision group after 1 to 2 years. Currently, there is not enough evidence to support excisional over ablative surgery to improve fecundity rates prior to IVF or ovarian stimulation and intrauterine insemination, although one study suggests that there may be an improved ovarian follicular response to ovarian stimulation in those patients who have undergone excisional surgery. However, excision of endometriomas prior to IVF may reduce the risk of tubo-ovarian abscess following follicle aspiration. Excision significantly reduces the endometrioma recurrence rate compared to ablation techniques. In comparison to ablative surgery, excisional surgery for endometriomas leads to improved outcomes in terms of recurrence of endometriomas, pain symptoms, spontaneous pregnancy rates, and probably ovarian response to ovarian stimulation. Therefore, excisional surgery should be the preferred surgical approach in the treatment of ovarian endometriomas.

Recurrence of ovarian endometriomas and dysmenorrhea has been shown to correlate with the total revised American Fertility Society score, but not the stage of endometriosis. If ovarian endometriomas do recur, repeat laparoscopic excision results in comparable outcomes compared to primary surgery in terms of pain symptoms, endometrioma recurrence, pregnancy rates, and the need for further medical or surgical treatment.

Infertility

For those patients who have minimal or mild endometriosis, surgical treatment is controversial, because the background fertility rate is higher in this group compared to those with severe disease. In one randomized controlled trial, infertile women with stage I or II disease had either laparoscopic excision or ablation versus a diagnostic laparoscopy alone. There was a significantly higher pregnancy rate in the endometriosis treatment group compared to the untreated controls at 9 months, 37.5% and 22.5%, respectively. Another similar randomized trial found no statistically significant differences in pregnancy outcomes after 1 year, although these patients had more disease and longer periods of infertility. A subsequent meta-analysis of these two trials did find a benefit to laparoscopic surgery.

In more advanced disease (stages III and IV), the baseline fertility rate is close to zero and hence surgery to improve fertility does show a benefit. In those patients who have previously undergone surgery for stage III or IV endometriosis, IVF has better pregnancy rates compared to repeat surgery. Compared to patients with tubal factor infertility, patients with severe endometriosis have statistically significantly poorer IVF outcomes with a reduced fertilization rate (40% vs. 70%), reduced pregnancy rate per cycle (10.6% vs. 22.4%), and reduced birth rate per cycle (6.7% vs. 16.6%).

In the setting of ovarian endometriomas, performing an ovarian cystectomy can result in a decrease in ovarian reserve but it does not appear to translate to decreased pregnancy rates postoperatively.

Bladder Symptoms

Small case series of laparoscopic excision of bladder endometriosis have shown significant improvement in urinary functional symptoms in 95% to 100% of patients after follow-up periods of 22 to 56 months, without evidence of recurrence. Success rates for lesions involving the base of the bladder are lower and require more radical excision, including a portion of the myometrium. Transurethral resection of the lesion may risk bladder perforation, and is rarely definitive by itself.

Adjuvant Medical Therapy

There is insufficient evidence to recommend preoperative hormonal treatment. According to the ESHRE guideline for the diagnosis and treatment of endometriosis, laparoscopy should not be performed during or within 3 months of hormonal treatment in order to avoid underdiagnosis, but surgery does not need to be specifically timed at a certain point in the menstrual cycle.

Postoperative hormonal suppression of endometriosis compared to surgery alone has demonstrated no benefit for long-term outcomes of pain or pregnancy rates but significantly reduces disease recurrence. Two randomized controlled trials have shown that postoperative medication results in decreased severity of pain and number of patients needing retreatment, while one trial did not demonstrate any difference in the degree of pain. A recent Cochrane review concluded that there is insufficient evidence that hormonal suppression in addition to surgery for endometriosis adds a significant benefit to surgery alone. However, the ESHRE guideline differs on this point, stating that postoperative medical therapy (combination oral contraceptives, danazol, progestins, and GnRH agonists) to suppress ovarian function for 6 months reduces endometriosis-related pain. A recent prospective study compared patients who had undergone a laparoscopic excision of an endometrioma and used oral contraceptive pills (OCP) postoperatively to those who underwent surgery alone and found that regular postoperative OCP use significantly reduced endometrioma recurrence rates. At 3 years, 94% of patients in the regular OCP group were free of endometriomas, versus 51% in those who never used OCPs. These data suggest that medical therapy suppresses the endometriotic lesions but once the patient discontinues the treatment, symptoms recur.

Conclusion

The goals of surgery for endometriosis are to provide symptom relief and restore normal anatomy. Surgery results in improved pain and fertility. Excision rather than ablation of ovarian endometriomas is recommended, because excisional surgery yields better outcomes and decreases recurrence rates. Conservative excisional or ablative surgery should be attempted prior to proceeding with radical surgery in terms of hysterectomy with or without oophorectomy. These complex operations often require a high degree of surgical skill and should be undertaken by surgeons who possess the requisite experience and level of comfort with these procedures.

Suggested Reading

Abbott J, Hawe J, Hunter D, Holmes M, Finn P, Garry R: Laparoscopic excision of endometriosis: a randomized, placebo-controlled trial, *Fertil Steril* 82(4):878-884, 2004.

Abbott JA, Hawe J, Clayton RD, Garry R: The effects and effectiveness of laparoscopic excision of endometriosis: a prospective study with 2-5 year follow-up, *Hum Reprod* 18(9):1922-1927, 2003.

Adamson GD, Pasta DJ: Surgical treatment of endometriosis-associated infertility: meta-analysis compared with survival analysis, *Am J Obstet Gynecol* 171:1488-1504, 1994.

Alborzi S, Momtahan M, Parsanezhad ME, Dehbashi S, Zolghadri J, Alborzi S: A prospective, randomized study comparing laparoscopic ovarian cystectomy versus fenestration and coagulation in patients with endometriomas, *Fertil Steril* 82:1633-1637, 2004.

Alborzi S, Ravanbakhsh R, Parsanezhad ME, Alborzi M, Alborzi S, Dehbashi S: A comparison of follicular response of ovaries to ovulation induction after laparoscopic ovarian cystectomy or fenestration and coagulation versus normal ovaries in patients with endometrioma, *Fertil Steril* 88(2):507-509, 2007.

American Society for Reproductive Medicine: Revised American Society for Reproductive Medicine classification of endometriosis: 1996, *Fertil Steril* 67:817, 1997.

Azem F, Lessing JB, Geva E, Shahar A, Lerner-Geva L, Yovel I, Amit A: Patients with stages III and IV endometriosis have a poorer outcome of in vitro fertilization-embryo transfer than patients with tubal infertility, *Fertil Steril* 72(6):1107-1109, 1999.

Beretta P, Franchi M, Ghezzi F, Busacca M, Zupi E, Bolis P: Randomized clinical trial of two laparoscopic treatments of endometriomas: cystectomy versus drainage and coagulation, *Fertil Steril* 70:1176-1180, 1998.

Busacca M, Riparini J, Somigliana E, Oggioni G, Izzo S, Vignali M, Candiani M: Postsurgical ovarian failure after laparoscopic excision of bilateral endometriomas, *Am J Obstet Gynecol* 195:421-425, 2006.

Chapron C, Dubuisson JB: Laparoscopic management of bladder endometriosis, *Acta Obstet Gynecol Scand* 78:887-890, 1999.

Chen CCG, Falcone T: Endoscopic management of endometriosis, *Minerva Ginecol* 58:347-360, 2006.

Eskenazi B, Warner ML: Epidemiology of endometriosis, *Obstet Gynecol Clin North Am* 24:234-258, 1997.

Fedele L, Bianchi S, Zanconato G, Berlanda N, Raffaelli R, Fontana E: Laparoscopic excision of recurrent endometriomas: long-term outcome and comparison with primary surgery, *Fertil Steril* 85:694-699, 2006.

Fedele L, Bianchi S, Zanconato G, Bergamini V, Berlanda N, Carmignani L: Long-term follow-up after conservative surgery for bladder endometriosis, *Fertil Steril* 83:1729-1733, 2005.

Fedele L, Parazzini F, Bianchi S, Arcaini L, Candiani GB: Stage and localization of pelvic endometriosis and pain, *Fertil Steril* 53:155-158, 1990.

Hart RJ, Hickey M, Maouris P, Buckett W: Excisional surgery versus ablative surgery for ovarian endometriomata, *Cochrane Database Syst Rev* 2:CD004992, 2008.

Hesla JS, Rock JA: Endometriosis. In Rock JA, Jones HW, editors: *Te Linde's Operative Gynecology*, ed 9, Lippincott Williams & Wilkins, Philadelphia, 2003.

Kennedy S, Bergqvist A, Chapron C, et al: ESHRE guidelines for the diagnosis and treatment of endometriosis, *Hum Reprod* 20(10):2698-2704, 2005.

Liu X, Yuan L, Shen F, Zhu Z, Jiang H, Guo S: Patterns of and risk factors for recurrence in women with ovarian endometriomas, *Obstet Gynecol* 109:1411-1420, 2007.

Marcoux S, Maheux R, Verube S: Laparoscopic surgery in infertile women with minimal or mild endometriosis. Canadian Collaborative Group on Endometriosis, *N Engl J Med* 337:217-222, 1997.

Muzii L, Bellati F, Palaia I, Plotti F, Manci N, Zullo MA, Angioli R, Panici PB: Laparoscopic stripping of endometriomas: a randomized trial of different surgical techniques. Part I: Clinical results, *Hum Reprod* 20(7):1981-1986, 2005.

Muzii L, Bianchi A, Bellati F, Cristi E, Pernice M, Zullo MA, Angioli R, Panici PB: Histologic analysis of endometriomas: what the surgeon needs to know, *Fertil Steril* 87:362-366, 2007.

Muzii L, Marana R, Caruana P, Catalano GF, Margutti F, Panici PB: Postoperative administration of monophasic combined oral contraceptives after laparoscopic treatment of ovarian endometriomas: a prospective, randomized trial, *Am J Obstet Gynecol* 183:588-592, 2000.

Namnoum AB, Hickman TN, Goodman SB, Gehlbach DL, Rock JA: Incidence of symptom recurrence after hysterectomy for endometriosis, *Fertil Steril* 64(5):898-902, 1995.

Pagidas K, Falcone T, Hemmings R, Miron R: Comparison of surgical treatment of moderate (Stage III) and severe (Stage IV) endometriosis-related infertility with IVF-ET, *Fertil Steril* 65:791-795, 1996.

Parazzini F: Ablation of lesions or no treatment in minimal-mild endometriosis in infertile women: a randomized trial. Gruppo Italiano per lo Studio dell'endometriosi, *Hum Reprod* 14:1332-1334, 1999.

Ragni G, Somigliani E, Benedetti F, Paffoni A, Vegetti W, Restelli L, Crosignani PG: Damage to ovarian reserve associated with laparoscopic excision of endometriomas: a quantitative rather than a qualitative injury, *Am J Obstet Gynecol* 193:1908-1914, 2005.

Saleh A, Tulandi T: Reoperation after laparoscopic treatment of ovarian endometriomas by excision and by fenestration, *Fertil Steril* 72(2):322-324, 1999.

Sampson JA: Peritoneal endometriosis due to menstrual dissemination of endometrial tissue into the peritoneal cavity, *Am J Obstet Gynecol* 14:422, 1925.

Shakiba K, Bena JF, McGill KM, Minger J, Falcone T: Surgical treatment of endometriosis: a 7-year follow-up on the requirement for further surgery, *Obstet Gynecol* 111:1285-1292, 2008.

Simpson JL, Elias S, Malinak LR, et al: Heritable aspects of endometriosis. I. Genetic studies, *Am J Obstet Gynecol* 137:325, 1980.

Stegmann BJ, Sinaii N, Liu S, Segars J, Merino M, Neiman LK, Stratton P: Using location, color, size, and depth to characterize and identify endometriosis lesions in a cohort of 133 women, *Fertil Steril* 89:1632-1636, 2008.

Stratton P, Winkel C, Premkumar A, Chow C, Wilson J, Hearns-Stokes R, Heo S, Merino M, Nieman LK: Diagnostic accuracy of laparoscopy, magnetic resonance imaging, and histopathologic examination for the detection of endometriosis, *Fertil Steril* 79(5):1078-1085, 2003.

Stratton P, Winkel C, Premkumar A, et al: Diagnostic accuracy of laparoscopy, magnetic resonance imaging, and histopathologic examination for the detection of endometriosis, *Fertil Steril* 79:1078-1085, 2003.

Stratton P, Winkel CA, Sinaii N, Merino MJ, Zimmer C, Nieman LK: Location, color, size, depth, and volume may predict endometriosis in lesions resected at surgery, *Fertil Steril* 78(4):743-749, 2002.

Sutton CJ, Ewen SP, Whitelaw N, Haines P: Prospective, randomized, double-blind, controlled trial of laser laparoscopy in the treatment of pelvic pain associated with minimal, mild, and moderate endometriosis, *Fertil Steril* 62:696-700, 1994.

Vercellini P, Somigliana E, Daguati R, Vigano P, Meroni F, Crosignani G: Postoperative oral contraceptive exposure and risk of endometrioma recurrence, *Am J Obstet Gynecol* 198:504.e1-504.e5, 2008.

Vercellini P, Trespidi L, De Giorgi O, Cortesi I, Parazzini F, Crosignani PG: Endometriosis and pelvic pain: relation to disease stage and localization, *Fertil Steril* 65:299-304, 1996.

Wheeler JM: Epidemiology of endometriosis-associated infertility, *J Reprod Med* 34:41-46, 1989.

Yap C, Furness S, Farquhar C: Pre and post operative medical therapy for endometriosis surgery, *Cochrane Database Syst Rev* (3):CD003678, 2004.

Zhao SZ, Wong JM, Davis MB, Gersh GE, Johnson KE: The cost of inpatient endometriosis treatment: an analysis based on the healthcare cost and utilization project nationwide inpatient sample, *Am J Manag Care* 4:1127-1134, 1998.

Laparoscopic Treatment of Pelvic Pain

12

Jeffrey M. Goldberg M.D.

 Video Clips on DVD

12-1 Laparoscopic Management of Chronic Pelvic Pain Secondary to Adhesions (6 minutes/15 seconds)

12-2 Laparoscopic Appendectomy for Right Lower Quadrant Pain (4 minutes/43 seconds)

12-3 Laparoscopic Presacral Neurectomy for Severe Midline Dysmenorrhea (4 minutes/38 seconds)

12-4 Laparoscopic Uterosacral Nerve Ablation (LUNA) for Severe Dysmenorrhea (2 minutes/21 seconds)

Introduction

Chronic pelvic pain (CPP) and dysmenorrhea are common presenting complaints to the gynecologist. Chronic pelvic pain is defined as pain below the umbilicus of at least 6 months duration that is severe enough to cause functional disability or require treatment. It affects 15% of US women, and accounts for approximately 10% of referrals to a gynecologist, 20% of hysterectomies, and at least 40% of gynecologic laparoscopies. No etiology for CPP is found in nearly two thirds of women, but in almost one third of cases, it is due to a gynecologic condition. Only about 4% of cases are due to a nongynecologic cause. Some of the more common causes are listed in Table 12-1.

Not uncommonly, patients may have more than one cause of pain. Those that do tend to have more severe pain than patients with a single diagnosis. It is important to involve gastroenterologists, urologists, physical therapists, and mental health professionals as indicated to evaluate and treat nongynecologic causes. Patients may also be referred to anesthesia pain management when no treatable cause can be found or when treatment of identifiable causes does not yield adequate pain relief.

Treatments for gynecologic causes include narcotic and nonsteroidal anti-inflammatory analgesics, antibiotics for pelvic inflammatory disease, ovarian suppression with oral contraceptives or GnRH analogues (especially if the pain is cyclic or patients have known or suspected endometriosis), hysterectomy for myomas or adenomyosis, ovarian cystectomy or oophorectomy for ovarian cysts, conservative surgical and nonsurgical options for myomas (myomectomy, uterine fibroid embolization, and MR-guided focused ultrasound), and lysis of adhesions. Endometriosis is the most common gynecologic cause of CPP and dysmenorrhea and its management is discussed in Chapter 11. This chapter addresses the role of adhesiolysis, appendectomy, and pelvic denervation procedures for the treatment of pelvic pain.

Adhesions

Adhesion formation is a normal physiologic response to peritoneal trauma. Adhesions give structural support, wall off inflammation and infection, and provide collateral

Table 12-1 Causes of Chronic Pelvic Pain

Gynecologic	*Musculoskeletal*
– Endometriosis	– Pelvic floor myalgia
– Pelvic inflammatory disease	– Myofascial pain
– Myomas	– Fibromyalgia
– Ovarian cysts or remnants	– Hernia
– Pelvic adhesions	
– Pelvic relaxation/prolapse	*Neurologic/Psychologic*
	– Neuralgias: iliohypogastric, ilioinguinal, genitofemoral, lateral femoral cutaneous, pudendal
Gastrointestinal	– Neuropathic pain
– Irritable bowel syndrome	– Depression
– Inflammatory bowel disease	– Somatization
– Diverticular disease	– History of physical/sexual abuse
– Celiac sprue	
Urologic	
– Interstitial cystitis	
– Recurrent cystitis	

circulation to devascularized tissue. Postoperative adhesions are also the bane of every surgeon who has had to perform a reoperative procedure, because they significantly increase surgical difficulty, operative time, and the risk of bleeding and enterotomy. Postoperative adhesions are the leading cause of bowel obstruction and may result in pain and infertility. Adhesion-related problems cost over one billion dollars annually in the United States.

The flow diagram in Figure 12-1 is an oversimplified explanation of the pathogenesis of adhesion formation. The inciting injury leads to bleeding and an inflammatory exudate, resulting in a fibrin matrix. Ultimately, the balance between plasminogen activators and plasminogen activator inhibitors determines whether fibrinolysis occurs with adhesion-free healing or the fibrin matrix persists and becomes incorporated with fibroblasts leading to permanent adhesions. Tissue ischemia is the main factor favoring adhesion formation by suppressing fibrinolytic activity. Angiogenic factors lead to neovascularization of the adhesions. Unlike skin, which heals inward from the edges, new peritoneal mesothelial cells originate from subperitoneal fibroblasts and/or mesenchymal stem cells. Thus, large defects heal as rapidly as small ones.

The best way to minimize postoperative adhesions is by observing the tenets of microsurgical technique. In spite of this, postoperative adhesions develop in approximately 85% of cases, even in the hands of leading infertility surgeons. Since laparoscopic surgery more closely conforms to microsurgical technique in that tissue handling and drying are minimized, there is no foreign body contamination from packs and sponges, there is no bleeding into the peritoneal cavity from the incision, and the laparoscope provides magnification, de novo adhesion formation has been shown to be less than after laparotomy.

While there has been an enormous volume of published literature over the past century, and no lack of ingenuity, no consistently efficacious treatment for adhesion prophylaxis has emerged. Initial encouraging results with most agents failed to be confirmed in subsequent studies that found them to be ineffective or actually deleterious. Of the available anti-adhesion adjuvants, Seprafilm (hyaluronic acid and carboxymethylcellulose) is a challenge to handle at laparotomy and is extremely difficult to apply laparoscopically. The Gore-Tex surgical membrane (expanded polytetrafluoroethylene) requires that it be sutured in place, making it impractical for laparoscopic use. Interceed (oxidized regenerated cellulose) is fairly easy to apply laparoscopically and adheres without sutures. Complete hemostasis is essential as Interceed is ineffective if it becomes impregnated with blood. Adept (4% icodextrin) 1500 mL is instilled into the peritoneal cavity at the conclusion of the case. Patients should be informed that the fluid may leak from their incisions and that labial edema may develop.

Figure 12-1. From Davey and Maher: *J Min Invas Gynecol* 14:15, 2007.

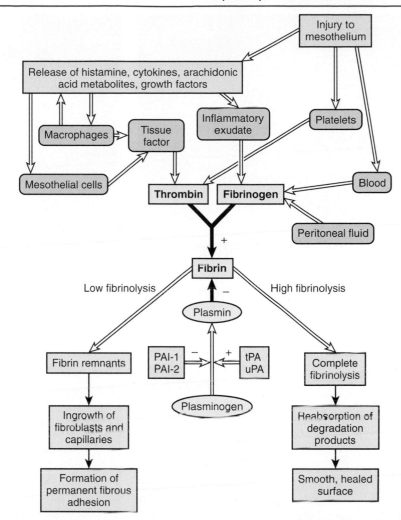

Case 1: Chronic Pelvic Pain Secondary to Adhesions

 View DVD: Video 12-1

NC is a 31-year-old nulligravida who presented with a 3.5-year history of primary infertility. She has had seven laparoscopic procedures for treatment of endometriosis and during the last one, 1.5 years ago, a midline laparotomy was made to repair a cystotomy. She has had chronic pelvic pain since then. An ultrasonogram was normal. Diagnostic hysteroscopy and laparoscopy with chromotubation was recommended instead of a hysterosalpingogram, due to the suspicion for adhesions as a cause of her pain. A 5-mm trocar was introduced through the left upper quadrant revealing extensive small bowel and omental adhesions to the anterior abdominal wall. Additional 5-mm ports were placed in both lower quadrants under direct vision. This facilitated rotating the camera, graspers, and scissors between the ports to achieve the best approach to the adhesions as the procedure progressed.

Once the bowel and omentum were completely released from the abdominal wall attachments, chromotubation disclosed bilateral proximal tubal occlusion. The tubes were successfully cannulated hysteroscopically. The uterine cavity was normal and minimal endometriosis was excised. Adept was instilled in the peritoneal cavity at the completion of the case in an effort to reduce adhesion re-formation. Her pain was relieved postoperatively and she is now attempting to conceive. This case illustrates that adhesions, especially dense bowel adhesions, may cause chronic pelvic pain that may be resolved with laparoscopic adhesiolysis. The video demonstrates some of these techniques.

Surgical Techniques

1. Adhesions should be excised, not just divided, using traction and countertraction to place the adhesions on stretch (Figures 12-2 and 12-3). Lysis of dense adhesions is difficult, because there are often no planes of cleavage and vascular adhesions may bleed easily. Adhesiolysis is carried out in a systematic fashion starting in an area

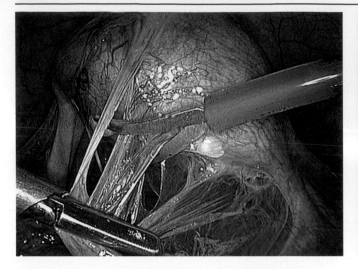

Figure 12-2. Traction is being applied to the adhesion while the uterus is anteverted with the uterine manipulator for countertraction. The adhesion is divided at the uterus for complete excision. Electrocautery is used for hemostasis if necessary.

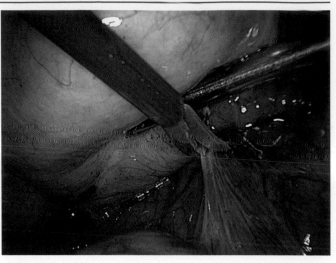

Figure 12-3. An ovary containing an endometrioma is adherent to the pelvic sidewall. The ovary is displaced upward with the suction/irrigation probe to put the adhesion on tension, enabling it to be lysed under direct vision. The cystectomy is performed after the ovary is fully mobilized.

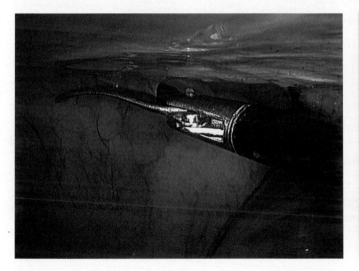

Figure 12-4. Placing the initial trocar in the left upper quadrant should be considered in patients who have had a prior laparotomy, especially with a midline incision. Here the scissor is in the left upper quadrant and the scope is in a left lower quadrant port. Moving the scope, scissors, and graspers to different ports may facilitate dissection of extensive adhesions between the omentum and anterior abdominal wall. Lysis begins in a relatively clear area, then the tissue is gently displaced downward away from the abdominal wall to put the adhesions on stretch and better visualize whether there is any bowel involvement.

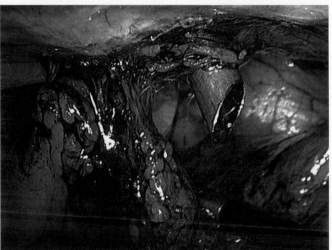

Figure 12-5. Once the adhesions are cleared from below the umbilicus, the umbilical trocar can be inserted under direct vision and the adhesiolysis completed.

of normal anatomy. When extensive adhesions are anticipated, a preoperative mechanical bowel prep may be considered and routine prophylactic antibiotics are administered intravenously. Initial trocar insertion in the left upper quadrant may provide safer entry into the peritoneal cavity (see Chapter 3). The scope, scissors, and graspers can be rotated between the ports to provide the best vantage point for lysing extensive bowel and omental adhesions to the anterior abdominal wall (Figures 12-4 and 12-5).

2. Dense bowel adhesions are taken down using small bites with the scissors. Monopolar cautery is to be avoided for this task (Figure 12-6). It is better to leave some of the adherent tissue on the bowel rather than the other way around. Once all of the

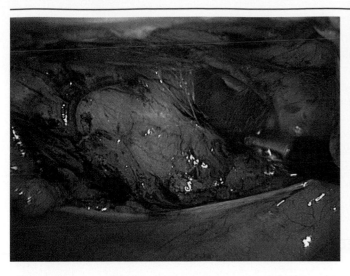

Figure 12-6. Downward traction helps to more clearly visualize the adhesions between this loop of small bowel and the abdominal wall.

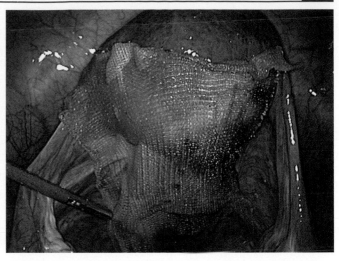

Figure 12-7. Interceed is applied to reduce postoperative adhesions. It is moistened to secure it in place. All fluid should be aspirated from the peritoneal cavity and the site of application should be hemostatic.

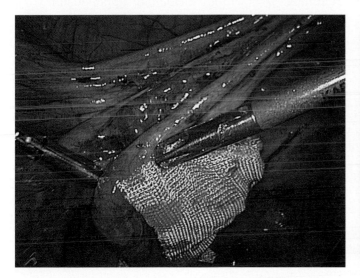

Figure 12-8. Interceed can also be used to wrap an ovary following a cystectomy.

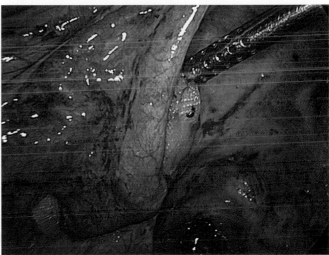

Figure 12-9. Interceed is moistened with a small amount of fluid to keep it in place.

adhesions are lysed, the areas are checked for any inadvertent injury and hemostasis.

3. Anti-adhesion adjuvants may be used at the conclusion of the case to reduce post-operative adhesion formation. Adept may be instilled into the peritoneal cavity through the suction/irrigator in one of the lower ports. It helps to close all the other ports first, because fluid leaking through the incisions makes closing them more difficult. Interceed may be applied after aspirating all irrigating fluid from the peritoneal cavity and when complete hemostasis is assured. The sheet is placed through a 10-mm trocar and positioned where desired using graspers. It is held in place by moistening it with a small amount of irrigating fluid (Figures 12-7 through 12-9). It is absorbed within about 2 weeks.

(See Video 12-1 📹)

Outcomes

It remains uncertain to what extent pelvic adhesions contribute to pelvic pain and infertility. Approximately 40% of women with CPP have adhesions, a figure that is similar to asymptomatic infertility patients. A conscious pain mapping study showed that filmy adhesions between mobile structures had the highest pain scores, while fixed or dense adhesions had lowest. However, another study that randomized 48 CPP patients to lysis of adhesions by laparotomy or no surgery found no significant difference except in cases of severe dense, fixed bowel adhesions. Another controlled trial randomized 100 CPP patients to laparoscopy with or without adhesiolysis and reported no significant difference. Lack of pain relief following adhesiolysis may be due to adhesion re-formation, or it may be that adhesions were not the cause of the pain. The only study to assess the effect of lysis of peritubal adhesions on infertility was a nonrandomized comparison of adhesiolysis at laparotomy in 69 patients versus diagnostic laparoscopy only in 78. The cumulative pregnancy rates were higher in the group that underwent lysis.

Laparoscopic Appendectomy

Appendectomy may be performed at the time of laparoscopy for patients with chronic pain, particularly when pain is in the right lower quadrant, or when the appendix is noted to be involved with endometriosis or another disease process. Although controversial, some recommend routinely performing incidental appendectomy at the time of any gynecologic surgery to prevent future appendicitis, eliminate the appendix in the differential diagnosis for pelvic pain, and remove undiagnosed pathology.

In patients with CPP, approximately half of visibly normal appendices were found to have pathology on histologic examination. The most common abnormality noted in women with right lower quadrant pain was fibrous obliteration of the lumen, which is related to neurogenic appendicopathy, a condition with proliferation and degeneration of neural elements and increased endocrine cells producing serotonin and regulatory peptides. Approximately 95% of patients experienced relief of right lower quadrant pain following removal of a grossly normal appendix. For those in whom the pain persists, the appendix is no longer on the list of differential diagnoses.

Case 2: Laparoscopic Appendectomy for Right Lower Quadrant Pain

 View DVD: Video 12-2

DB is a 33-year-old single nulligravida with constant chronic right lower quadrant pain for 16 years. She had been on continuous oral contraceptives for the past 4 years with some relief. She also has fibromyalgia and irritable bowel syndrome with alternating diarrhea and constipation. She is uncertain about future fertility. An ultrasonogram showed a 3.3 × 2.3 cm right adnexal cyst. Diagnostic laparoscopy with appendectomy was recommended. At surgery, the pelvis and appendix were grossly normal except for some superficial endometriosis on the bladder flap and posterior cul-de-sac, which was treated. The pathology report on the appendix noted fibrous obliteration of the lumen. She remains pain-free. She was advised to stay on oral contraception to prevent recurrence and progression of endometriosis until she is ready to conceive. Even if her pain had persisted, the appendix is off the differential diagnosis list.

Surgical Techniques

1. Prophylactic antibiotics are routinely given, but a bowel prep is unnecessary. A 10-mm trocar is placed in the umbilicus for specimen removal and a 5-mm trocar is inserted in each lower quadrant. Any concurrent procedures are performed first so that the potentially contaminated trocars will not have to be used following the appendectomy.

2. The mesoappendix is serially coagulated with bipolar cautery, then cut with scissors from the tip to the base of the appendix. A tripolar, Ligasure, or harmonic scalpel could also be used for this step (Figure 12-10).

3. Once the base of the appendix has been skeletonized, two 0-PDS Endo-loops are placed at the base (Figures 12-11 and 12-12). A third Endo-loop is placed about a centimeter distal to these, and the appendix is divided between them (Figures 12-13 and 12-14).

4. The appendix is grasped at the suture end and withdrawn through the 10-mm umbilical port (Figure 12-15). The stump of the appendix is copiously irrigated (Figure 12-16).

5. Anti-adhesion adjuvants such as Interceed and Adept are contraindicated if an appendectomy has been performed, due to the risk for infection.

(See Video 12-2 📹)

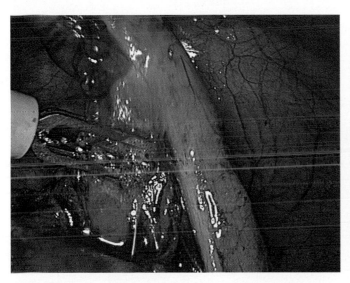

Figure 12-10. The mesoappendix is serially coagulated with bipolar and cut with scissors. A tripolar or Ligasure may also be used for this step. Adhesiolysis to mobilize the appendix may need to be performed first.

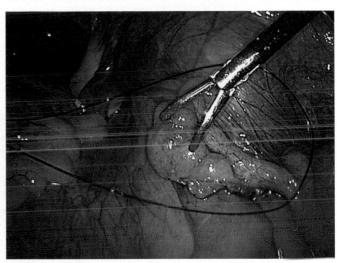

Figure 12-11. The appendix is grasped through an Endo-loop. The base of the appendix has been well skeletonized.

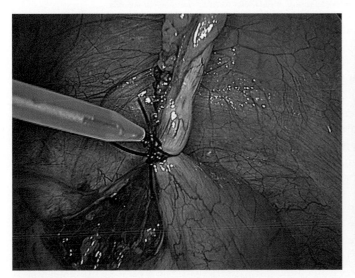

Figure 12-12. Two 0-PDS Endo-loops are placed at the base of the appendix.

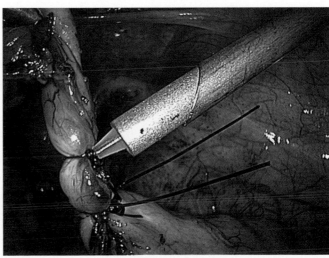

Figure 12-13. A third Endo-loop is placed distally.

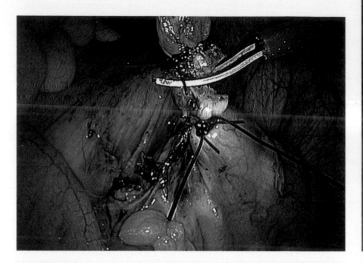

Figure 12-14. The appendix is excised with scissors or monopolar cautery.

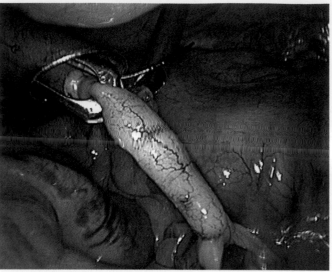

Figure 12-15. The luminal end of the appendix is grasped with a 10-mm Allis forceps for removal through the 10-mm umbilical port while viewing through a 5-mm laparoscope placed through one of the lower ports.

Figure 12-16. The abdomen is copiously irrigated and the stump checked for hemostasis and leaks. It is not cauterized or oversewn.

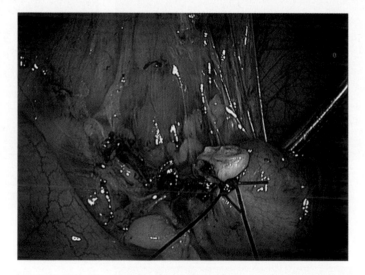

Laparoscopic Presacral Neurectomy and Uterosacral Nerve Ablation

Afferent pain fibers from the cervix, uterus, and proximal fallopian tubes course with the sympathetic nerves through the uterosacral ligaments to the Frankenhauser pelvic plexus, then to the superior hypogastric plexus in the loose areolar tissue overlying the fifth lumbar vertebra before entering the spinal cord at T10-L1. The effectiveness of treatment of midline dysmenorrhea with surgical disruption of the sensory afferent nerves supplying the uterus by presacral neurectomy (PSN) or laparoscopic uterosacral nerve ablation (LUNA) remains controversial. Studies have been compromised by lack of randomization, small sample size, no standard pain scoring system, different surgical techniques, and concurrent treatment of pelvic pathology. Also, the results of uncontrolled trials with follow-up of 6 months or less should be viewed with skepticism due to a very significant placebo effect. Because pain fibers from the ovaries and distal tubes travel along the infundibulopelvic ligaments to the aortic and renal plexuses, lateral pelvic pain is not improved with PSN or LUNA.

Case 3: Presacral Neurectomy for Severe Midline Dysmenorrhea

 View DVD: Video 12-3

ML is a 31-year-old woman, para 1031. She had a cesarean section and three spontaneous abortions. She presented with secondary infertility, recurrent pregnancy loss, and irregular 29- to 54-day cycles with severe midline dysmenorrhea. She denied any other pain, bowel symptoms, or urinary symptoms. Her laboratory evaluation for anovulation and recurrent pregnancy loss was normal. Review of her hysterosalpingogram films revealed patent tubes and multiple intrauterine filling defects consistent with air bubbles. Her physical examination was normal except for obesity, with a BMI of 36.5. A transvaginal ultrasonogram was also normal. She was scheduled for a diagnostic hysteroscopy and laparoscopic uterosacral nerve ablation or presacral neurectomy.

The uterine cavity was normal, and superficial endometriosis on the posterior aspect of the uterus, left pelvic sidewall, and posterior cul-de-sac was treated with bipolar cautery. A presacral neurectomy was performed because it has been reported to be more successful in treating dysmenorrhea than uterosacral nerve ablation in the presence of endometriosis. The procedure was uneventful but was made technically more difficult due to increased retroperitoneal fat and decreased lateral mobility of the sigmoid.

The pathology report noted fibroadipose tissue with proliferation of nerves, many showing perineural fibrosis. Her cycles were regulated with clomiphene citrate postoperatively, with resolution of her dysmenorrhea. It is uncertain whether this effect is due to treatment of the endometriosis or to the presacral neurectomy. Bowel and bladder function remained normal.

Surgical Techniques

1. The patient is placed in steep Trendelenburg. Tilting the table to the patient's left may help to displace the sigmoid colon away from the sacral promontory.

2. A standard three-port setup with 5-mm trocars in the umbilicus and lower quadrants is used. Care must be taken to keep the anatomic landmarks visualized throughout, to avoid bleeding complications.

3. The peritoneum is opened in the midline over the sacral promontory to the aortic bifurcation. The right common iliac forms the border on the right and the left common iliac and inferior mesenteric vessels form the left border (Figure 12-17).

4. The peritoneal edges are grasped with Allis forceps and the subperitoneal fat containing the nerve plexus is gently swept off the peritoneum towards the midline (Figure 12-18). The tissue is coagulated proximally and distally with bipolar cautery, then excised. The peritoneal defect is left open (Figure 12-19).

(See Video 12-3)

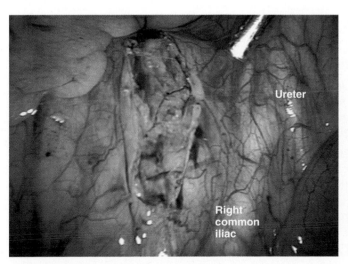

Figure 12-17. The peritoneum is incised vertically from the sacral promontory to the aortic bifurcation. The right common iliac forms the right border and the inferior mesenteric vessels the left border.

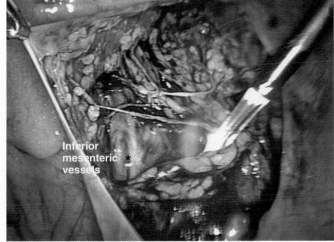

Figure 12-18. The subperitoneal tissue containing the presacral nerve plexus is gently mobilized off the peritoneum on both sides, taking care to avoid injury to the vascular borders and the middle sacral vessels.

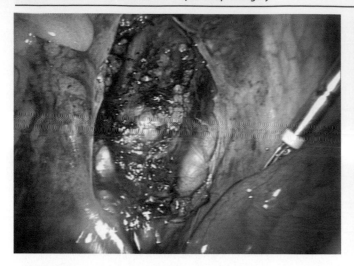

Figure 12-19. The tissue is excised and the peritoneal defect is left open.

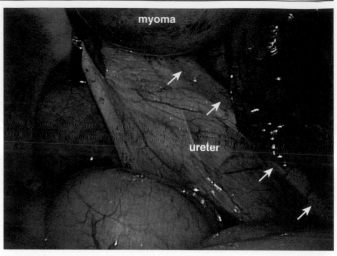

Figure 12-20. No relaxing incision is necessary when the ureter is clearly visualized away from the uterosacral ligament. The ligament is still retracted medially as current is applied.

Case 4: Laparoscopic Uterosacral Nerve Ablation (LUNA) for Severe Dysmenorrhea

 View DVD: Video 12-4

LP is a 29-year-old nulligravida with primary infertility since discontinuing oral contraceptives (OCs) 2 years ago in order to conceive. She had been on OCs since age 16 due to severe dysmenorrhea, which has been getting progressively worse off OCs. She has regular 28- to 30-day menstrual cycles with severe midline dyspareunia causing her to miss 2 days of work each month despite the use of high doses of nonsteroidal anti-inflammatory analgesics and heat. She has no pain during the remainder of the cycle. She has had no prior surgery and denies any sexually transmitted diseases. Her pelvic

examination and a transvaginal ultrasonogram were normal. Her husband has a normal semen analysis.

Due to her severe dysmenorrhea, a decision was made to proceed to diagnostic laparoscopy with chromotubation and diagnostic hysteroscopy instead of performing a hysterosalpingogram. She consented presacral neurectomy or LUNA depending on the pelvic findings. The uterine cavity was normal, both tubes were patent, and there was no evidence of any pelvic pathology, including adhesions or endometriosis. A LUNA procedure was performed. Her dysmenorrhea has resolved and she is currently undergoing treatment with controlled ovarian stimulation and intrauterine insemination for unexplained infertility.

Surgical Techniques

1. A uterine manipulator is placed to antevert the uterus and put the uterosacral ligaments on stretch.

2. A 5-mm port is inserted in the umbilicus and an additional port is placed suprapubically in the midline.

3. If the ureters can be visualized transperitoneally at a safe distance from the uterosacral ligaments, the uterosacral ligament is grasped with the bipolar forceps at the cervical insertion and coagulated (Figure 12-20).

4. In cases where the ureters are not visualized transperitoneally, or where they are noted to be close to the uterosacral ligaments, a relaxing incision is made lateral to the uterosacral ligaments and the ureters are retracted laterally as the uterosacral ligaments are coagulated (Figures 12-21 and 12-22). Pulling the uterosacral ligaments medially with the bipolar forceps as current is applied further increases the distance from the ureters.

5. The uterosacral ligaments are then divided (Figure 12-23). The intervening cervical serosa is incised to transect any nerves that may be running between the ligaments, to improve the effectiveness of the procedure (Figures 12-24 and 12-25).

(See Video 12-4 📹)

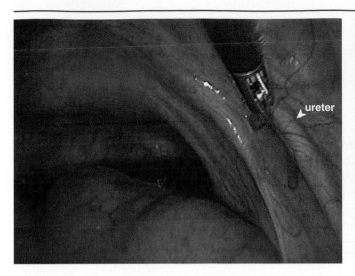

Figure 12-21. A relaxing incision is made lateral to the uterosacral ligament in cases where the ureter is in close proximity, as is shown here.

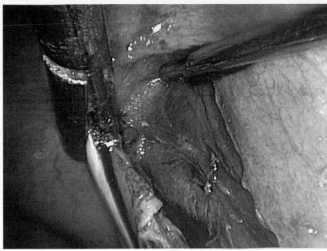

Figure 12-22. The uterosacral ligament is grasped and retracted medially, while the ureter is displaced laterally away from the uterosacral ligament as current is applied.

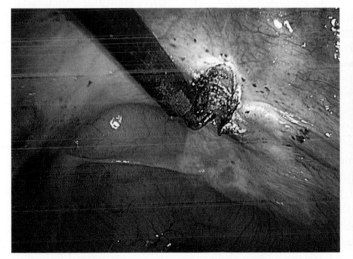

Figure 12-23. The uterosacral ligament is divided with the monopolar hook. Scissors or harmonic scalpel could also be used.

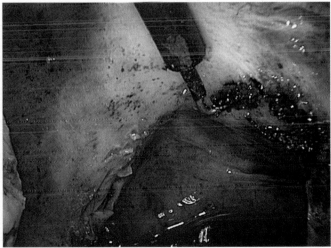

Figure 12-24. The intervening posterior cervical serosa is also incised to improve treatment outcome.

Figure 12-25. This is the appearance of the completed procedure.

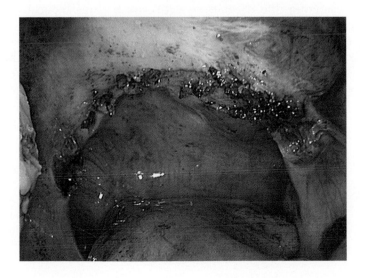

Outcomes

Two randomized trials evaluated the addition of PSN to conservative surgical treatment of endometriosis for relief of dysmenorrhea. PSN was effective in one study but not the other. In both studies, constipation occurred in 14% to 37% and urinary urgency in 5% to 10%, in the PSN groups only. There are no randomized studies comparing PSN to a control group for relief of primary dysmenorrhea.

Johnson and coworkers, performed a randomized controlled double-blind trial of LUNA in 67 women with endometriosis and 56 women without disease. Dysmenorrhea was significantly reduced at 12 months with LUNA in patients without endometriosis but was not significantly different in the endometriosis group. Chronic pelvic pain, dyspareunia, and dyschezia were not significantly different in either group. Two other randomized trials of laparoscopic treatment of endometriosis with or without the addition of LUNA found no difference in dysmenorrhea.

Chen and colleagues randomized, 68 patients with primary dysmenorrhea to treatment with PSN or LUNA. There was no difference at 3 months postoperatively, but at 1 year, the PSN group had significantly better pain relief. However, PSN required 20 to 40 minutes to complete versus 5 to 10 minutes for LUNA, and is an inherently riskier procedure. Also, 93.9% in the PSN group developed constipation while none in the LUNA group did.

In a recent study by Juang and coauthors, 74 women with severe dysmenorrhea were randomly assigned to LUNA only or LUNA combined with PSN if no pelvic pathology was found (i.e., primary dysmenorrhea). Sixty-seven were available for follow-up analysis. At 3 months, 69% of the LUNA group had significant improvement versus 73% in the combined LUNA/PSN group (P = .9). The results were unchanged at 6 and 12 months. Patients in the combined group had greater postoperative pain and significantly more short-term and long-term constipation, 53.1% versus 14.2% and 15.6% versus 0%, respectively. It was concluded that LUNA is as effective as PSN for primary dysmenorrhea and avoids the well-known complications of PSN.

Collectively, the aforementioned studies support the effectiveness of LUNA for primary dysmenorrhea but not for dysmenorrhea associated with endometriosis. PSN appears to be effective for relief of primary dysmenorrhea as well as dysmenorrhea in patients with endometriosis, but may result in constipation and/or urinary frequency.

Appendectomy should be performed if there is gross pathology of the appendix as well as for patients with right lower quadrant pain with a grossly normal-appearing appendix. Microscopic disease is frequently found and patients often get pain relief. LUNA and presacral neurectomy have both been shown to improve primary dysmenorrhea, and presacral neurectomy may also be effective for treating dysmenorrhea associated with endometriosis.

SUMMARY: Considering the frequency with which adhesiolysis is performed and the hundreds of publications relating to intraperitoneal adhesions over several decades, data on adhesions as the cause of pain or infertility, and the effectiveness of adhesiolysis for treating these conditions, are essentially nonexistent. In spite of this, meticulous surgical technique should be used and anti-adhesion adjuvants considered to help reduce postoperative adhesion formation/re-formation. Performing procedures by laparoscopy has been shown to reduce de novo adhesions.

Suggested Reading

Chronic Pain

Howard FM: The role of laparoscopy in chronic pelvic pain: promise and pitfalls, *Obstet Gynecol Surv* 48:357, 1993.

Mathias SD, Kuppermann M, Liberman RF, et al: Chronic pelvic pain: prevalence, health-related quality of life, and economic correlates, *Obstet Gynecol* 87:321, 1996.

Reiter RC: A profile of women with chronic pelvic pain, *Clin Obstet Gynecol* 33:130, 1990.

Zondervan KT, Yudkin PL, Vessey MP, et al: Chronic pelvic pain in the community—symptoms, investigations, and diagnoses, *Am J Obstet Gynecol* 184:1149, 2001.

Appendectomy

AlSalilli M, Vilos GA: Prospective evaluation of laparoscopic appendectomy in women with chronic right lower quadrant pain, *J Am Assoc Gynecol Laparosc* 2:139-142, 1995

Bryson K: Laparoscopic appendicecetomy, *J Gynecol Surg* 7:93, 1991.

Daniell JF, Kurtz BR, McTavish G, et al: Incidental appendectomy: preventive and therapeutic, *Gynaecol Endosc* 3:221-223, 1994.

Martin LC, Puente I, Sosa JL, et al: Open versus laparoscopic appendectomy: a prospective randomised comparison, *Ann Surg* 222:256-262, 1995.

Nezhat C, Nezhat F: Incidental appendectomy during videolaseroscopy, *Am J Obstet Gynecol* 165:559-564, 1991.

O'Hanlan KA, Fisher DT, O'Holleran MS: 257 incidental appendectomies during total laparoscopic hysterectomy, *J Soc Laparoendosc Surg* 11:428-431, 2007.

Adhesions

Davey AK, Maher PJ: Surgical adhesions: A timely update, a great challenge for the future, *J Min Invas Gynecol* 14:15-22, 2007.

Demco L: Pain mapping of adhesions, *J Am Assoc Gynecol Laparosc* 11:181-183, 2004.

Peters AAW, Trimbos-Kemper GCM, Admiraal C, Trimbos JB: A randomized clinicial trial on the benefits of adhesiolysis in patients with intraperitoneal adhesions and chronic pelvic pain, *Br J Obstet Gynaecol* 99:59-62, 1992.

Ray NF, Denton WG, Thamer M, Henderson SC, Perry S: Abdominal adhesiolysis: inpatient care and expenditures in the United States in 1994, *J Am Coll Surg* 186:1-9, 1998.

Swank DJ, Swank-Bordewijk SCG, Hop WCJ, et al: Laparoscopic adhesiolysis in patients with chronic abdominal pain: a blinded randomized controlled multi-center trial, *Lancet* 361:1247-1251, 2003.

Tulandi T, Collins JA, Burrows E, Jarrell JF, McInnes RA, Wrixon W, et al: Treatment-dependent and treatment-independent pregnancy among women with periadnexal adhesions, *Am J Obstet Gynecol* 162:354-357, 1990.

Pelvic Denervation

Candiani GB, Fedele L, Vercellini P, Bianchi S, Di Nola G: Presacral neurectomy for the treatment of pelvic pain associated with endometriosis: a controlled study, *Am J Obstet Gynecol* 167:100-103, 1992.

Chen FP, Chang SD, Chu KK, Soong YK: Comparison of laparoscopic presacral neurectomy and laparoscopic uterine nerve ablation for primary dysmenorrhea, *J Reprod Med* 41:463-466, 1996.

Fedele L, Marchini M, Acaia B, Garagiola U, Tiengo M: Dynamics and significance of placebo response in primary dysmenorrhea, *Pain* 36:43-47, 1989.

Johnson NP, Farquhar CM, Crossley Y, Yu AM, Van Peperstraten AM, Sprecher M, et al: A double-blind randomised controlled trial of laparoscopic uterine nerve ablation for women with chronic pelvic pain, *Br J Obstet Gynaecol* 111:950-959, 2004.

Juang CM, Chou P, Yen MS, et al: Laparoscopic uterosacral nerve ablation with and without presacral neurectomy in the treatment of primary dysmenorrhea. A prospective efficacy analysis, *J Reprod Med* 52:591-596, 2007.

Lee TTM, Yang LC: Pelvic denervation procedures: a current reappraisal, *Int J Gynecol Obstet* 101:304-308, 2008.

Sutton C, Pooley AS, Jones KD, Dover RW, Haines P: A prospective, randomized, double-blind controlled trial of laparoscopic uterine nerve ablation in the treatment of pelvic pain associated with endometriosis, *Gynaecol Endosc* 10:217-222, 2001.

Vercellini P, Aimi G, Busacca M, Apolone G, Uglietti A, Crosignani PG: Laparoscopic uterosacral ligament resection for dysmenorrhea associated with endometriosis: results of a randomized, controlled trial, *Fertil Steril* 80:310-319, 2003.

Zullo F, Palomba S, Zupi E, Russo T, Morelli M, Cappiello F, Mastrantonio P: Effectiveness of presacral neurectomy in women with severe dysmenorrhea caused by endometriosis who were treated with laparoscopic conservative surgery: a 1-year prospective randomized double-blind controlled trial, *Am J Obstet Gynecol* 189:5-10, 2003.

Robotic Surgery

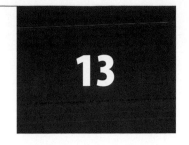

13

Gouri B. Diwadkar M.D.
Tommaso Falcone M.D.

 Video Clips on DVD

13-1 Appropriate Steps for Setting up the Robot (8 minutes/23 seconds)
13-2 Robotic-Assisted Hysterectomy (7 minutes/52 seconds)
13-3 Robotic-Assisted Myomectomy: Example #1 (7 minutes/45 seconds)

13-4 Robotic-Assisted Myomectomy: Example #2 (10 minutes/2 seconds)
13-5 Robotic-Assisted Sacral Colpopexy (12 minutes/17 seconds)
13-6 Robotic-Assisted Tubal Reanastomosis (5 minutes/19 seconds)

Introduction

The use of robotics in gynecologic surgery has gained increasing popularity over the past decade. First introduced in 1994, AESOP (Automated Endoscopic System for Optimal Positioning) (Computer Motion Inc., Goleta, CA), a voice-activated robotic arm that operated the camera during laparoscopic surgery, allowed surgeons to use both hands while operating. In 2003, the surgical console was introduced, with Zeus (Computer Motion Inc., Goleta, CA), a system comprised of AESOP and two robotic instrument arms attached to the siderails of the surgical table telemanipulated by the surgeon at a workstation, or console. Currently, the only Food and Drug Administration–approved robotic system in production for gynecologic surgery is the da Vinci surgical system (Intuitive Surgical, Sunnyvale, CA). The da Vinci system includes three components: a console from where the surgeon sits and operates the system remotely, the patient-side cart comprised of three to four robotic arms that hold the EndoWrist instruments (Intuitive Surgical, Sunnyvale, CA), and the InSite vision system (Intuitive Surgical, Sunnyvale, CA) that provides 3-D vision through two optical channels of the endoscope (Figure 13-1). A second generation of the da Vinci system, the da Vinci S system, was released in 2006. Compared to the original da Vinci system, this system provides longer instruments, narrower robotic arms, increased flexion-extension and lateral excursion, and subwindows on the surgeon's 3-D screen.

The aim of this chapter is to describe the techniques for performing the most common robotic-assisted gynecologic procedures with the latest da Vinci S robotic system, including total hysterectomy, myomectomy, sacral colpopexy, and tubal reanastomosis.

Indications and Patient Selection

Similar to conventional laparoscopic surgery, robotic surgery offers the many advantages of minimally invasive surgery, such as decreased blood loss, faster recovery periods, shorter hospital stay, decreased postoperative pain, and improved cosmesis.

Figure 13-1. Components of the surgical robot: **A,** Surgeon seated at the surgical console. **B,** The surgical tower that is placed at the bedside. **C,** The video tower that holds the computer interface between the patient and the console.

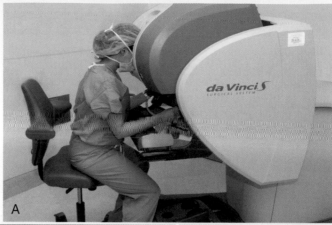

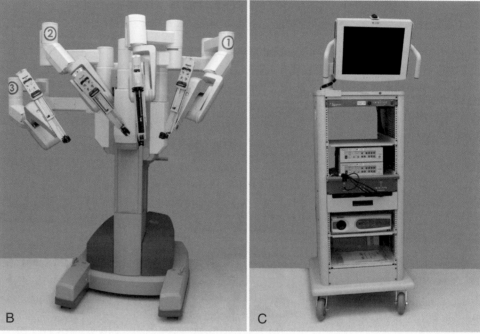

Further, robotic-assisted surgery offers several advantages over conventional laparoscopy. The robot system includes various scales for downscaling movements. For a scale of 10:1, for every 10 cm of handle movement from the console, the robotic instruments move 1 cm at the surgical site, also leading to tremor filtration. Intuitive hand movement refers to the movement of the robotic instruments in the same direction the surgeon's hands move at the console, whereas with conventional laparoscopy, the movements are counterintuitive. The 3-D vision assists with difficult dissections and microsurgery. In addition, the robotic instruments have seven degrees of instrument articulation similar to the human wrist. The ergonomics are also improved, as the surgeon sits comfortably at the console while performing the surgery. Due to these advantages, robotic surgery may have a shorter learning curve compared to conventional laparoscopy and has become an option for gynecologists who have not mastered conventional laparoscopic skills, such as suturing. Myomectomy and sacral colpopexy, two procedures that require extensive suturing and dissection, have been increasingly performed with robotic assistance. In addition, the stereoscopic imaging and tremor filtering facilitate procedures that require accurate, precise suturing, as in tubal reanastomosis.

The primary disadvantage of the robotic system is the absence of tactile or haptic feedback. The lack of haptics can result in increased tissue trauma, breaking suture, and not tying knots securely. It is partially compensated by visual cues. However, lack of tactile feedback is advantageous in morbidly obese patients because the surgeon does

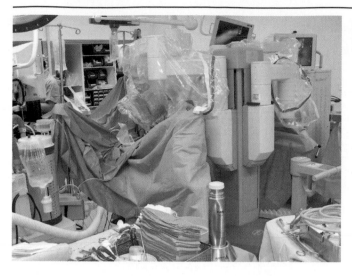

Figure 13-2. The surgical tower around the patient: view from the legs.

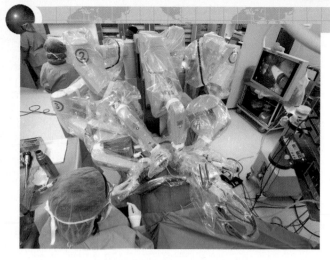

Figure 13-3. The surgical tower around the patient: view from the head.

not feel any resistance of the robotic instruments against the thick abdominal wall as experienced with conventional laparoscopy. Another disadvantage of the robot is its size. The bulkiness of the robot impedes the surgical assistant from easily moving around the surgical table during the surgery (Figures 13-2 and 13-3). However more recent versions of the robot can be "side docked" which allows easier access of assistants to the vagina for uterine manipulation. Once the robot is docked between the patient's legs and the arms are attached to the trocars, it is extremely difficult to access the perineum and lower abdomen. In cases such as sacral colpopexy in which manipulation of the vagina and rectum are essential for assisting with dissection, a second surgical assistant often sits in between the legs at the perineum with the robot docked behind and above the assistant. The robot must be disconnected and redocked in order to move the operating table, such as to decrease Trendelenburg if the anesthesiologist is having difficulty ventilating the patient.

Contraindications to using the robot are similar to those for conventional laparoscopic surgery, including insufficient knowledge of the robot or procedure, severe adhesions that preclude safe entry, or medical conditions that prevent appropriate positioning. Prior to surgery, patients should be adequately counseled about the risks of conversion to conventional laparoscopy or laparotomy.

Preoperative Preparation and Patient Positioning (Table 13-1)

Bowel preparation with an agent of the surgeon's choice may be given on the day and/ or night prior to surgery in order to decompress the bowel prior to hysterectomy, myomectomy, and sacral colpopexy. Prophylactic antibiotics should be administered within 30 minutes of making the initial incision for all procedures discussed below. The patient should be placed in low dorsal lithotomy position with well-padded stirrups. The patient's arms should be tucked and protected with padding to provide sufficient room for the surgical assistant. The patient should be secured to the operating table because steep Trendelenburg position is required for all of the surgeries. A Foley catheter should be inserted for continuous bladder drainage.

Trocar Insertion and Robot Docking

View DVD: Video 13-1

Proper trocar placement is essential in facilitating any robotic surgery. Inaccurate placement can lead to collision between the robotic arms, difficulty reaching the operative site, and therefore delays in the surgery. Port placement for hysterectomy, myomectomy, sacral colpopexy, and tubal reanastomosis is similar.

Table 13-1   Tips for Robotic Gynecologic Surgery

- The patient's arms should be tucked and protected with padding to provide sufficient room for the surgical assistant.
- Shoulder pads or other devices should be used to prevent the patient from slipping on the table, because steep Trendelenburg position is required throughout most surgeries.
- Insert appropriate vaginal instruments prior to docking the patient side-cart.
- Proper trocar placement is essential in facilitating any robotic surgery.
- In a patient with an enlarged uterus, the distance between the pubic symphysis and the port for the endoscope may need to be adjusted up to 25 cm to allow sufficient distance between the endoscope and uterus.
- A full hand's-breadth or 8 cm between the ipsilateral port sites is important to prevent robotic arm collision.
- The fourth robotic arm is always helpful for retraction, exposure, and tension on suture.

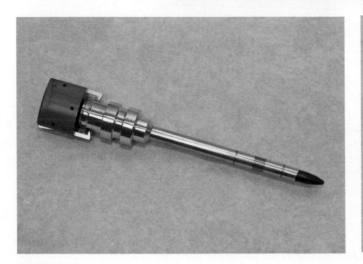

Figure 13-4. The 8-mm trocars used for the robotic arms.

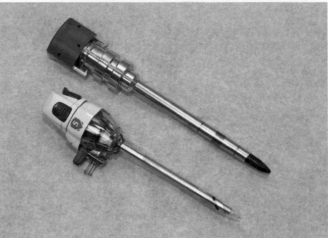

Figure 13-5. Relative size with a 5-mm trocar.

1. The first port is created 20 to 25 cm superior to the pubic symphysis at the midline. A Veress needle can be inserted to obtain pneumoperitoneum, although we prefer to use a 5 mm conventional laparoscopic trocar. Twenty centimeters corresponds to the level of the umbilicus. With a large uterus, this distance may need to be adjusted to 25 cm to allow sufficient distance between the endoscope and uterus, although this may restrict access to the pelvis. Insertion of the conventional 5-mm endoscope through this port allows visualization of the pelvis for adhesions and confirmation of anatomic findings prior to creating a larger incision for the robotic endoscope. With this method, the conventional laparoscopic trocar eventually needs to be replaced with a 12- or 15-mm trocar to accommodate the robotic endoscope. Alternatively, a 12- or 15-mm trocar can be inserted from the start.

2. For patients with suspected adhesions at the umbilicus due to prior abdominal or pelvic surgery, a left upper quadrant port can be created initially, 1 cm below the costal margin at the midclavicular line, followed by trocar insertion at the umbilicus once the area is confirmed to be free of adhesions.

3. The patient is placed in steep Trendelenburg position to retract the bowels cephalad.

4. The 8-mm reusable robotic trocars are inserted (Figures 13-4 and 13-5). The ports are placed in a "W" configuration. Bilaterally, a trocar is inserted 10 cm lateral of the umbilical trocar and 15 to 30 degrees caudad, with a full hand's-breadth between the port site and iliac crest (Figure 13-6). For sacral colpopexy, the robotic trocars are often placed 15 degrees cephalad rather than caudad to access the sacral promontory.

5. A third robotic trocar is inserted 8 to 10 cm lateral and 4 to 5 cm cephalad of the robotic port on either side, to which the fourth robotic arm is attached once the robot is docked. A full hand's-breadth or 8 cm between the ipsilateral port sites is important to prevent robotic arm collision (Figure 13-7).

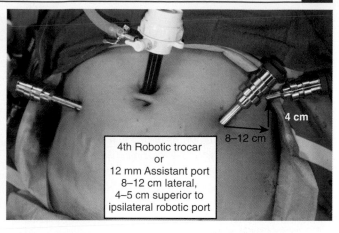

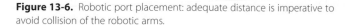

Figure 13-6. Robotic port placement: adequate distance is imperative to avoid collision of the robotic arms.

Figure 13-7. The placement of the fourth arm trocar is critical to its proper use. Typically it should be placed on the side of the dominant hand.

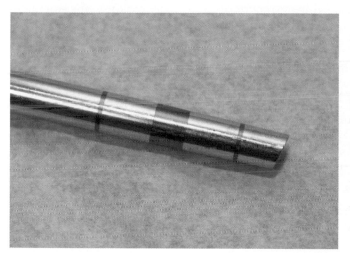

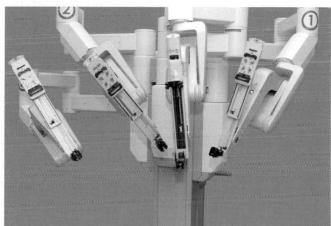

Figure 13-8. The trocar should be advanced until the thick black line is seen.

Figure 13-9. The robotic arms are numbered so as to correctly communicate where instrument changes should occur.

6. An optional 12-mm assistant port can be created using similar measurements on the contralateral side, allowing suture introduction, further retraction, and irrigation (see Figure 13-7).

7. The umbilical trocar is converted from 5 mm to 12 mm to accommodate the 12-mm robotic endoscope.

8. The robotic trocar is inserted until the marked thick black line is visualized, representing the focal point of the trocar (Figure 13-8).

9. The robotic side-cart (Figure 13-9) is docked by manually navigating the system between the patient's legs. The arms of the robot are adjusted at the appropriate angles, such that they can be snapped onto the robotic trocars. The arms should be adjusted to allow full range of motion during surgery.

10. The Endowrist instruments and endoscope are inserted through the appropriate ports, and the surgeon can then begin the surgery from the console. Both straight (0-degree) and angled (30-degree) tip scopes are available, although we prefer to use the straight scope.

(See Video 13-1)

Case 1: Robotic-Assisted Total Hysterectomy

 View DVD: Video 13-2

A 40-year-old female presents with complaints of worsening dysmenorrhea and menorrhagia refractory to oral contraceptives. Several months prior, the patient underwent a diagnostic laparoscopy for pelvic pain and was found to have an enlarged uterus and dense, extensive adhesions from the lower segment of the uterus to the anterior abdominal wall. The adhesions were in close proximity to the bladder and were not taken down by the surgeon. Her surgical history includes three low transverse cesarean sections. A transvaginal ultrasound reveals a uterus measuring 12 cm in greatest dimension with multiple intramural fibroids. She has completed her childbearing and desires a hysterectomy via a minimally invasive approach. After a thorough discussion about risks and benefits, informed consent is obtained for a robotic-assisted total hysterectomy.

Robotic hysterectomy is an appropriate approach to this patient's findings. The dense adhesions from the uterus and bladder to the anterior abdominal wall increase the risk for cystotomy. The robot's 3-D-vision system and enhanced dexterity may be advantageous in dissecting tissue planes.

Surgical Techniques

The steps and technique to performing a robotic-assisted hysterectomy are similar to those used for conventional laparoscopic hysterectomy.

1. Robotic instruments recommended for this procedure include monopolar cautery scissors (Figure 13-10A), bipolar forceps (Figure 13-10B), monopolar hook, and needle-drivers.

2. A Koh colpotomizer (Cooper Surgical, Trumbull, CT) and RUMI (Cooper Surgical, Trumbull, CT) uterine manipulator are inserted vaginally prior to docking the robot if a total hysterectomy is to be performed. The Koh cup assists with delineating the vaginal fornices. For a supracervical hysterectomy, a Koh cup is not required, but a uterine manipulator is recommended.

3. Trocars are placed and the robotic side-cart is docked as described earlier.

4. The round ligaments are cauterized with the bipolar forceps and divided with the scissors, with countertraction from the fourth arm or surgical assistant.

5. The anterior and posterior leaves of the broad ligament are divided with the tips of the monopolar cautery scissors, opening the retroperitoneal space. The internal and external iliac vessels and the course of the ureter can be identified with gentle blunt dissection.

6. If the ovaries are to be left in place, the utero-ovarian ligaments are cauterized with the bipolar forceps and divided. If the ovaries are to be removed, the infundibulo-pelvic ligament needs to be identified, cauterized, and transected in the standard fashion after the ureter's course has been identified.

7. The peritoneal incision is extended anteriorly to the bladder reflection with the monopolar scissors, and the avascular plane of loose areolar tissue between the posterior bladder and anterior cervix is identified. Using the scissors, this plane is sharply dissected, pushing the bladder caudad.

8. The uterine vessels are skeletonized using the monopolar scissors, cauterized with the bipolar forceps in consecutive segments, and divided.

9. The cardinal ligaments are cauterized with the bipolar forceps and transected with the monopolar scissors.

10. Once the inferior margin of the cervix is reached, the monopolar scissors are replaced with the monopolar hook, and the hook is used to amputate the cervix from the vagina by making a circumferential incision at the proximal margin of the Koh cup. The bipolar forceps should be available in the opposite arm in case small vessels are encountered during the amputation. The assistant at the bedside removes the uterine manipulator and amputated uterus and inserts the balloon occluder to maintain pneumoperitoneum.

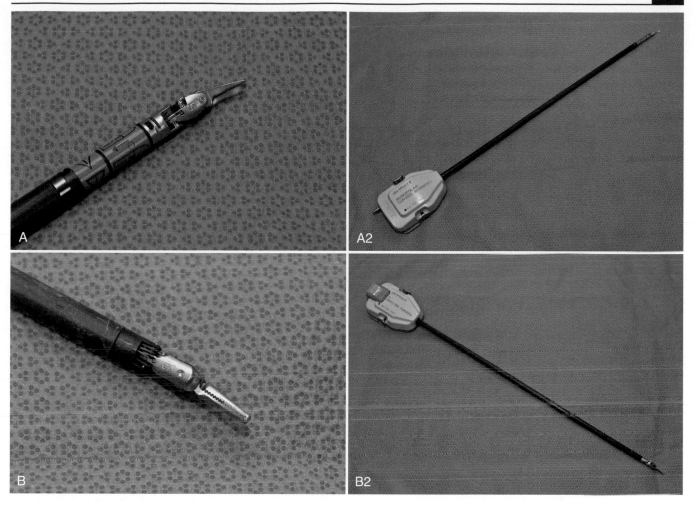

Figure 13-10. A and B, Close up of the tip and complete Instrument of the unipolar scissors and bipolar grasper.

11. The bipolar forceps and monopolar hook are exchanged for two robotic needle drivers. A 0-Vicryl suture is introduced through the assistant port via a laparoscopic needle-driver. The surgeon reapproximates the cuff with interrupted or figure-of-eight stitches using intracorporeal knot-tying. The needle is cut and removed by the assistant. (If a cutting needle driver is used, the surgeon can cut the needle.) The camera should follow the needle as it is pulled out by the assistant, in case it dislodges from the driver and falls into the surgical field.

12. In the case of a supracervical hysterectomy, the monopolar hook or scissors are used to transect the cervix. Morcellation is performed via conventional laparoscopy after the robot side-cart is undocked.

13. To prevent future apical prolapse, we often place a McCall's culdoplasty stitch using 0-Prolene suture. The robotic needle-drivers are used to place the stitch through one of the remaining uterosacral ligaments, followed by a bite through the posterior vaginal cuff or cervical stump (in the case of a supracervical hysterectomy), and then through the contralateral uterosacral ligament. The stitch is then tied using intracorporeal knot-tying, functioning to suspend the vaginal cuff to the uterosacral ligaments. The stitch should be placed on the medial aspect of the uterosacral ligaments to prevent kinking the ureters.

14. It is essential that a cystoscopy be performed to assess the bladder for any evidence of cystotomy and the ureters for patency. Indigo carmine dye is administered by anesthesiologist the anesthesiologis intravenously. After approximately 10 to 15 minutes, bilateral spill of dye should be visible from the ureteral orifices in a patient with normal renal function.

15. All areas are examined for hemostasis.

16. All fascial incisions greater than 5 mm are reapproximated after the robotic side-cart is undocked.

    (See Video 13-2 📹)

Case 2: Robotic-Assisted Myomectomy

 View DVD: Videos 13-3 and 13-4

A 37-year-old female is referred for a second opinion regarding symptomatic uterine fibroids. She is mostly troubled by heavy pressure and bloating, and states that she is unable to work because of the discomfort. She prefers a minimally invasive approach and desires to retain her uterus for future childbearing. She has not had any prior surgeries, but has been told in the past that she may have endometriosis. On ultrasound, she has an 8-cm fundal, intramural fibroid. An MRI confirms these findings. After a thorough discussion including the risk for conversion to conventional laparoscopy or laparotomy, the patient consents to a robotic-assisted myomectomy.

This patient is an ideal candidate for a robotic approach. Our selection criteria for robotic myomectomy of intramural leiomyomata are uterine size less than 16 cm, dominant fibroid size less than 15 cm in greatest dimension, and a maximum of five fibroids. Due to lack of haptic feedback with robotic surgery, preoperative imaging with MRI is recommended to delineate the location, number, and size of each leiomyoma. In addition, the presence of endometriosis may require precise dissection surrounding the pelvic sidewalls, ureters, and bladder.

Surgical Techniques

The steps and principles of a robotic-assisted myomectomy are similar to those of conventional laparoscopy.

1. Robotic instruments recommended for this procedure are monopolar scissors (Figure 13-10A), bipolar forceps (Figure 13-10B), monopolar hook, needle drivers, and a tenaculum.

2. Trocars are placed and the robotic side-cart is docked as described earlier.

3. The surgical assistant uses the assistant port to inject dilute vasopressin (20 units/100 mL) into the fibroid to control bleeding.

4. The surgeon begins by making an incision into the uterine serosa overlying the leiomyoma with the monopolar hook or monopolar scissors, cauterizing bleeding vessels along the incision line. The dissection is carried down through the myometrium to the level of the leiomyoma. The assistant inserts a conventional laparoscopic tenaculum to grasp the leiomyoma and provide countertraction, while the surgeon dissects the surrounding myometrium off with blunt and sharp dissection. Alternatively, a tenaculum in the fourth arm can be used for retraction (Figure 13-11).

5. Once the fibroid has been completely enucleated, hemostasis over the myometrial bed is achieved using the bipolar cautery.

6. The dissecting forceps and monopolar hook instruments are exchanged for two needle drivers. A/O-Vicryl suture is introduced through the laparoscopic port by the assistant. The surgeon places figure-of-eight stitches in the deepest layer of the myometrium using intracorporeal knot-tying. The needle is cut and removed by the assistant. (If a cutting needle driver is used, the surgeon can cut the needle.) The camera should follow the needle as it is pulled out by the assistant, in case it dislodges from the driver and falls into the surgical field.

7. A 0-PDS suture is introduced and the myometrium is further reapproximated with a running stitch. We prefer PDS suture for a running stitch because it is easier to manipulate through the tissue and tie with the robotic instruments. Interrupted stitches can also be used. A grasper in the stationary fourth robotic arm is used to grasp the suture at one end to assist in holding up the uterus. In the case of

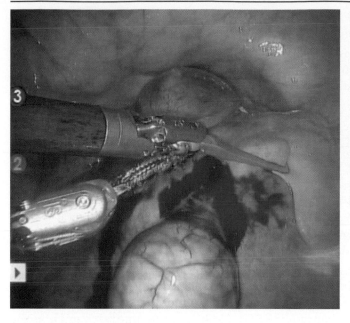

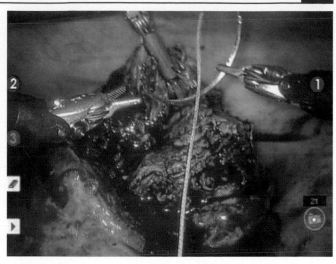

Figure 13-12. Use of the fourth arm to hold the uterus in a proper place while the other two arms are used for suturing the defect in the myometrium after myomectomy.

Figure 13-11. Robotic tenaculum: its size limits enucleation of large myomas.

posterior fibroids, the fourth arm may also be used to hold up the uterus to provide further visualization (Figure 13-12).

8. The serosa is reapproximated with interrupted stitches or running 2-0 or 3-0 PDS suture.

9. Once hemostasis is achieved, the robotic arms are released from the trocars and the robot is disengaged.

10. Either the assistant port or one of the robotic ports is extended to 15 mm in order to allow insertion of a uterine morcellator. The leiomyoma is carefully morcellated, and all fragments of tissue are removed from the pelvis.

11. All fascial incisions greater than 5 mm are reapproximated after the robotic side-cart is undocked.

(See Videos 13-3 and 13-4)

Case 3: Robotic-Assisted Sacral Colpopexy

View DVD: Video 13-5

A 55-year-old postmenopausal female is referred by her primary care physician to a urogynecologist for urinary voiding difficulties and vaginal prolapse. The patient reports discomfort from the "bulge" between her legs and has to manually reduce the prolapse in order to empty her bladder. She tried a pessary in the past but developed a vaginal erosion and now requests other options for management. Her history includes a total abdominal hysterectomy 15 years ago. Examination reveals stage III prolapse of the apical vaginal wall. The patient is very interested in a minimally invasive option because she would like to return to her desk job as quickly as possible. Robotic sacral colpopexy is a reasonable option because it tremendously simplifies the laparoscopic suturing required for this procedure when compared to conventional laparoscopic sacral colpopexy.

Surgical Techniques

1. Robotic instruments recommended for this procedure are bipolpar forceps (Figure 13-10A), monopolar scissors (Figure 13-10B), needle drivers, and a bowel grasper.

2. Two surgical assistants increase the efficiency of this procedure. The first assistant is at the bedside, while the second assistant sits between the patient's legs to manipulate the vaginal instruments. The robot is docked after the second assistant is comfortably seated between the patient's legs.

3. Trocars are placed and the robotic side-cart is docked as described earlier.

4. A bowel grasper in the fourth robotic arm on the left side is used to retract the rectum to the left, exposing the sacral promontory.

5. The second assistant inserts an EEA (end-to-end anastomosis) sizer into the vagina to determine the length and width of the vagina. Using the monopolar scissors, the peritoneum overlying the vaginal apex is incised transversely by the surgeon. Countertraction is provided by a grasper in the robotic arm on the opposite side or by the first assistant. The bladder and rectum are carefully dissected off the vagina using the monopolar scissors and blunt dissection. The second assistant manipulates the EEA sizer in various directions to facilitate the dissection.

6. Using the monopolar scissors in one hand and a bipolar grasper in the other, the tissue overlying the sacral promontory is dissected off, taking care to not deviate laterally or caudad where heavy bleeding may occur from the lateral sacral venous plexus. The course of the right ureter is identified, and the peritoneal incision is extended caudad towards the vagina.

7. The mesh strips are then tailored to fit the distance between the vaginal apex and sacral promontory. The monopolar scissors and bipolar grasper are exchanged for two needle drivers. A full-length 0-Prolene stitch is introduced through the assistant port, and the surgeon places an interrupted stitch into the anterior vagina at the most distal point dissected free from the bladder, without entering the mucosa. The mesh is introduced into the pelvis by the first assistant, and intracorporeal knots are placed securing the mesh to the anterior vagina. Two to three pairs of interrupted sutures are placed symmetrically into the mesh and vagina to fix the mesh to the anterior vagina.

8. The posterior strip of mesh is introduced by the first assistant. Similarly, two to three pairs of interrupted stitches of 0-Prolene are placed into the posterior vagina and mesh starting at the most distal region free from the rectum. Other permanent suture, such as Ethibond, may also be used by the surgeon instead of Prolene.

9. The second assistant places gentle traction on the vaginal EEA sizer, bringing the vaginal apex towards the sacrum. The two strips of mesh are extended cephalad towards the sacral promontory. The first assistant introduces 0-Prolene suture. The suture is threaded through the two strips of mesh, into the anterior longitudinal ligament, threaded back through the mesh, and tied down fastening the mesh to the sacrum. A similar second stitch is placed approximately 1 cm caudad or cephalad of the first, avoiding the middle sacral vessels and other surrounding structures.

10. If needed, the mesh is trimmed proximal to the sacral stitches, and the fragments of mesh are removed by the assistant.

11. A 0-Vicryl suture is used by the surgeon to reapproximate the peritoneum over the mesh in a running fashion or via figure-of-eight stitches.

12. All port sites greater than 5 mm are reapproximated after the robotic side-cart is undocked.

(See Video 13-5 🎞️)

Case 4: Robotic-Assisted Tubal Reanastomosis

View DVD: Video 13-6

A 31-year-old female presents for consultation for tubal ligation reversal. Her most recent vaginal delivery was 6 years ago and was followed by a tubal ligation with Falope rings. She is now with a new partner and desires pregnancy. She is healthy and has not had any other surgeries. Partner had a normal semen analysis. After discussing options and pregnancy rates following tubal reversal, the patient is consented for a robotic-assisted tubal reanastomosis.

The magnification and three-dimensional visualization provided with the robotic system facilitates the microsurgery of tubal reanastomosis. Additionally, with the minimally invasive approach, patients are discharged home within hours of completing the procedure.

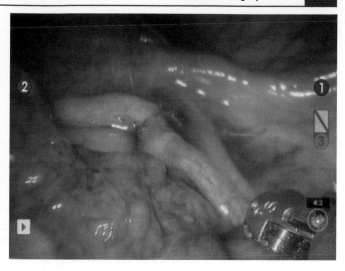

Figure 13-13. Robotic tubal anastomosis: 8-0 Vicryl has been introduced into the proximal tube through the serosa into the lumen.

Figure 13-14. Completed anastomosis.

Surgical Techniques

1. Robotic instruments recommended for this procedure are monopolar cautery hook or monopolar cautery scissors (Figure 13-10A), bipolar graspers (Figure 13-10B), and two needle drivers. The fourth robotic arm is not required for this procedure. A uterine manipulator that allows injection of dye is required and should be inserted prior to docking the robotic side-cart.

2. Trocars are placed and the robotic side-cart is docked as described earlier.

3. The surgical assistant injects dilute vasopressin into the mesosalpinx bilaterally

4. The monopolar hook with cautery is used to open the proximal and distal anastomotic sites. Countertraction is provided with an atraumatic grasper in the opposite arm. Extensive use of cautery should be avoided to prevent future adhesions.

5. Indigo carmine dye is injected transcervically and the proximal end is confirmed to be patent, as evidenced by efflux of dye. The assistant injects dye into the distal tube using a laparoscopic needle to confirm patency of the distal end.

6. The monopolar hook and grasper are replaced with two needle drivers. Using 6-0 Vicryl suture, the mesosalpinx is reapproximated with interrupted stitches.

7. Interrupted stitches of 8-0 Vicryl suture are placed at the 12-, 3-, 6-, and 9-o'clock positions to reapproximate the mucosal and muscularis layers of the divided segments of fallopian tube (Figure 13-13).

8. After the sutures are placed, indigo carmine dye is injected transcervically to check for patency and leaks (Figure 13-14). Additional interrupted stitches may be required at the locations where leaks are noted.

9. All fascial incisions greater than 5 mm are reapproximated after the robotic side-cart is undocked.

(See Video 13-6 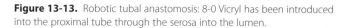)

Outcomes and Complications

Reports on outcomes and complications from robotic-assisted surgeries are sparse because the robotic system was introduced relatively recently. The majority of published data has been from retrospective studies of less than 50 patients, with few large comparative studies to date.

Most gynecologic robotic data report on robotic-assisted hysterectomy outcomes. Reynolds and Advincula reported on 16 patients who underwent robotic-assisted laparoscopic hysterectomy or supracervical hysterectomy. There were no conversions to laparotomy. The robot was advantageous in performing the hysterectomy despite scarred and obliterated surgical planes from prior surgeries in 13 of the patients. Kho and coauthors reviewed 91 patients, with a mean uterine weight of 135.5 grams, who underwent robotic hysterectomy. Additional procedures included salpingo-oophorectomy, appendectomy, and lysis of adhesions. Mean total operative time was 128 minutes, and mean estimated blood loss was 79 mL. The only intraoperative complication was an enterotomy which was repaired robotically. One study noted that the incidence of vaginal cuff dehiscence was four times higher than with laparoscopic hysterectomy and 15 times higher than with vaginal hysterectomy. Therefore it is important to introduce the needle into the vaginal cuff in an area that does not have tissue necrosis from the energy form used to incise the vagina.

Myomectomy outcomes have only been reported by Advincula and colleagues in a series of 35 cases. Two cases (8.6%) were converted to laparotomy due to difficulty enucleating the myomas from lack of haptic feedback. The mean operative time was 230.8 ± 83 minutes, and the mean estimated blood loss was 169 ± 198.7 mL. A mean of 1.6 myomas were removed, and the mean diameter was 7.9 ± 3.5 cm.

Falcone and coworkers performed the first robotic-assisted tubal reanastomosis in 1999, using the Zeus robotic system. There was an 89% tubal patency rate on hysterosalpingogram at 6 weeks and a 50% pregnancy rate at 12 months. Most recently, Rodgers and colleagues compared tubal reanastomosis via outpatient minilaparotomy to robotic-assisted surgery. Intrauterine and ectopic pregnancy rates were not different between the two groups. Operative time was greater in the robotic group (229 vs. 181 minutes). Hospitalization time was not different between the groups, but convalesence time was shorter by 1 week in the robotic surgery group. Robotic surgery was more costly by $1446 USD. These costs were calculated solely for the hospital care.

In 2006, Elliott and coworkers reported the findings of 30 women undergoing robotic-assisted sacral colpopexy, the largest series to date. Only 21 patients had follow-up at 1 year. One patient had recurrence of vault prolapse, and one patient had a recurrent rectocele. Two patients had vaginal mesh extrusion. Despite these adverse outcomes, all patients were satisfied with the surgery.

In a 2007 study of 15 patients undergoing laparoscopic and robotic-assisted surgery for myomectomy, sacral colpopexy, total laparoscopic hysterectomy, supracervical hysterectomy, and treatment of endometriosis, Nehzat and colleagues reported difficulties with the robot due to lack of haptic feedback, lack of vaginal access, awkward exchange of instruments, and costs. This is one of the few studies to date reporting negative feedback after use of the robotic system.

SUMMARY: Robotic-assisted surgery is another technique for performing common surgical procedures in gynecology. The advantages of three-dimensional vision, improved dexterity, and improved ergonomics give it an edge over conventional laparoscopy. Although the intuitive movement of the robot may allow inexperienced laparoscopic surgeons to perform procedures in a minimally invasive fashion, robotic training and experience are essential to become a proficient robotic surgeon. A study by Lenihan and coworkers that included 115 patients concluded that the learning curve to stabilize operative times for robotic surgery for benign gynecologic conditions is 50 cases, in the hands of an experienced laparoscopic surgeon. Robotic technology also has a role in telementoring and telesurgery, during which a robotic specialist guides a physically remote surgeon through a surgery or performs the surgery from a remote location, respectively. Several feasibility studies have been published over the past 10 years supporting the robot. However, large randomized studies comparing clinical outcomes and cost-effectiveness for laparoscopic surgery with and without robotic assistance are essential to determine the proper indications for using the robot. As seen by the rapid progression in minimally invasive technology over the past decade, there will most definitely be further advances in improving ease, efficiency, and accuracy of robotic technology.

Suggested Reading

Advincula AP, Song A: The role of robotic surgery in gynecology, *Curr Opin Obstet Gynecol* 19(4):331-336, 2007.

Advincula AP, Song A, Burke W, Reynolds RK: Preliminary experience with robot-assisted laparoscopic myomectomy, *J Am Assoc Gynecol Laparosc* 11:511-518, 2004.

Kho RM, Akl MN, Cornella JL et al: Incidence of characteristics of patients with vaginal cuff dehiscence after robotic procedures, *Obstet Gynecol* 114:231-235, 2009.

Dharia Patel SP, Steinkampf MP, Whitten SJ, Malizia BA: Robotic tubal anastomosis: surgical technique and cost effectiveness, *Fertil Steril* 90:1175-1179, 2008.

Elliott DS, Krambeck AE, Chow GK: Long-term results of robotic assisted laparoscopic sacrocolpopexy for the treatment of high grade vaginal vault prolapse, *J Urol* 176(2):655-659, 2006.

Falcone T, Goldberg JM, Margossian H, Stevens L: Robotic-assisted laparoscopic microsurgical tubal anastomosis: a human pilot study, *Fertil Steril* 73(5):1040-1042, 2000.

Kho RM, Wesley SH, Hentz JG, Matibay PM, Magrina JF: Robotic hysterectomy: technique and initial outcomes, *Am J Obstet Gynecol* 197:113.e1-113.e4, 2007.

Lenihan JP, Covanda C, Seshadri-Kreaden U: What is the learning curve for robotic assisted gynecologic surgery? *J Min Invasive Gynecol* 15:589-594, 2008.

Magrina JF: Robotic surgery in gynecology, *Eur J Gynaecol Oncol* 28(2):77-82, 2007.

Magrina JF, Kho RM, Weaver AL, Montero RP, Magtibay PM: Robotic radical hysterectomy: comparison with laparoscopy and laparotomy, *Gynecol Oncol* 109(1):86-91, 2008.

Nezhat C, Saberi NS, Shahmohamady B, Nezhat F: Robotic-assisted laparoscopy in gynecological surgery, *JSLS* 10(3):317-320, 2006.

Reynold RK, Advincula AP: Robot-assisted laparoscopic hysterectomy: technique and initial experience, *Am J Surg* 191:555-560, 2006.

Rodgers AK, Goldberg JM, Hammel JP, Falcone T: Tubal anastomosis by robotic compared with outpatient minilaparotomy, *Obstet Gynecol* 109(6):1375-1380, 2007.

Sroga J, Dharia-Patel S, Falcone T: Robotics in reproductive medicine, *Front Biosci* 13:1308-1317, 2008

Laparoscopic and Robotic Advances in Gynecologic Malignancies

Amanda Nickles Fader M.D.
Pedro Escobar M.D.
Leigh G. Seamon D.O.
Jeffrey M. Fowler M.D.

 Video Clips on DVD

14-1 Robotic Hysterectomy and Lymphadenectomy for Endometrial Carcinoma (8 minutes/20 seconds)

14-2 Robotic radical hysterectomy for cervical or endometrial carcinomas (14 minutes/2 seconds)

Introduction

The role of conventional and robotic-assisted laparoscopy in the management of gynecologic malignancies has increased considerably in the past decade. The ability to perform minimally invasive surgical staging procedures has revolutionized care and quality-of-life outcomes for women with suspected or known cancer of the female reproductive tract. Herein, we describe the role of laparoscopy in the treatment of endometrial and cervical cancers. A review of conventional and robotic laparoscopic techniques will be demonstrated in the approach to each of these cancers.

Endometrial Cancer

Endometrial carcinoma, the fourth most common cancer in women and the most common invasive neoplasm of the female genital tract, is a cancer of the developed world. In the United States, it is estimated that nearly 40,100 cases of endometrial cancer will have been diagnosed in 2008. The majority of patients present with early-stage disease that can be cured, in a large percentage of patients, by surgery, with or without adjuvant therapy. Well-established risk factors for this disease include obesity, diabetes mellitus, hypertension, late menopause, chronic anovulation, and exogenous estrogen use. In 1983, Bokhman proposed a dualistic model of endometrial oncogenesis based on clinical observations and clinicopathologic correlations. Approximately 80% of these carcinomas are "sporadic carcinomas" or type I endometrial cancers, and are mediated by an estrogen-driven pathway. Histologically, type I endometrial carcinomas are of the "endometrioid subtype", are low-grade in nature and exhibit an indolent clinical behavior. By contrast, type II carcinomas are characterized by an aggressive tumor biology and a poor prognosis. Histologically, these high-grade lesions are most often of the serous and clear cell types and are not estrogen mediated. At present, the most common phenotypes of the type I and II endometrial carcinomas (endometrioid and serous subtypes, respectively), are characterized by distinctive types of genetic instability and molecular alterations. Four major molecular mechanisms that play a role in type I tumorigenesis are: (1) silencing of the PTEN tumor suppressor gene; (2) the presence of microsatellite instability due to alterations of the mismatch repair genes; (3) mutation of the K-ras proto-oncogene; and (4) alteration of the β-catenin gene. On the other hand, p53 mutations and overexpression of the Her2/neu oncogene are two major genetic alterations in type II carcinomas. Endometrial carcinomas may rarely present with hybrid features of both type I and type II cancers.

Staging describes the extent or spread of the disease at the time of diagnosis, and helps determine the choice of adjuvant therapy and assign prognosis (Figure 14-1). Despite the prevalence of this disease, the optimal surgical management of endometrial cancer remains controversial. Standard-of-care management for early-stage disease includes a primary surgical staging procedure (an adequate midline vertical incision, peritoneal washings, exploration of the abdominal and pelvic cavities, total abdominal hysterectomy, bilateral salpingo-oophorectomy, and a bilateral pelvic and para-aortic lymph node assessment). In 1988, the International Federation of Gynecology and Obstetrics (FIGO) changed the staging of endometrial cancer to include pelvic and para-aortic lymphadenectomy in recognition that the lymph node status is one of the most important prognostic factors. Whether to perform a comprehensive surgical staging procedure on every early-stage patient is controversial. Because of the unreliability of both intraoperative endometrial cavity inspection and frozen section analysis, it is our opinion that thorough surgical staging is essential for the treatment of surgically-fit patients with early-stage endometrial cancer.

The role of minimally invasive surgery in the management of endometrial cancer is evolving. Laparoscopy is rapidly becoming an alternative standard of care for the

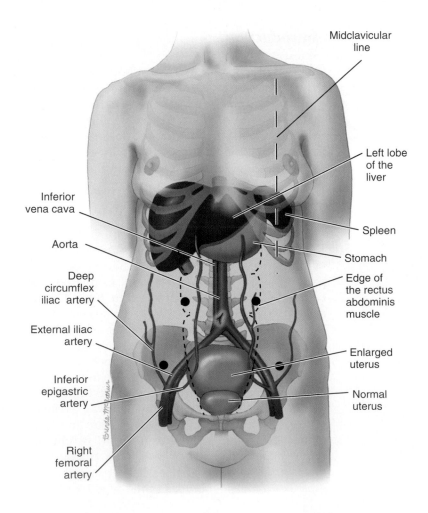

Figure 14-1. Port sites for conventional laparoscopic oncologic procedures: Trocar distribution for endometrial cancer staging procedure. Trocars are placed in the right and the left lateral lower quadrants, along with 12 mm trocars 1.5 to 2.0 cm superior and to the right of the umbilicus and 1.5 to 2.0 cm superior and to the left of the umbilicus.

management of type 1, early-stage endometrial cancer. Numerous studies have reported their findings on the laparoscopic approach. These studies collectively demonstrate that endometrial cancer patients who undergo minimally invasive surgery have a similar or increased number of lymph nodes removed, with comparable operating time, shorter hospital stay, improved quality of life, faster return to daily activities and work, and similar perioperative morbidity. More importantly, long-term recurrence and survival outcomes do not appear to be different. Preliminary data from the largest, randomized trial conducted to date (the LAP2 study from the Gynecologic Oncology Group) demonstrates that operative morbidity is significantly decreased and quality-of-life outcomes are significantly improved in the first 6 months after surgery in patients who undergo staging by laparoscopy versus laparatomy.

Upwards of 50% to 80% of women with endometrial cancer are obese, and many possess obesity-driven comorbidities including heart disease, hypertension, diabetes, renal disease, and arthritis. The performance of an endometrial cancer surgical staging procedure can be technically challenging in a morbidly obese woman. Moreover, a patient's comorbidities put her at significant risk for perioperative morbidity. Therefore, a surgical procedure that minimizes duration under anesthesia and operative morbidity for a patient is preferable in this patient cohort. Most of these women can be safely managed with minimally invasive surgery with overall excellent surgical outcome, shorter hospitalization, and less postoperative pain than those managed through laparotomy.

However, in a recent survey of gynecologic oncologists to evaluate treatment patterns for endometrial cancer, only 49% of gynecologic oncologists that responded to the survey stated that they used laparoscopy to stage endometrial cancer, and less than 8% regularly employed laparoscopy to stage their patients. Some concerns cited for the limited use of laparoscopy in this setting included longer operative times, a steep learning curve to adopt minimally invasive techniques, and a lack of training for surgeons who had already completed formal medical training. An alternative technology to help overcome many of the perceived obstacles of conventional laparoscopy is robotic-assisted technology. The da Vinci Surgical System (Intuitive Surgical Inc., Sunnyvale, California) is currently the only robotic surgical platform commercially available and FDA-approved for performing gynecologic oncology procedures. Introduced in 1999, the da Vinci is comprised of three elements: the surgical cart, the vision system, and the surgeon console. The surgical cart is composed of three to four arms for controlling a 12-mm camera and three surgical instruments. The improved optics, three-dimensional imaging, and increased dexterity with wristed instruments offer some advantages to the surgeon compared to conventional laparoscopy, although there are many gynecologic oncologists trained in minimally invasive techniques who still perform staging via conventional laparoscopic means. Here we describe a case of an endometrial cancer patient who was treated by conventional laparoscopic surgery.

Case 1: Laparoscopic Management of Endometrial Cancer

 View DVD: Video 14-1

A 65-year-old woman, gravida 2 para 2002, with a BMI of 30 and a history of hypertension, presents to her gynecologist with vaginal bleeding of 3 months duration. Pertinent history includes annual, normal Pap smears and a family history significant for breast cancer in a maternal grandmother. Her medications include a beta-blocker and multivitamin, she does not smoke or drink alcohol, and she does not exercise regularly. On physical examination, her vital signs are within normal limits. On speculum examination, the vaginal mucosa is smooth and normal in appearance, the cervix is without lesions and there is some blood in the vaginal vault. Her uterus is 6 to 8 weeks in size and nontender, and rectovaginal examination reveals no parametrial thickening, or cul-de-sac nodularity. A pelvic ultrasound evaluation demonstrates a thickened endometrial lining measuring 16 mm. An endometrial biopsy and endocervical sampling are performed, revealing a moderately-differentiated (grade 2) adenocarcinoma of the endometrium, endometrioid type, with negative endocervical currettings. A serum CA-125 is 15. The natural history and biology of the disease are discussed with the patient in detail. The rationale, risks, benefits, and alternatives of a total

Continued

Case 1: Laparoscopic Management of Endometrial Cancer—cont'd

laparoscopic hysterectomy, bilateral salpingo-oophorectomy, washings, and pelvic and para-aortic lymph node dissection are discussed with the patient.

Preoperative Evaluation

Preoperative testing includes a complete blood count and serum chemistries, as indicated by the patient's age and medical comorbidities. Any obesity-related and other comorbidities should be optimized preoperatively, and a screening ECG and chest x-ray are recommended in all women older than 50 years old.

Measurement of the serum tumor marker CA-125 is a clinically useful test for predicting more advanced-stage endometrial cancer, but is not a sensitive preoperative marker of extrauterine disease. In a prospective nonrandomized study of women with a diagnosis of endometrial cancer referred for staging, a CA-125 level of greater than 20 U/mL, a grade 3 tumor, or both, correctly identified 75% to 87% of women requiring lymphadenectomy. These results have been confirmed by others, but the optimal threshold (e.g., >20, >35,

or >40 U/mL) has not been determined. If initial serum CA-125 levels are elevated in a patient, the tumor marker may be most useful in following patients after initial treatment. An elevated preoperative value may prompt further evaluation by imaging with an abdominal-pelvic computed tomography scan (CT) or magnetic resonance imaging (MRI). Finally, we recommend bowel-prepping all patients undergoing laparoscopy where there is a likelihood of cancer, because it may facilitate decompression of the rectosigmoid colon, resulting in improved pelvic exposure during the case. This is especially important in morbidly obese women who may have significant visceral adiposity that makes pelvic exposure more difficult. A recent Cochrane review, however, questioned its utility in decreasing the frequency of bowel anastomosis breakdown or decreasing the frequency of peritoneal infection. All patients are at high risk for venous thromboembolism (VTE) and are therefore placed on unfractionated heparin (5000 units every 8 hours) or low-molecular-weight heparin (5000 units of dalteparin or enoxaparin 40 mg) and intermittent pneumatic compression devices.

Surgical Techniques

1. It is our practice to perform gynecologic oncology laparoscopic procedures in minimally invasive surgery suites (MISS). These are large operating rooms equipped with high-definition cameras, ceiling-mounted high-definition screens, and laparoscopic towers. These suites allow surgeons to perform complex laparoscopic operations and procedures like high para-aortic node dissections with minimal operating room flow disruption.

2. Proper patient positioning is critical. The patient must be secured to the operating table with a positioning pad, such as back-bubble padding, gel padding, a bean bag, or shoulder padding blades to prevent slippage on the table during steep Trendelenburg position. The steep Trendelenburg position is tested to ensure the patient does not move and can tolerate the position in terms of mechanical ventilation.

3. To enhance surgeon ergonomics and prevent patient injury, the patient's arms are tucked against her sides, palms turned inward with arm-extenders. Extra padding at the elbows and wrists provides support and helps prevent neuropathies.

4. Yellofins are used to position the legs in a dorsal lithotomy position. We ensure that the patient's buttocks are positioned at least 2 inches beyond the end of the bed so that uterine manipulation and access to the vagina can be accomplished with greater ease. Padding is used to protect tucked arms, hands, elbows, and knees.

5. A uterine exam under anesthesia or preoperative pelvic ultrasound can help determine the proper Koh tip to use for the case.

6. The patient is then prepped and draped. An orogastric tube is inserted in order to decompress the stomach. A Foley catheter is placed into the bladder. An exam under anesthesia is performed and the uterus is sounded and dilated.

7. Depending on the size of the cervix, a KOH colpotomizer (Cooper Surgical, Trumbull, CT) and Rumi uterine manipulator are then placed on the cervix.

8. The abdominal/peritoneal cavity is then entered. The initial camera trocar is placed 1.5 to 2.0 cm above the base of the umbilicus or 20 to 25 cm from the symphysis pubis. Because the majority of our endometrial cancer patients are

obese, we recommend using either an open Hasson entry technique or direct insertion technique to place the 12 mm camera trocar. Three additional trocars, 5- to 12-mm in size, are then placed under direct laparoscopic visualization, with two trocars about 20 degrees and 10 cm away from the camera trocar, and a left paraumbilical trocar (Figure 14-2).

9. Washings are performed. The entire peritoneal cavity is inspected. The dissection begins by transecting the round ligament to access the retroperitoneal space. The paravesical and pararectal spaces are developed and the retroperitoneal structures identified.

10. The ureter is identified and dissected away from the ovarian ligament/vessels. Then the infundibulopelvic ligament of the ovary is skeletonized and transected. The laparoscopic hysterectomy is performed in the usual fashion (see Chapter 8).

11. It is our practice to stage all patients with endometrial cancer, when medically feasible. The anatomical margins for the pelvic lymph node dissection are the following: medially, the ureter; laterally, the body of the psoas muscle and genitofemoral nerve; posteriorly, the obturator nerve; inferiorly, the circumflex iliac vein; and cephalad, 2 cm above the bifurcation of the common iliac artery (Figure 14-3).

12. The dissection begins by identifying the external iliac artery (Figure 14-3). The nodal tissue should be gently handled with atraumatic graspers (see Video 14-1 📹). Maryland graspers or a surgical aspirator are useful to help develop the retroperitoneal planes. The energy source utilized during the node dissection as well as technique varies widely among surgeons and will depend on a surgeon's skill and level of comfort with the energy modality. It is our practice to utilize either the harmonic scalpel or monopolar endoshears for node dissection.

13. The uppermost boundary of the para-aortic dissection is usually at the level of the inferior mesenteric artery, but for high-risk endometrial lesions, higher aortic dissections, omentectomy, and peritoneal biopsies are recommended. The aortic

Figure 14-2. Potential sites of nodal involvement in endometrial and cervical cancers.

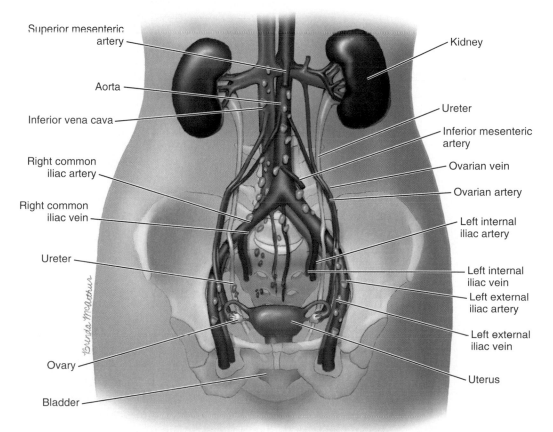

Superior mesenteric artery

Aorta

Inferior vena cava

Right common iliac artery

Right common iliac vein

Ureter

Ovary

Bladder

Kidney

Ureter

Inferior mesenteric artery

Ovarian vein

Ovarian artery

Left internal iliac artery

Left internal iliac vein

Left external iliac artery

Left external iliac vein

Uterus

Figure 14-3. Pelvic and para-aortic lymphadenectomy: The borders of the lymph node dissection are defined by specific anatomic sites. From lateral to medial: psoas muscle (with the genitofemoral nerve), external iliac vessels, and obturator space (with obturator nerve); from caudad to cephalad: the circumflex iliac vessels to 2 cm above the bifurcation of the common iliac artery. The uppermost boundary of the para-aortic dissection is usually at the level of the inferior mesenteric artery.

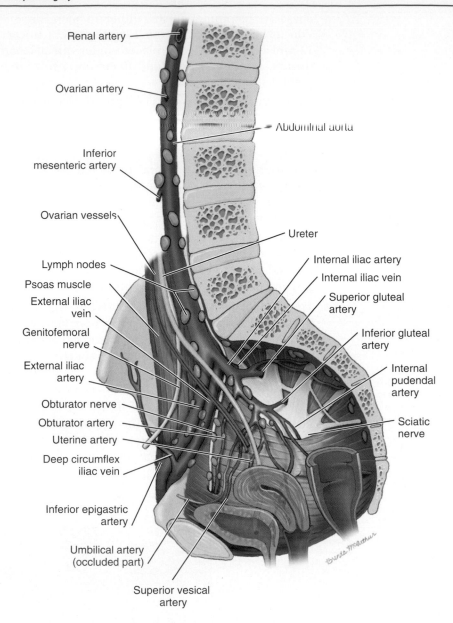

dissection (see Video 14-1 📹) begins by carefully dissecting on top of the lower aorta after identifying the pertinent anatomy. The dissection proceeds cephalad, usually to the level of the inferior mesenteric artery.

14. The nodal specimens are removed in separate Endocatch bags and are identified by region (pelvic vs. para-aortic) and by hemipelvis (right vs. left).

(See Video 14-1 📹)

Cervical Cancer

Cervical cancer is the second most common malignancy in women worldwide, and it remains a leading cause of cancer-related death for women in developing countries. In the United States, cervical cancer is relatively uncommon. The incidence of invasive cervical cancer has declined steadily in the U.S. over the past few decades; however, it continues to rise in many developing countries. The change in the epidemiological trend domestically has been attributed to mass screening with Papanicolaou tests. Internationally, 500,000 new cases of cervical cancer are diagnosed each year, 11,000 of which are detected in the U.S. The most common sign of cervical cancer is a grossly visible lesion upon a vaginal speculum examination. In addition, more than 50,000 cases of carcinoma in situ are diagnosed each year domestically. Of the 11,150 U.S. patients with cervical cancer, 3670 will die from their disease each year. This represents 1.3% of all cancer deaths and 6.5% of deaths from gynecologic cancers.

Treatment for early-stage cervical cancer involves either a simple or radical hysterectomy (most commonly, type II or III) and pelvic ± para-aortic lymphadenectomy. Radical hysterectomy is indicated for patients with FIGO stage IA2 to IIA cervical cancer who are surgically fit enough to tolerate an aggressive surgery and wish to avoid the long-term adverse effects of radiation therapy. Prospective randomized trials have validated equal curative rates from radical surgery and radiotherapy (overall survival similar at 83%). Radical hysterectomy refers to the excision of the uterus en bloc with the parametrium (i.e., the round, broad, cardinal, and uterosacral ligaments), and the upper one third to one half of the vagina (Figure 14-4). In addition to a radical hysterectomy, ovarian preservation with extrapelvic oophoropexy is often performed in premenopausal women if there is no evidence of metastatic disease to the ovaries. In postmenopausal women, it is common practice to perform a bilateral salpingo-ooporectomy at the time of hysterectomy.

During the past decade, however, there have been several studies demonstrating that total laparoscopic or robotic-assisted radical hysterectomy are both feasible and safe in selected cervical cancer patients. Laparoscopic radical hysterectomy was ini-

Figure 14-4. Tissue removed en bloc at the time of a radical hysterectomy, note that it includes the upper vagina and the tissue around the uterus (*dashed lines*).

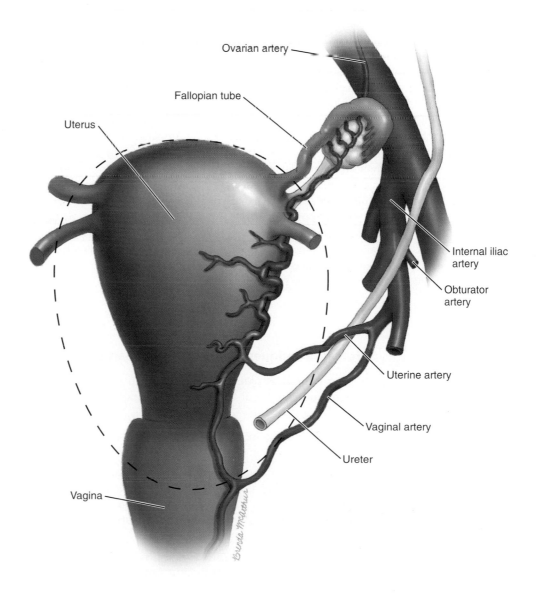

tially described by Canis and coworkers and Nezhat and colleagues in the 1990s. Numerous reports since that time have shown that hospital stay, quality of life, and operative morbidity are improved with minimally invasive versus open hysterectomy techniques, without compromising long-term oncologic outcomes. Although radical hysterectomy can be safely performed by conventional laparoscopy by experienced surgeons, there are advantages to performing the procedure robotically. The three-dimensional view, tremor control, and articulating instruments can enhance the surgical precision required for this procedure.

Case 2: Laparoscopic Radical Hysterectomy

 View DVD: Video 14-2

A 45-year-old woman, gravida 5 para 5, with a history of smoking and no regular gynecologic care for the past 10 years, presents to the office complaining of vaginal bleeding after intercourse and a foul vaginal odor. She denies fevers, chills, abdominal pain, dysuria or hematuria, back or leg pain, and reports other than postcoital bleeding, regular 28-day menstrual cycles with normal flow. She has no other medical problems and no past surgical history; she does recall having an abnormal Pap smear during her last pregnancy, but did not follow up with a physician postpartum. Her BMI is 23 and her vitals are normal. She is well-appearing, her skin is without rashes or lesions, and her neck and supraclavicular region are without adenopathy. Her lung, heart, and abdominal exams are unremarkable. Her external genitalia, urethral meatus, and anus appear normal, but on speculum exam, a 2 × 2 cm fungating lesion is visualized on the anterior lip of the cervix. On rectovaginal exam, the lesion appears confined to her firm but mobile cervix and there is no evidence of parametrial thickening or pelvic masses. A cervical biopsy reveals a moderately differentiated squamous cell cancer. A pelvic ultrasound reveals no hydronephrosis and no pelvic masses. A PET-CT scan reveals FDG uptake only in the cervix. The patient is diagnosed with Stage IB1 cervical carcinoma and is

counseled on primary therapy with a radical hysterectomy and pelvic lymphadenectomy. She is an excellent candidate for total laparoscopic radical hysterectomy and consents to the procedure.

Preoperative Evaluation

Preoperative testing includes a complete blood count and serum chemistries, as indicated by the patient's age and medical comorbidities. Any comorbidities should be optimized preoperatively, and a screening ECG and chest x-ray are recommended in all women older than 50 years. Either CT, MRI, or PET-CT scan is recommended to assess the cervical tumor size and evaluate for metastatic disease. Whereas MRI is the most sensitive tool for visualizing the cervical tumor, a PET-CT is most sensitive for identifying 1-cm nodal metastases. Furthermore, if a PET-CT is not performed, a chest x-ray is also recommended in premenopausal women to rule out lung metastases. Any evidence of metastatic disease would likely result in aborting the radical hysterectomy procedure, although there is accumulating data that primary excision of bulky lymph nodes can improve outcomes for patients. A technique for conventional laparoscopic type III radical hysterectomy and pelvic lymphadenectomy is described here. A technique for robotic-assisted radical hysterectomy is illustrated in Video 14-2 .

Surgical Techniques: Conventional Laparoscopic Radical Hysterectomy

1. The patient is placed in the dorsal lithotomy position in Allen stirrups, with her arms positioned at her sides, as described earlier for endometrial cancer.

2. A Rumi-Koh or V-Care uterine manipulator and Foley catheter are placed.

3. The anesthesiologist places an orogastric or nasogastric tube to decompress the stomach.

4. A 12-mm, direct-entry trocar is placed at the level of the umbilicus or 1.5 to 2.0 cm superior and to the right of the umbilicus. (Note: in patients with a prior midline vertical incision, initial access into the abdominal cavity is achieved at the umbilicus through an open Hasson technique or in the left upper quadrant with a direct or Veress needle technique.

5. Three additional 12-mm trocars are placed under direct visualization in the left paraumbilical region and right and left lower quadrants, as described in endome-

trial cancer staging section. If performed as a robotic radical hysterectomy, trocar distribution is demonstrated in Figure 14-7 and Video 13-1.

6. The patient is placed in steep Trendelenburg position and the abdominal cavity and pelvis are explored to rule out extracervical disease.

7. The round ligaments are ligated and divided bilaterally with either a harmonic scalpel or monopolar Endoshears, and the peritoneum lateral to the infundibulo-pelvic ligament is incised to gain access to the retroperitoneal space.

8. The ureter is visualized and a pelvic lymphadenectomy is performed bilaterally, as previously described for the endometrial cancer staging procedure. The lymph node–bearing tissue from each hemipelvis is placed in separate Endocatch bags and removed through one of the lower quadrant ports. Any suspicious-appearing nodes are sent for frozen section analysis.

9. If any lymph nodes are positive for metastatic disease, the procedure is aborted.

10. The paravesical and pararectal spaces are then developed (Figure 14-5).

11. Bilateral ureterolysis is performed, and the uterine artery and vein in each hemipelvis are identified crossing over the distal ureter and ligated at their origin from the anterior division of the internal iliac vessels (Figure 14-6).

12. A bladder flap is created and it is mobilized inferiorly.

13. The ureters are dissected until their insertion into the bladder bilaterally, and any uterine or parametrial tissue medial to this is resected en bloc with the uterus. The vesicouterine peritoneum is further mobilized to obtain adequate vaginal margins.

14. The utero-ovarian ligaments are transected if ovarian preservation is performed.

15. The uterus is then anteflexed with the manipulator and the peritoneum overlying the rectovaginal junction is incised. The rectovaginal space is developed.

16. The uterosacral ligaments are then divided at their midpoint, exactly halfway between the sacrum and their origin in the posterior uterus.

17. The en bloc specimen (uterus, cervix parametria, upper one third of vagina) is removed by making a circumferential colpotomy along the distal aspect of the Koh colpotomizing cup.

18. The vaginal cuff is sutured laparoscopically with 4 or 5 interrupted 0-Vicryl sutures.

Surgical Techniques: Robotic-Assisted Radical Hysterectomy

1. Perform steps 1 through 3 as described earlier for conventional laparoscopy.

2. A 12-mm direct-insertion trocar is placed in the midline, approximately 2 cm above the umbilicus (Figure 14-7).

3. CO_2 gas is attached to the trocar once intraperitoneal access is confirmed, and the patient is placed in steep Trendelenburg position.

4. Two 8-mm robotic trocars are placed 10 cm to the left and right of the supraumbilical port and 15 degrees more inferiorly. A 12-mm assistant trocar and an 8 mm robotic trocar are then placed in the right and left lower quadrants, respectively, at least 10 cm away from and 15 degrees more inferiorly to the two previously-placed robotic trocars. These lower quadrant trocars should be placed as laterally as possible to maximize instrument mobility in the pelvis.

5. The robotic surgical cart is then positioned between the patient's legs and the robotics arms and camera are docked. An Endowrist monopolar shears is placed in the right robotic trocar and an Endowrist Maryland bipolar instrument is placed in the left robotic trocar. An atraumatic Endowrist tool can be placed in the trocar of the fourth robotic arm.

6. Steps 6 through 18 are performed as described for the conventional laparoscopic radical hysterectomy.

(See Video 14-2 📹)

Figure 14-5. A, The dissection of the paravesical space (*green shading*) has specific anatomic landmarks that include the obliterated umbilical artery medially, the obturator muscle and vessels laterally, the cardinal ligament posteriorly, and the pubic symphysis anteriorly. **B,** The dissection of the pararectal space has specific anatomic landmarks including the rectum and ureter laterally, the internal iliac artery laterally, the sacrum posteriorly, and the cardinal ligaments anteriorly. This space (*green*) is usually dissected bluntly.

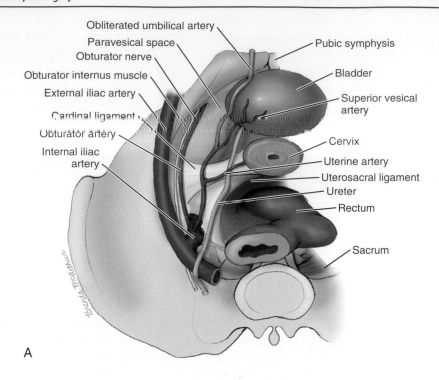

A

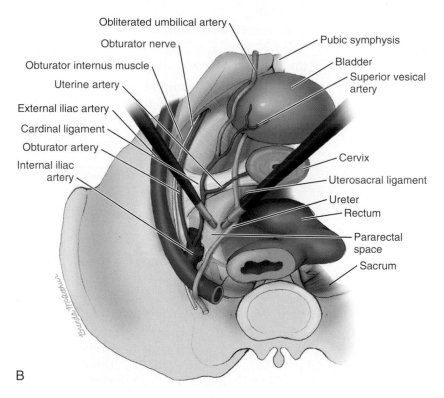

B

Figure 14-6. The uterine artery should be ligated or coagulated at its origin on the anterior division (trunk) of the internal iliac artery.

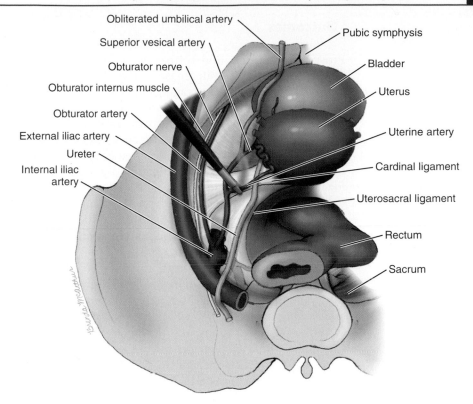

Obliterated umbilical artery
Superior vesical artery
Obturator nerve
Obturator internus muscle
Obturator artery
External iliac artery
Ureter
Internal iliac artery

Pubic symphysis
Bladder
Uterus
Uterine artery
Cardinal ligament
Uterosacral ligament
Rectum
Sacrum

Figure 14-7. Port placement for robotic laparoscopic surgery. The robotic trocar for the introduction of the laparoscope is placed 2 to 3 cm above the umbilicus—typically 20 to 25 cm from the pubic symphysis.

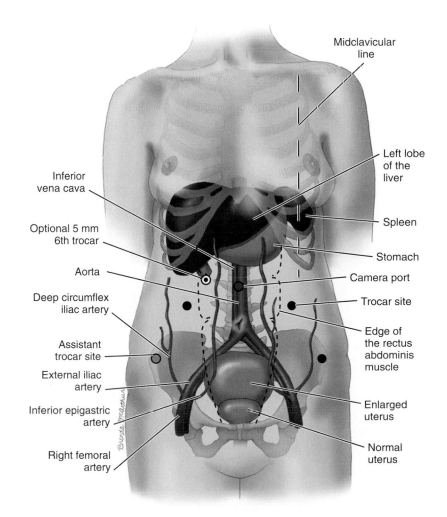

Midclavicular line

Inferior vena cava
Optional 5 mm 6th trocar
Aorta
Deep circumflex iliac artery
Assistant trocar site
External iliac artery
Inferior epigastric artery
Right femoral artery

Left lobe of the liver
Spleen
Stomach
Camera port
Trocar site
Edge of the rectus abdominis muscle
Enlarged uterus
Normal uterus

Outcomes

Prospective studies and retrospective reviews have demonstrated consistent patient benefit in the form of decreased morbidity with similar oncologic outcomes for those treated by laparoscopic staging versus open staging procedures. Simple and radical hysterectomies as well as pelvic and para-aortic lymph node dissection have been shown to be feasible when performed by conventional or robotic-assisted techniques. However, there is a steep learning curve to master these techniques. The complication rates for laparoscopic and robotic hysterectomy were detailed in previous chapters of this text. Seamon and colleagues recently reported on the learning curve and outcomes for the first 105 endometrial cancer patients who underwent robotic hysterectomy and pelvic-aortic lymphadenectomy at The Ohio State University and determined that 20 procedures are needed to acquire proficiency with this technique. However, these were gynecologic oncologists with extensive experience performing this procedure with both open and conventional laparoscopy.

The question also remains that if laparoscopy is evolving into an alternative standard of care for the treatment of endometrial and cervical cancers, what is the optimal laparoscopic approach? This matter is particularly relevant in morbidly-obese women, in whom surgery of any type can be challenging. In a retrospective review of various laparoscopic approaches performed in 100 obese endometrial cancer patients at the Cleveland Clinic, Fader and coworkers demonstrated that total laparoscopic hysterectomy may be more feasible to perform (in terms of operative time and blood loss) than laparoscopic-assisted vaginal hysterectomy. Furthermore, Boggess and coauthors recently compared outcomes in women who underwent endometrial cancer staging by either laparotomy (TAH, n = 138), total laparoscopic hysterectomy (TLH, n = 81) or by robotic-assisted techniques (TRH, n = 103). Despite the TRH patients having a higher BMI than the TLH patients ($P = .0008$), the lymph node yield was highest for TRH ($P < .0001$) and hospital stay ($P < .0001$) and estimated blood loss ($P < .0001$) were lowest for this cohort. Operative time was longest for TLH (213.4 minutes), followed by TRH (191.2 minutes), and then TAH (146.5 minutes; $P < .0001$. However, postoperative complication rates were lower for TRH compared with TAH (5.9% vs. 29.7%; $P < .0001$). Conversion rates for the robotic and laparoscopic groups were similar. The group concluded that TRH with staging is feasible and preferable over TAH, and may be preferable over TLH in women with endometrial cancer.

SUMMARY: In conclusion, laparoscopy is an exciting alternative surgical approach for the treatment of gynecologic malignancies. Its overall safety and efficacy as a surgical method have been well-documented, but further study is necessary to determine the optimal laparoscopic approach in both thin and obese women and to determine long-term oncologic outcomes.

Suggested Reading

American Cancer Society: Cancer Facts & Figures 2008. Atlanta, American Cancer Society, 2008.

Bats AS, Chatellier G, Clément D, Larousserie F, Lefrère-Belda MA, Lecuru F, Nos C: Comparison of different approaches in surgical management of early endometrial cancer, *Bull Cancer* 94:1003-1007, 2007.

Bell MC, Torgerson J, Seshadri-Kreaden U, Suttle AW, Hunt S: Comparison of outcomes and cost for endometrial cancer staging via traditional laparotomy, standard laparoscopy and robotic techniques, *Gynecol Oncol* 111:407-411, 2008.

Benedet JL, Odicino F, Maisonneuve P, et al: Carcinoma of the cervix uteri, *J Epidemiol Biostat* 6:7-43, 2001.

Boggess J, Gehrig P, Cantrell L, et al: A comparative study of 3 surgical methods for hysterectomy with staging for endometrial cancer: robotic assistance, laparoscopy, laparotomy, *Am J Obstet Gynecol* 199:360.e1-9, 2008.

Bokhman JV: Two pathogenetic types of endometrial carcinoma, *Gynecol Oncol* 15:10-17, 1983.

Campion MJ: Preinvasive disease. In: Berek JS, Hacker NF: *Practical Gynecologic Oncology*, ed 4, Elsevier, Philadelphia, PA, 2005.

Chee JJ, Ho TH, Tay EH, Low JJH, Yam KL: Endometrioid adenocarcinoma of the uterus: surgico-pathological correlations and role of pelvic lymphadenectomy, *Ann Acad Med Singapore* 32:670-675, 2003.

Creasman WT, Zaino RJ, Major FJ, et al: Early invasive carcinoma of the cervix (3 to 5 mm invasion): risk factors and prognosis, a Gynecologic Oncology Group study, *Am J Obstet Gynecol* 178:62-65, 1998.

Eltabbakh GH, Shamonki MI, Moody JM, Garafano LL: Hysterectomy for obese women with endometrial cancer: laparoscopy or laparotomy? *Gynecol Oncol* 78:329-335, 2000.

Fader AN, Michener CM, Frasure HE, et al: Total laparoscopic hysterectomy versus laparoscopic-assisted vaginal hysterectomy in endometrial cancer: surgical and survival outcomes, *J Minim Invasive Gynecol* 16:333-339, 2009.

Franco EL, Duarte-Franco E, Ferenczy A: Cervical cancer: epidemiology, prevention and the role of human papillomavirus infection, *CMAJ* 164:1017-1025, 2001.

Gehrig PA, Cantrell LA, Shafer A, Abaid LN, Mendivil A, Boggess JF: What is the optimal minimally-invasive surgical procedure for endometrial cancer staging in the obese and morbidly obese woman? *Gynecol Oncol* 111:41-45, 2008.

Greenlee RT, Hill-Harmon MB, Murray T, Thun M: Cancer statistics, 2001, *CA Cancer J Clin* 51:15-36, 2001.

Jemal A, Murray T, Ward E, et al: Cancer statistics, 2005, *CA J Clin* 55:10-30, 2005.

Kalogiannidis I, Lambrechts S, Amant F, Neven P, Van Gorp T, Vergote I: Laparoscopy-assisted vaginal hysterectomy compared with abdominal hysterectomy in clinical stage I endometrial cancer: safety, recurrence, and long-term outcome, *Am J Obstet Gynecol* 196:248.e1-e8, 2007.

Landoni F, Maneo A, Colombo A, et al: Randomised study of radical surgery versus radiotherapy for stage Ib-IIa cervical cancer, *Lancet* 350:535-540, 1997.

Liu FS: Molecular carcinogenesis of endometrial cancer, *Taiwan J Obstet Gynecol* 46:26-32, 2007.

Nezhat F, Yadav J, Rahaman J, Gretz H, Cohen C: Analysis of survival after laparoscopic management of endometrial cancer, *J Minim Invasive Gynecol* 15:181-187, 2008.

Pecorelli S, Benedet JL, Creasman WT, Shepherd JH: FIGO staging of gynecologic cancer, 1994 1997 FIGO Committee on Gynecologic Oncology, International Federation of Gynecology and Obstetrics, *Int J Gynaecol Obstet* 64:5-10, 1999.

Scribner DR Jr, Mannel RS, Walker JL, Johnson GA: Cost analysis of laparoscopy versus laparotomy for early endometrial cancer, *Gynecol Oncol* 75:460-463, 1999.

Seamon LG, Cohn D, Richardson DL, et al: Robotic hysterectomy and para-aortic lymphadenectomy for endometrial cancer, *Obstet Gynecol* 112:1207-1213, 2008.

Spirtos NM, Schlaerth JB, Kimball RE, et al: Laparoscopic radical hysterectomy (type III) with aortic and pelvic lymphadenectomy, *Am J Obstet Gynecol* 174:1763-1767, 1996.

Complications of Laparoscopic Surgery

15

Jeffrey M. Goldberg M.D.
Chi Chiung Grace Chen M.D.
Tommaso Falcone M.D.

 Video Clips on DVD

15-1 Laparoscopic Management of Cystotomy (2 minutes/40 seconds)

15-2 Laparoscopic Ureteral Reimplantation (11 minutes/9 seconds)

Introduction

Intraoperative or perioperative complications from laparoscopic gynecologic surgery are uncommon, with overall rates ranging from 0.1% to 10%. A meta-analysis of 27 prospective randomized, controlled trials, comparing 1809 women treated by laparoscopy with 1802 treated by laparotomy for benign gynecologic conditions, found no greater rate of major or minor complications in the laparoscopic group. Given the rare occurrence of major complications, a randomized controlled trial would need over 10,000 subjects in each treatment arm to achieve 90% power to detect a difference in complications. Over half of these complications are related to the entry technique, and 20% to 25% of intraoperative complications were not detected intraoperatively.

Risk factors that lead to increased perioperative complication rates include extremes of body weight and any patient characteristics that could potentially increase the risk associated with anesthesia, such as a history of cardiopulmonary disease. Other factors that could potentially distort pelvic anatomy leading to a more complicated surgery include a past history of abdominopelvic surgery and the presence of intra-abdominal diseases such as endometriosis, pelvic inflammatory disease, or pelvic adhesions. Complication rates were found to be higher for operative or major laparoscopic procedures than for diagnostic or minor laparoscopic procedures, 0.1% to 18% versus 0.1% to 7%, respectively.

As expected, complication rates are also related to the surgeon's experience, with one study demonstrating a three-fold to five-fold increase in inadequately trained urologic surgeons incurring at least one complication, compared with surgeons with more training. Another study reported that the major complication rate decreased from 1.59% [95% CI 1.07%–2.36%] in 1507 gynecologic laparoscopic surgeries performed from 1992 through 1999 to 0.72% [95% CI 0.51%–1.02%] in 4307 undergoing surgery between 2000 and 2006. Additionally, surgeons without a skilled surgical assistant or those in single practice were also five and eight times more likely to incur a complication, respectively.

Finally, faulty instrumentation can predispose to unnecessary injury. Dull trocars require greater force to enter the peritoneal cavity, increasing the risk of injury. Anything that compromises visualization, such as damaged laparoscope lenses, broken fiberoptic cables in the scope or light cable, and low-resolution monitors, places the patient in peril. Low-flow insufflators and cracked gaskets can lead to loss of pneumoperitoneum and reduced exposure. All electrosurgical instruments should be checked for defects in insulation that can cause an unrecognized bowel burn.

Anesthetic Considerations

The CO_2 pneumoperitoneum and Trendelenburg position induce numerous physiologic responses that are generally well tolerated by young healthy patients but which may be hazardous to those with compromised cardiopulmonary function. All patients should be monitored with blood pressure, temperature, ECG, pulse oximetry, end-tidal CO_2, minute ventilation, airway pressure, urine output, and muscle relaxation. Patients with cardiopulmonary disease may also require central hemodynamic and arterial blood gas monitoring.

Managing fluid balance may be difficult, as some patients start off dehydrated following a bowel prep and being NPO preoperatively. Blood loss is difficult to estimate, because bleeding looks magnified through the laparoscope and is also mixed with large volumes of irrigating fluid. The irrigating fluid may be absorbed leading to fluid overload. In addition, the pneumoperitoneum reduces the glomerular filtration rate and urine output by about 50% due to decreased renal cortical perfusion and increased antidiuretic hormone. The irrigating fluid should be warmed and a forced-air warming blanket placed over the patient's head and chest to prevent hypothermia. Hypothermia can predispose to hypokalemia and respiratory depression. The use of warmed humidified CO_2 for insufflation has been shown to reduce the incidence of hypothermia.

The pneumoperitoneum causes an increase in systemic and pulmonary vascular resistance. Intra-abdominal pressures above 15 mm Hg may compress the vena cava, leading to venous stasis in the lower extremities, reduced cardiac preload, and reduced cardiac output. Thus, both hypertension and hypotension may occur. The intra-abdominal pressure should be kept below 15 mm Hg whenever possible. Mechanical stretching of the peritoneum, as well as Veress needle or trocar insertion and manipulation of the pelvic organs, may cause vagal stimulation leading to significant bradycardia and bradyarrthymias. The procedure should be interrupted, the pneumoperitoneum released, and atropine administered.

The pneumoperitoneum also restricts diaphragmatic excursion and lung expansion, causing the peak inspiratory and mean airway pressures to increase. Pulmonary compliance and functional residual capacity are reduced. The above-mentioned changes can lead to ventilation-perfusion mismatch and intrapulmonary shunting with hypercapnea and hypoxemia. Intravascular absorption of the CO_2 pneumoperitoneum further adds to the hypercapnea, requiring an increase in the minute ventilation to prevent respiratory acidosis. Hypercapnea stimulates the sympathetic nervous system resulting in increases in systemic vascular resistance and blood pressure and heart rate, and sensitizes the myocardium to catecholamines, which may lead to tachyarrhythmias. Most of these changes are avoided with gasless laparoscopy using a mechanical lifting device.

The steep Trendelenburg position increases cardiac preload by elevating the lower extremities. The Trendelenburg position further increases intrathoracic pressure and compromises respiratory status. Obese patients and those with impaired pulmonary function tolerate Trendelenburg poorly. It may be necessary to reverse the Trendelenburg position and release the pneumoperitoneum if anesthesia is having difficulty adequately ventilating the patient. Lastly, the increased intra-abdominal pressure and Trendelenburg position predispose to aspiration of gastric contents, which is why all patients undergoing laparoscopy under general anesthesia require endotracheal intubation and an orogastric tube.

Two complications that impact anesthesia care are subcutaneous emphysema and CO_2 embolism. Subcutaneous emphysema results from preperitoneal insufflation. Increased CO_2 absorption from the large surface area may result in significant hypercapnea and respiratory acidosis requiring higher minute ventilation. When subcutaneous emphysema is detected over the neck and face by crepitus under the skin, there is concern that the gas can extend into the thorax leading to pneumoperitoneum and pneumomediastinum. Most cases can be managed by releasing the pnemoperitoneum, but a chest tube may be required in more severe cases, as this can lead to significant hypotension and cardiac arrest.

CO_2 embolism in gynecologic surgery is usually caused by insufflation of a large volume of gas through the Veress needle into a large vein. The air lock in the vena cava or right atrium results in inflow obstruction to the right heart causing sudden profound hypotension, hypoxia with cyanosis, and dysrhythmias or asystole. A precordial mill-wheel murmur may be auscultated. The following steps must be taken to prevent a lethal outcome. The pneumoperitoneum is released and 100% oxygen is administered with hyperventilation. The patient is placed in left lateral decubitus position in Trendelenburg, so the gas bubbles collect at the apex of the right ventricle and do not enter the pulmonary artery. The gas may be aspirated through a central venous catheter and cardiopulmonary resuscitation performed.

Neurologic Injury

Neurologic complications during laparoscopic surgery are uncommon, and primarily consist of peripheral nerve compression or stretch from improper positioning during the case. Risk factors for these complications include the duration of surgery, with one study suggesting that each additional hour in lithotomy increases the risk for lower extremity neuropathy by 100-fold. Other risk factors for neurologic compromise include patients with a body mass index of less than 20 kg/m² and pre-existing systemic conditions such as diabetes.

Upper extremity neuopathies from brachial plexus injury are estimated to occur in 0.16% of advanced laparoscopic cases. The use of shoulder braces with steep Trendelenburg position places downward force on the shoulder, which can result in Erb palsy or damage to the upper trunk, manifesting as weakness of the upper arm and sensory deficits extending to the lateral forearm. Hyperabduction of the arm can result in Klumpke palsy or damage to the lower trunk, manifesting as weakness of the hand and sensory deficits extending to the medial forearm.

To avoid upper extremity nerve injury, it is advisable to tuck the patient's arms at her side instead of keeping them outstretched on arm boards during laparoscopic cases. Sleds can be used if the patient is obese to ensure that the arms are tucked securely against the patient and will not fall off the operative table. Additionally, the use of shoulder braces should be avoided. However, if these braces must be used to secure the patient's position in steep Trendelenburg position, they should be positioned on the shoulder as laterally as possible on the acromioclavicular joint.

Lower extremity nerve injuries result primarily from improper patient positioning during lithotomy, leading to sensory and motor deficits in approximately 1.5% and 0.03%, respectively, of all surgical cases performed in lithotomy position. Specifically, the femoral nerve can be stretched and compressed as it passes under the inguinal ligament because of prolonged hip flexion, abduction, and external rotation. This can lead to decreased sensation of the anterior thigh and medial lower leg, with possible weakness of the quadriceps and absent patellar reflex. Patients with femoral neuropathies can also present with inability to extend the knee and difficulty with external rotation and abduction of the thigh. These patients can have difficulty standing from a seated position without using their arms and hands. Because the lateral femoral cutaneous nerve travels in a similar path to the femoral nerve, it can also be injured as it passes under the inguinal ligament. This is a solely sensory nerve and damage results in anesthesia and sometimes parethesias to the lateral thigh.

Another sensory nerve that may be damaged is the genitofemoral nerve, which lies on the belly of the psoas muscle. Injury to the genitofemoral nerve results in decreased sensation and paresthesia to the labia majora and upper medial thigh. Both of these nerves may be susceptible to injury during any lateral pelvic wall dissection, such as excision of a large pelvic mass adherent to the pelvic sidewall or external iliac lymph node dissection. Additionally, these nerves may also be damaged during mobilization of the sigmoid colon where the physiologic attachment of the sigmoid to the sidewall is released.

The obturator nerve can be stretched at the obturator foramen from prolonged hip flexion and abduction. This is sometimes seen after laparoscopic-assisted vaginal hysterectomy if the vaginal portion is difficult and prolonged. Direct injury to this nerve can also happen during laparoscopic obturator lymph node dissection, excision of retroperitoneal endometriosis implants, and dissection within the space of Retzius such as during paravaginal defect repairs or Burch colposuspension procedures. Damage to the obturator nerve can lead to decreased sensation of the medial thigh and inability to adduct the thigh resulting in ambulatory/gait difficulties.

The common peroneal nerve can be injured in lithotomy, either by direct compression of the lateral knee where the nerve wraps around the lateral fibula, or the nerve can be stretched from extended flexion of the knee with external hip rotation. Damage to this nerve can manifest as numbness over the anterior and lateral lower leg and dorsum of the foot as well as decreased dorsiflexion resulting in foot drop. Although uncommon, the sciatic nerve can also be compromised from prolonged hyperflexion and external rotation of the hips with the knees extended. Injury can lead to decreased sensation to the calf and lateral foot. Motor deficits can include foot drop and inability to flex the knee.

The key to preventing lower extremity peripheral nerve injury is attention to patient positioning. For most gynecologic laparoscopic procedures, the patients are placed in low lithotomy, with the legs placed in boot stirrups where the foot and posterior lower leg are cushioned and inadvertent external pressure to the legs can be avoided. Correct lithotomy position includes making sure that the hip is not hyperflexed, so the trunk to thigh angle should be between 60 and 170 degrees. The knee should be flexed and not extended, so that the thigh to calf angle is between 90 and 120 degrees. There should be minimal external hip rotation and the angle of the hip abduction should be no more than 90 degrees as measured between the inner thighs (Figure 15-1).

Besides compression and stretch of upper and lower extremity nerves from improper patient positioning, the ilioinguinal and iliohypogastric nerves can also be entrapped or injured during placement of lateral lower quadrant secondary laparoscopic ports. In a cadaveric study, the ilioinguinal nerve was found to enter the abdominal wall between the internal and external abdominal oblique muscles an average of 3.1 cm medial and 3.7 cm inferior to the anterior superior iliac spine. The iliohypogastric nerve travels along the anterior abdominal wall an average of 2.1 cm medial and 0.9 cm inferior to the anterior superior iliac spine. These patients usually present with burning pain from the incision radiating to the suprapubic, labial, or upper inner thigh area.

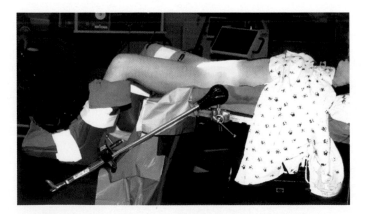

Figure 15-1. The patient's arms are tucked at her sides, there is minimal hip flexion and abduction, and the weight of the legs rests on the bottom of the feet in Allen stirrups. The hands and legs may require additional padding to avoid compression injuries. In addition to reducing neurologic injuries, this position affords the surgeon maximal access to the patient. Avoiding arm boards allows the surgeon to assume a comfortable stance. Keeping the hips in a neutral position eliminates interference with the thighs, particularly when operating cephalad to the pelvis such as when performing appendectomy, lysis of abdominal wall adhesions, or closing the umbilical port with the endo-stitch technique.

We recommend making the incisions for laparoscopic lower quadrant trocars approximately 2 cm cephalad and 2 cm medial to the anterior superior iliac spine. Also, whenever possible, the lower quadrant trocars should be limited to 5 mm. Closing the fascial incisions of larger trocar sites may cause nerve entrapment.

Most neurologic injuries from compression or stretch mechanisms can be conservatively managed and will usually resolve with supportive care. Patients suffering from isolated sensory loss without paresthesias, pain, or motor deficits can be reassured. Those that have paresthesias or pain can be administered tricyclic antidepressants, anticonvulsants, serotonin, and norepinephrine reuptake inhibitors, and/or GABA antagonists. Pain from injury to the iliohypogastric or ilioinguinal nerves can be managed with a nerve block with a local anesthetic. If this provides temporary relief, permanent relief can be attained from surgical resection of the nerves. A retrospective series reported complete pain relief in 70% of patients after this procedure. Motor deficits from nerve injury will usually warrant a neurologic consult. Treatment options often include physical therapy and the use of braces to assist in ambulation and to prevent additional injury.

Case 1: Neurologic injury

AB is a 29-year-old nulligravida with primary infertility. She had a laparoscopic treatment of stage III endometriosis several years ago for pelvic pain. A recent ultrasonogram revealed bilateral complex ovarian cysts measuring 5 to 6 cm consistent with endometriomas. Diagnostic hysteroscopy and laparoscopic ovarian cystectomies, extensive adhesiolysis, excision of peritoneal endometrosis, and chromotubation was performed.

At the time of surgery, the patient was positioned with her arms outstretched on arm boards due to obesity. The case took 4 hours and progressed without complications. Patient was discharged home the same day. On postoperative day 1, she called with new onset persistent numbness over the fourth and fifth fingers of the right hand and difficulty making a fist with the right hand. She was found to have decreased sensation over the medial forearm and hand to light touch and pin prick with 3/5 hand-squeeze strength. She also had 3/5 strength with wrist extension and elbow flexion. She was diagnosed with brachial plexus neuropathy, likely a mild Klumpke palsy. She was referred to occupational therapy. On her 6-week postoperative visit, her neuropathy symptoms were completely resolved and her neurologic examination was normal.

Discussion of Case

Although neurologic complications during laparoscopic surgery are uncommon, they primarily consist of peripheral nerve compression or stretch from improper positioning during surgery. The above scenario illustrates the importance of proper positioning of upper and lower extremities during laparoscopy, especially long cases. This patient should have had her arms tucked at her sides. If the arms cannot be tucked securely because of her large size relative to the size of the bed, sleds should be used.

Most neurologic complications resulting from stretch or compression of peripheral nerves can be managed conservatively. Mild motor deficits such as the above will usually improve or resolve with occupational or physical therapy. Mild sensory deficits will usually resolve with supportive care. Pharmacotherapy including tricyclic antidepressants, anticonvulsants, serotonin, and norepinephrine reuptake inhibitors, and/ or GABA antagonists can be used for paresthesias or pain symptoms. If the neurologic deficit is severe or cannot be explained, a neurologic consultation should be obtained.

Vascular Injury

The most frequent vascular injury is laceration of the superficial or inferior epigastric vessels during insertion of the lateral ancillary trocars. The inferior epigastrics can usually be visualized transperitoneally and the superficial epigastrics can be seen by transilluminating the abdominal wall with the laparoscope. The trocars are then inserted under direct vision, to avoid the vessels (Figure 15-2). Injury to the vessels can result in bleeding along the trocars into the operative field as well as abdominal wall hematoma formation.

Hemostasis may sometimes be achieved by using bipolar cautery through another port. Another option is to place a suture around the vessel above and below the port by using an Endo-close needle. The suture is then tied over the fascia but under the skin. This is the technique we recommend (Figure 15-3). Similarly, a large Keith needle

Figure 15-2. Trocar insertion in the right lower quadrant showing the trocar in relation to the abdominal wall anatomy.

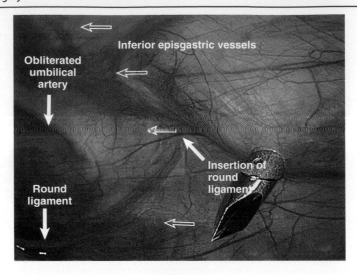

Figure 15-3. An Endo-close needle is used to place a suture around a lacerated abdominal wall vessel. The suture is tied with the trocar in place.

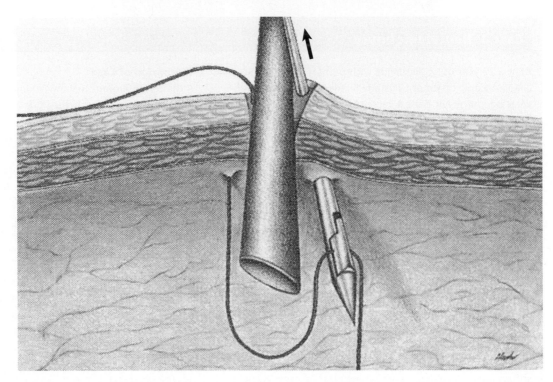

can be inserted through the abdominal wall, then, using a laparoscopic grasper, push the needle back out through the abdominal wall on the other side of the vessels. The suture is tied over a surgical sponge and removed at the end of the case while observing that there is no further bleeding.

Another alternative is to place a Foley catheter through the trocar and inflate the balloon. A Kelly clamp is then placed across the catheter at the abdominal wall so that the inflated balloon is pulled tight against the abdominal wall, compressing the vessels. It is quick and effective but use of that trocar site is lost (Figure 15-4). The surgeon should not leave the Foley in place to be removed postoperatively because the vessels may start bleeding again. Complete hemostasis must be assured at the end of the case and injured vessels completely occluded if persistent bleeding is noted. Because the inferior epigastric vessels are deep to the fascia, intraperitoneal bleeding may occur, with significant blood loss.

Pelvic bleeding can almost always be managed laparoscopically. Suction and irrigation will demonstrate the bleeding source to be coagulated. A 4 × 4 surgical sponge may be inserted through a 10-mm trocar to apply pressure to tamponade brisker bleeding within the pelvis. This will often stop the bleeding or at least provide better iden-

Figure 15-4. A Kelly clamp across the catheter maintains compression of the Foley balloon on the abdominal wall.

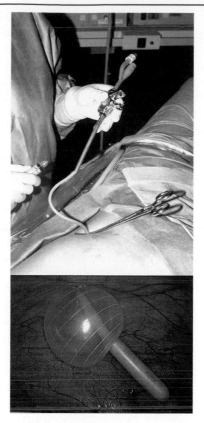

tification of the source for precise surgical control. Ligation of the uterine artery at its origin will usually control persistent bleeding. The anterior division of the internal iliac artery may also be ligated if necessary. It is important to always reduce the intraperitoneal pressure at the end of the case to assure hemostasis. Higher pressures from the pneumoperitoneum may compress small vessels which begin to bleed as the pressure decreases.

Injury to major vessels—aorta, vena cava, iliacs, and mesenteric vessels—is approximately 0.8% based on large series, but is likely to be underreported. Whereas the risk is fairly low, the mortality rate has been reported to be as high as 17%. Nearly all of the injuries occurred with initial insertion of the Veress needle or trocar. Major vessel injury is usually recognized by bleeding through the Veress needle or intraperitoneal bleeding. An expanding retroperitoneal hemorrhage may not be immediately obvious but should be at the top of the differential diagnosis list when a previously stable patient becomes hypotensive and tachycardic. Although there are case reports of laparoscopic management of major vessel injuries, the standard course of action is to perform an immediate laparotomy with a midline incision, apply direct pressure to the bleeding area, begin blood transfusion, and consult a vascular surgeon.

Bowel Injury

Bowel injuries are uncommon during laparoscopy, occurring at estimated rates of 0% to 0.5% with approximately one third to one half of these injuries incurring at the time of trocar insertion. Not surprisingly, injuries are more frequent in cases where the bowel is distended or there is a risk of bowel being adherent to the anterior abdominal wall, such as after prior laparotomy or pelvic inflammatory disease. Initial trocar entry in the left upper quadrant should be considered in these situations. An orogastric tube should always be inserted and the gastric contents aspirated to reduce the risk of GI injury. A small trocar perforation of the stomach may be managed with only nasogastric suction for 48 hours, as the stomach heals rapidly. The conventional wisdom of using a preoperative bowel prep has been challenged by the weight of evidence-based medicine.

The risk of bowel injury is also higher when dissection directly involves the bowel or the rectovaginal septum. In a series, from our institution, of laparoscopic excisions of rectovaginal or colorectal lesions, the perioperative complication rate was 10.3%, similar to what has been reported in the literature. The most common complication was inadvertent rectal injury at the time of rectovaginal dissection, despite the lack of endometriosis in the rectum itself. Bowel injuries are one of the most common causes of postoperative mortality from gynecologic laparoscopy because approximately two thirds of those injuries are unrecognized intraoperatively and there is often also a delay in postoperative diagnosis.

If not recognized intraoperatively, enterotomies from sharp dissection will usually manifest in 12 to 36 hours, whereas electrosurgical injuries will often not become evident for several days. Often patients with bowel injury after laparoscopic surgery may not present with the typical signs and symptoms of ruptured viscera. In a review of 266 laparoscopic urologic cases of bowel injury, Bishoff and colleagues found that most patients presented with low-grade temperature elevations, decreased or normal white blood cell counts, abdominal distention, and increasing abdominal pain or pain at the trocar sites. These patients may actually have normal bowel sounds with diarrhea. Peritoneal signs and gastrointestinal complaints such as nausea or vomiting were uncommon. Imaging modalities such as an upright abdominal radiograph, often useful for demonstrating free subdiaphragmatic air in the presence of perforated viscera, may not be useful after laparoscopy as it is often normal to see free air in the abdomen. Therefore, bowel injury should be suspected in any patient that presents with increased temperature, increasing abdominal pain and distention, other signs or symptoms of ileus, or increasing free air on consecutive upright abdominal radiographs after operative laparoscopy.

When a bowel injury is suspected or recognized, a colorectal or general surgeon should be consulted for assistance with management. The reported laparotomy rates in the literature for repair of bowel injuries diagnosed during or after laparoscopy is 52% to 90%. The route of repair will often depend upon the surgeon's experience and expertise, especially if the diagnosis is made intraoperatively. Injuries that are recognized postoperatively are generally managed with a laparotomy because the chances of further bowel injury from laparoscopic entry may be higher due to potentially dilated loops of bowel. However, cases of laparoscopy using the open entry have been successfully performed for repair of enterotomies.

Generally, serosal abrasions need not be repaired. Trauma to the muscularis or mucosa is usually repaired with a two-layered imbricating closure though some use a single layer closure. To avoid decreasing the caliber of the bowel lumen, the suture lines should be perpendicular to the long axis of the bowel. During electrosurgery, because the electrothermal damage is often wider than the actual enterotomy, care should be taken to make sure that at least a 1- to 2-cm margin of tissue is resected around the enterotomy to ensure the reapproximation of healthy tissue. Most cases of small or large bowel injury can either be repaired laparoscopically or by minilaparotomy, including segmental resection and primary reanastomosis, depending on the extent of injury. Even in cases of large bowel injury where the patient has not received a bowel preparation, a diverting colostomy is generally not indicated.

As bowel injury is often not recognized intraoperatively and may have an atypical presention postoperatively, it is one of the most common causes of postoperative mortality from laparoscopy. It is paramount that we improve our recognition of intraoperative bowel traumas. The bowel should be run laparoscopically if an injury is suspected. If an injury is noted, check the back wall to rule out a through and through injury. A proctosigmoidoscopy should be performed before removing the laparoscopic instruments in cases where the chance for sigmoid or rectal injury is increased, such as in cases of endometriosis involving the rectovaginal septum.

Another technique to check for sigmoid/rectal injury is to insert a large Foley catheter with a 30 cc balloon transanally and inflate the balloon. The proximal sigmoid is occluded with a bowel grasper and the patient placed in reverse Trendelenburg position. The pelvis is then filled with irrigating fluid so that the distal sigmoid/rectum is submersed. Air is then insufflated to distend the distal sigmoid/rectum. The presence of air bubbles in the fluid indicates a lack of bowel integrity. In a series of 262 patients that underwent operative laparoscopy for rectosigmoid endometriosis, 44 patients sustained a bowel injury. Although all the injuries were recognized intraoperatively, four injuries were identified only on performing the proctosigmoidoscopy.

Case 2: Bowel injury

LK is a 40-year-old woman, para 3003, undergoing total laparoscopic hysterectomy for symptomatic uterine fibroids. A laparoscopic myomectomy was performed 4 years ago and an open appendectomy 25 years ago. Ultrasound revealed an enlarged uterus, measuring 16 cm, with multiple fibroids within the myometrium distorting the endometrial canal. At the time of surgery, the uterus was 16 weeks size with multiple intramural and subserosal fibroids and there were small bowel adhesions to the uterine fundus. The small bowel was sharply dissected off the uterus and bowel integrity confirmed. The remainder of the hysterectomy was performed in the usual fashion using LigaSure (Valleylab, Boulder, CO) and monopolar scissors.

After the uterine vessels were secured, the uterus was amputated using a monopolar hook to better maneuver the remaining uterus and cervix. After dissecting down the bladder, an anterior colpotomy was performed and extended circumferentially until the remaining uterus and cervix were disconnected from the upper vagina. A morcellator was used to decrease the size of the uterus until the entire uterus and cervix were able to be removed from the abdomen through the vagina. At the completion of the case, the pelvis was carefully examined and noted to be hemostatic. A proctosigmoidoscopy was performed and the rectum and distal sigmoid noted to be intact and without injuries.

The patient did well postoperatively and was discharged home on postoperative day 1 after tolerating a regular diet. She presented to the emergency room on postoperative day 5 complaining of increased abdominal pain, nausea, vomiting, and subjective fevers and chills. She was found to have a temperature of 39° C with a heart rate of 120, respiratory rate of 30, and blood pressure of 80/50. Her abdomen was distended and extremely tender with guarding and rebound. Her white blood count was elevated with a left shift. General surgery was consulted and the decision was made to proceed with emergency laparotomy. This revealed multiple dilated loops of small bowel. After running the bowel,

a perforation, with leakage of bowel contents, was found in the ileum. The area of the enterotomy was surrounded by necrotic tissue. This segment of bowel was excised and healthy portions were reanastomosed. There were no complications. The patient did well from this surgery with normalization of vital signs and other objective parameters. She was discharged in stable condition on postoperative day 5.

Discussion of Case

Bowel injuries during laparoscopy are unusual. When they do occur, it is estimated that only one third of these injuries are recognized intraoperatively. The risk of bowel injury is higher if the operative dissection involves the bowel, the bowel is adherent near the operative area, or the dissection involves the rectovaginal septum. If unrecognized intraoperatively, enterotomies from sharp dissection will usually manifest in 12 to 36 hours, whereas electrosurgical injuries will not become apparent until several days later. In the above case, the patient did not become symptomatic from the enterotomy until a few days after surgery, indicating that the perforation was most likely due to an electrosurgical injury during the hysterectomy.

Although many patients with unrecognized bowel injury can present in an insidious or atypical manner, this patient presented classically with an acute abdomen. In this case, the patient was taken for emergency laparotomy without the need for confirmatory imaging studies. Most bowel injuries, except for small punctures from the Veress needle, will require repair. Sharp injury at the time of laparoscopy can usually be repaired by reapproximating the cut edges. However, because the area of electrothermal damage is often wider than the apparent injury, extra tissue should be resected around the margins to ensure reapproximation of healthy tissue. If the injury is not recognized until the postoperative period, usually segmental resection of bowel with primary reanastomosis is required, due to the wide extent of bowel edema and inflammation. In the presence of an abscess, a diverting colostomy or ileostomy should be considered.

Surgical Techniques

1. Once the full extent of the injury has been identified, it is closed with two layers of delayed absorbable suture perpendicular to the long axis of the bowel so the lumen is not constricted. The first layer incorporates the mucosa and muscularis and may be run or interrupted (Figure 15-5). Next, the seromuscular layer is imbricated over the first layer with interrupted sutures (Figure 15-6).

2. After completing the repair of a rectal or distal sigmoid injury, the sigmoid is cross-clamped with a bowel grasper, the pelvis is filled with irrigating fluid, and air is injected transanally through a proctoscope or large Foley catheter with a 30 cc balloon. An airtight closure is assured if no bubbles appear (Figure 15-7).

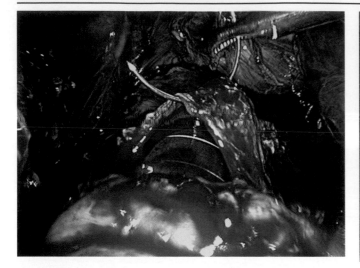

Figure 15-5. Interrupted sutures are placed through the mucosa and muscularis, perpendicular to the long axis of the bowel so as not to constrict the lumen. A rigid sigmoidoscope is in place.

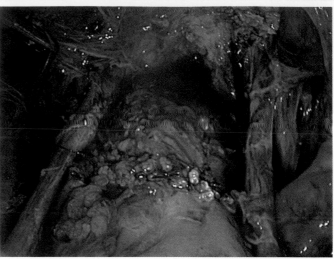

Figure 15-6. A second layer of interrupted sutures to close the serosa has been completed.

Figure 15-7. The pelvis is filled with irrigating fluid and the sigmoid colon is cross-clamped with a bowel grasper to occlude the lumen. Air is inflated through the sigmoidoscope. The presence of bubbles would indicate that the closure is not airtight.

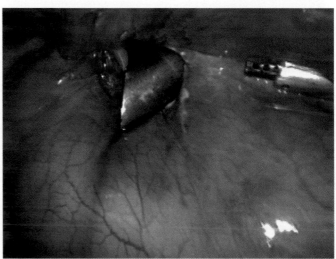

Figure 15-8. In this case, the patient underwent a prior midline laparotomy for a myomectomy and the bladder is adherent high on the abdominal wall. Retrograde filling of the bladder demonstrates a probable perforation from the midline suprapubic trocar.

Urinary Tract Injury

The incidence of damage to the urinary tract is estimated to be 0.02% to 3%, with bladder injuries being more common than ureteral injuries. Approximately a third of these injuries are not identified intraoperatively. Bladder damage was more likely to be found intraoperatively, whereas ureteral injuries were more likely to be missed. In a retrospective analysis of 126 total laparoscopic hysterectomies performed at our institution, the urinary tract injury rate was 4% (95% CI 1.7%–9.0%) with 75% of these injuries (two cystotomies and one ureteral obstruction) detected only with intraoperative cystoscopy.

Bladder Injury

Bladder injuries commonly occur at the time of secondary trocar insertion, especially the suprapubic trocar (Figure 15-8). This can be avoided by continuous bladder drainage with Foley catheter and by placing secondary trocars at least 2 to 3 cm cephalad of the pubic symphysis. Electrothermal compromise of the bladder can also occur during excision of endometriotic implants within the vesicouterine fold or dissection of the bladder flap at the time of laparoscopic hysterectomy. Blood and/or gas in the Foley catheter bag is suspicious for bladder injury. If bladder damage is suspected intraoperatively, retrograde filling of the bladder with indigo carmine, methylene blue, or sterile infant formula can be used to facilitate identification of a cystotomy. Cystoscopy can also be performed.

If not recognized intraoperatively, these patients will often present with hematuria; oliguria; elevated blood urea nitrogen, creatinine, and white blood cell counts; elevated temperatures; and other signs and symptoms of urinary ascites such as abdominal pain, distention with nausea and vomiting, and even peritoneal signs. Imaging modalities such as a cystogram (CT or plain film) can be obtained to demonstrate leakage of contrast from the bladder. During the postoperative evaluation of bladder injury, it is often necessary to eliminate the possibility of isolated or concomitant ureteral injury. Intravenous pyelogram (IVP) can be helpful to assess the integrity of the upper as well as lower urinary tract.

When bladder or ureteral damage is suspected, the decision as to whether or not to consult an urologist or urogynecologist will depend on the experience of the primary surgeon, as will the decision to commence with repair via laparoscopy or laparotomy. Small extraperitoneal injuries to the bladder can be managed with Foley catheter drainage for 5 to 7 days. Intraperitoneal bladder injuries can be repaired in one or two layers using delayed absorbable suture. Care should be taken to make sure that ureteral orifices are not being compromised. Cystoscopy should be performed to assure a watertight seal and demonstrate ureteral patency. If the bladder repair is near the ureteral orifices, retrograde placement of ureteral stents should be performed. As the bladder generally re-epithelializes in 3 to 4 days, an indwelling Foley catheter is placed for continuous bladder drainage for approximately 1 week. Although not always necessary, in complicated cases, a CT or plain film cystogram can be obtained to confirm integrity of repair prior to removing the catheter.

Case 3: Cystotomy

 View DVD: Video 15-1

MM is a 32-year-old nulligravida with pelvic pressure and urinary frequency due to a large myomatous uterus She was recently married and desires future fertility. An ultrasonogram was performed to assess the size, number, and location of the myomas to determine the best route of access for performing the myomectomy. An 8-cm subserosal myoma was noted at the anterior lower uterine segment. A laparoscopic approach was planned. It was necessary to fully displace the bladder off of the lower uterine segment.

After the myoma was removed, retrograde filling of the bladder with dilute indigo carmine through the Foley catheter demonstrated a small cystotomy. This was repaired with a two-layer closure using 2-0 delayed absorbable suture. Retrograde filling showed the closure was watertight. Cystoscopy confirmed that the injury was limited to the dome of the bladder and it was adequately repaired with no compromise of the ureters. The patient was discharged home the following morning with a Foley catheter to keep the bladder decompressed during healing. A cystogram may be performed when the catheter is removed 7 to 10 days later to assure that no leak is present.

Surgical Techniques

1. If a bladder injury is suspected, retrograde filling with dilute indigo carmine through the Foley catheter can help identify the lesion (see Figure 15-9).

2. The bladder is mobilized to facilitate the repair. Cystoscopy will demonstrate the luminal defect and assure that the ureters are not involved (Figure 15-10).

3. The defect is repaired in one or two layers with delayed absorbable suture (Figure 15-11). Permanent sutures are to be avoided because they may lead to calculus formation within the bladder mucosa.

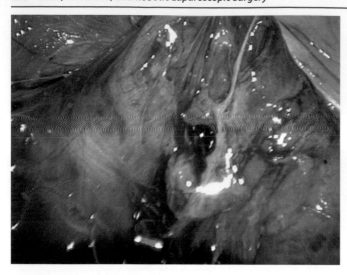

Figure 15-9. The bladder is mobilized from the abdominal wall to better delineate the injury.

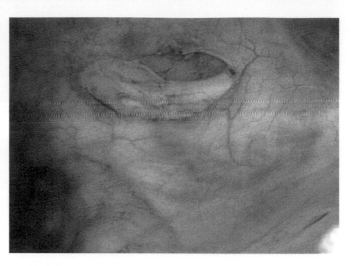

Figure 15-10. Cystoscopy shows the damage is limited to the dome.

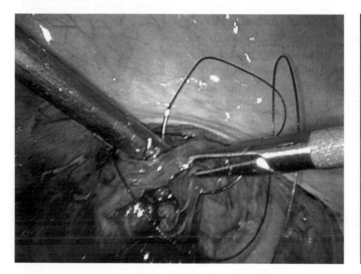

Figure 15-11. This small defect is closed with interrupted sutures through the muscularis. A second imbricating layer may also be performed.

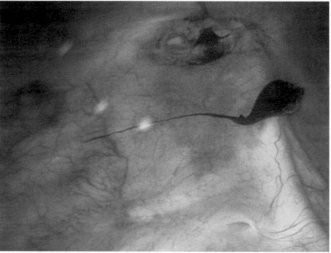

Figure 15-12. Cystoscopy following the repair shows no suture in the bladder and bilateral ureteral patency. Note the ureteral orifice in the lower part of the picture. The patient is discharged with a Foley catheter which will be removed in a week.

4. Cystoscopy is again performed at the completion of the repair to assure that the ureters have not been compromised (Figure 15-12).

(See Video 15-1 📷)

Ureteral Injury

Ureteral injuries are rare in minor laparoscopic cases, but can be as high as 8% in cases of laparoscopic management of malignancy or of benign disease such as endometriosis where the pelvic anatomy is distorted and there is extensive fibrosis within the retroperitoneal space. The most definitive method to avoid ureteral injury is to directly observe and identify the entire course of the ureter within the operative field. It is often necessary to enter the retroperitoneal space and dissect out the pelvic ureter in order to retract it away from the operative field, such as during cases of laparoscopic uterosacral ligament suspension. Ureteral stents are often not helpful for identification or dissection in the face of extensive fibrosis. However, lighted stents may facilitate identification. In order of descending frequency, the ureter is most commonly injured at the pelvic brim where it courses beneath the infundibulopelvic ligament, at the level of the internal cervical os where it passes under the uterine arteries, and at the ureteral canal where it enters the bladder lateral to the vaginal fornices. The most common types of ureteral injuries reported were transection followed by laceration, obstruction, stenosis, fistula formation, and resection/electrothermal trauma. Cystoscopy with administration of intravenous indigo carmine can be performed if damage is suspected intraoperatively. The absence of blue dye effluxing from the ureteral orifices cystoscopically or the presence of blue dye within the peritoneal cavity in the absence of a cystotomy would indicate ureteral injury. Of note, intravenous administration of methylene blue should be cautioned as it may precipitate methemoglobinemia in susceptible patients. If the ureteral injuries are not identified intraoperatively, these patients may have flank pain postoperatively and may present in a similar manner to patients with cystotomies, as outlined earlier. They may also have a serum creatinine increase of greater than or equal to 0.3 mg/dL compared with preoperative values. However, up to 50% of patients with unilateral ureteral obstructions may be asymptomatic. Therefore, because many patients with ureteral injuries will either have nonspecific symptoms or will be asymptomatic, and because many of these injuries are not recognized intraoperatively, imaging modalities such as IVP may assist in postoperative diagnosis. If there is concern for ureteral obstruction, an ultrasonogram may also demonstrate hydronephrosis.

Intraoperative management of ureteral injuries will depend on the expertise of the primary surgeon. In the literature, most ureteral injuries diagnosed postoperatively were repaired via laparotomy, although laparoscopic ureteral anastomosis has also been reported. If there is a small focal ureteral injury without complete transection caused by sharp dissection, some experts have advocated retrograde placement of a ureteral stent to allow for spontaneous healing without the need for reapproximation of the defect. If there is evidence of hydronephrosis, or if the risk of ureteral stenosis is high, such as with ureters that are clamped or ligated, ureteral stents can also be placed after the obstruction has been removed. The ureteral stents are usually left for 2 to 4 weeks, followed by an IVP to confirm ureteral integrity and patency before removal. In contrast, in cases of injury caused by electrosurgery, even without obvious defect, the damaged ureteral portion should be resected and reimplanted or reanastomosed depending upon the location of the injury.

The decision to perform a ureteroureterostomy versus a ureteroneocystostomy ultimately depends upon whether the repair can be performed in a tension-free manner. However, it is important to note that the incidence of ureteral stricture and obstruction is higher after ureteroureterostomy than ureteroneocystostomy. Traditionally, if the injury occurs above the pelvic brim, a ureteroureterostomy is advocated if a ureteroneocystostomy cannot be performed in a tension-free manner. The ureteral ends are spatulated to increase the surface area being sutured. Generally, a one-layer closure is performed with 4-0 absorbable suture. Ureteral stents are placed for 2 to 4 weeks, and IVP is performed before stent removal. Often a Jackson-Pratt drain is placed adjacent to the ureteral repair for drainage of any potential urine leakage within the peritoneal cavity. It can be removed if the drainage is less than approximately 50 mL over 24 hours. A Foley catheter should be maintained as long as the urine remains bloody, and if there is any worry for urinary retention.

If the ureteral injury occurs below the pelvic brim, generally a ureteroneocystostomy is performed in a similar manner as described above for the ureteroureterostomy. If there is not enough ureteral length for a tension-free repair, a psoas hitch can be performed where the bladder is mobilized and secured to the psoas tendon, or a Boari flap can be created where the bladder is elongated. Ureteral stents are placed along with a Jackson-Pratt drain. The postoperative management is similar to after ureteroureterostomy except that a Foley catheter is usually left for the duration of the ureteral stent. In a prospective study of nine patients who underwent laparoscopic ureteroureterostomy, seven subjects experienced successful repairs without further complications. One patient had a mild ureteral stricture which was relieved with transvesical ureteral dilation. The other patient experienced ureteral stricture distal to the anastomotic site, which required a reoperation.

Case 4: Ureteral Transection

 View DVD: Video 15-2

DS is a 16 year old para 2002 who presented with chronic left lower quadrant pain for 18 months, which was worse with physical activity and during her menses. She also complained of continuous spotting throughout the month. She denied associated urinary or GI symptoms. She had a normal endometrial biopsy, and a sonohysterogram demonstrated a complex 2 cm left ovarian cyst. She underwent a laparotomy with lysis of adhesions as well as endometrial ablation for menorrhagia 2 months previously. A left hydrosalpinx with dense adhesions to bowel and pelvic sidewall was noted but not treated. She had a history of pelvic inflammatory disease in the past. Laparoscopic hysterectomy with left salpingo-oophorectomy and lysis of adhesions was planned.

Laparoscopy revealed extensive pelvic adhesive disease. The uterus was approximately 8 weeks size and the right tube and ovary were normal. A left tubo-ovarian complex was densely adherent to the pelvic sidewall. In addition, the left ovary contained an endometrioma. A 5-mm trocar was inserted through the umbilicus and 12-mm trocars were placed under direct visualization cephalad and medial to the anterior superior iliac spine bilaterally. An additional 5 mm trocar was placed along the midclavicular line at the level of the umbilicus on the left side. Extensive lysis of adhesions was performed with blunt and sharp dissection with scissors, and bipolar cautery was used to obtain hemostasis. While attempting to separate the left adnexa from the pelvic sidewall the ureter was completely transected. This was confirmed by giving intravenous indigo carmine with spillage of blue dye into the peritoneal cavity. The remainder of the case was completed by excising the left tubo-ovarian complex and performing the hysterectomy. A urologist then performed a laparoscopic end-to-end ureteral anastomosis over a stent. Cystoscopy was performed at the completion of the case after intravenous administration of indigo carmine was given and bilateral spill was noted from both ureters. A Jackson-Pratt drain was placed near the uretero-ureteral reanastomosis and removed on postoperative day 3 when the patient was discharged. The stent was removed cystoscopically 2 months later.

Surgical Techniques

1. If a ureteral injury is suspected, 5 mL of indigo carmine may be administered intravenously to help identity the site of the lesion (Figure 15-13).

2. The proximal and distal segments need to be fully mobilized so that they can be brought together without tension (Figure 15-14).

3. The transected ends are freshened and spatulated to increase the area for anastomosis (see Figure 15-14).

4. A double-J ureteral stent is inserted into the ureteral orifice cystoscopically. The catheter is then fed into the proximal end and advanced into the renal pelvis (Figure 15-15).

5. The anastomosis is performed with interrupted 4-0 delayed absorbable sutures (Figure 15-16).

6. A Jackson-Pratt drain is placed through one of the lower quadrant ports to detect the presence of intraperitoneal urine (Figure 15-17).

(See Video 15-2)

Port-Site Hernia

Midline ports may be placed at the umbilicus and suprapubically. Port-site hernias at these locations are uncommon. Omental herniation may occur at the umbilical site. It is recommended to close the fascia in midline ports that are greater than 8 mm.

Lateral ports have a far higher incidence of herniation and typically occur with diameters greater than or equal to 10 mm. The fascia of these ports should always be closed, although closing the lateral port sites presents a risk of chronic pain from entrapping the ilioinguinal and iliohypogastric nerves. Hernias may present acutely with a postoperative small bowel obstruction or chronically with a bulge at the site (Figure 15-18). An acute postoperative hernia is a surgical emergency and surgical exploration is necessary.

Figure 15-13. The transected ureter is identified. Intravenous indigo carmine can be seen spilling from the proximal end.

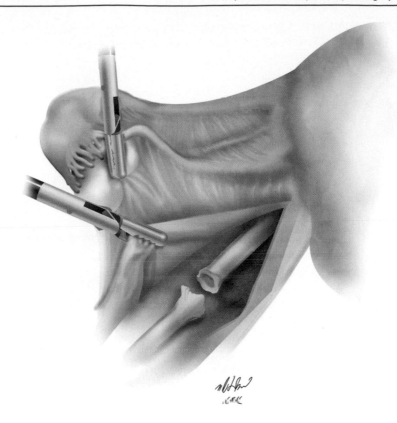

Figure 15-14. The ureter is mobilized throughout the pelvic course and the ends are freshened. They may be spatulated to increase the area for closure.

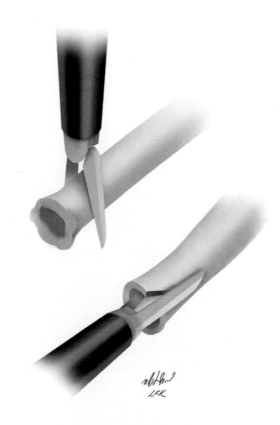

Figure 15-15. A double-J ureteral catheter is placed in retrograde fashion through a cystoscope and then manipulated into the proximal opening and advanced into the renal pelvis.

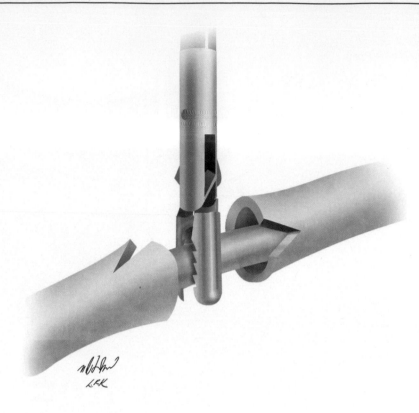

Figure 15-16. The anastomosis is performed with interrupted 4-0 delayed reabsorbable suture using intracorporeal knot-tying.

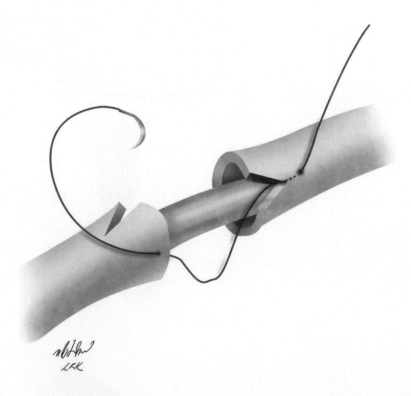

Figure 15-17. The completed repair. A Jackson-Pratt drain may be placed to assure there is no urine leak.

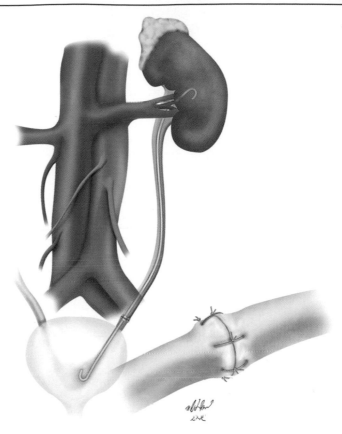

Figure 15-18. Abdominal CT showing a small bowel hernia at the right lower quadrant port site resulting in small bowel obstruction.

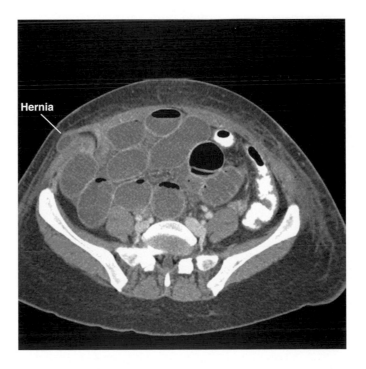

There are different types of trocars. A conventional trocar is pyramidal and cuts into fascia. Radially expanding trocars spread tissue and, in theory, have a decreased incidence of hernia formation. However, most studies are underpowered to detect a difference in hernia rates. It is controversial whether or not to close the fascia of these 10-mm radially expanding trocar ports.

Conclusions

Fortunately, complications of laparoscopic gynecologic surgery are uncommon, with most of the complications occurring at the time of the initial trocar insertion. The complication rates are directly related to the general medical condition of the patient, the complexity of the case, and the extent of anatomic distortion. Most complications are avoidable and/or can be recognized intraoperatively, allowing for immediate correction to avert further potentially severe consequences. Emphasis must be placed on prevention and intraoperative detection of complications.

The key to preventing most neurologic injuries is proper patient positioning with the arms tucked and the legs in low lithotomy with minimal hip flexion, external rotation, and abduction. The stomach should be decompressed with an orogastric tube and an indwelling Foley catheter placed in the bladder prior to trocar insertion. Attention should be paid to anatomic landmarks to reduce vascular and neurologic injuries when inserting the trocars. Placement of the initial trocar in the left upper quadrant should be considered when there is a risk of bowel adhesions to the anterior abdominal wall.

If there is any suspicion of a potential bowel injury, the bowel should be run laparoscopically. Rectal injuries may be diagnosed by proctosigmoidoscopy or by cross-clamping the sigmoid and distending the rectum with air after filling the pelvis with fluid, to check for air bubbles indicating a perforation. Indigo carmine may be given intravenously to detect intraperitoneal spill from a ureteral laceration as well as to document ureteral patency while performing cystoscopy. Cystoscopy can also be performed to check for bladder injury. The bladder may also be filled in retrograde fashion with indigo carmine, methylene blue, or sterile milk to rule out a bladder perforation.

Most laparoscopic complications may be treated immediately by laparoscopy including bladder, ureter, bowel, and minor vascular injuries. Major vascular injuries are still best managed by emergent laparotomy. One of the main advantages of laparoscopic surgery is a rapid postoperative recovery. There should be a high index of suspicion for an unrecognized complication if postoperative pain is getting worse or the patient has any problems with bladder or bowel function.

Suggested Reading

Chapron C, Querleu D, Mage G, et al: Complications of gynecologic laparoscopy: multicentre study of 7604 procedures [in French], *J Gynecol Obstet Biol Reprod* 21:207-213, 1992.

Coleman RL, Muller CY: Effects of a laboratory-based skills curriculum on laparoscopic proficiency: a randomized trial, *Am J Obstet Gynecol* 186:836, 2002.

Harkki-Siren P, Kurki T: A nationwide analysis of laparoscopic complications, *Obstet Gynecol* 89:108-112, 1997.

Jansen FW, Kapiteyn K, Trimbos-Kemper T, Hermans J, Trimbos JB: Complications of laparoscopy: a prospective multicentre observational study, *BJOG* 104:595-600, 1997.

Magrina JF: Complications of laparoscopic surgery, *Clin Obstet Gynecol* 45:469-480, 2002.

Merlin TL, Hiller JE, Maddern GJ, Jamieson GG, Brown AR, Kolbe A: Pneumoperitoneum in laparoscopic surgery, *Br J Surg* 90: 668-679, 2003.

Saidi MH, Vancaillie TG, White AJ, Sadler RK, Akright BD, Farhart SA: Complications of major operative laparoscopy. A review of 452 cases, *J Reprod Med* 41:471-476, 1996.

See WA, Cooper CS, Fisher RJ: Predictors of laparoscopic complications after formal training in laparoscopic surgery, *JAMA* 270:2689, 1993.

Shirk GJ, Johns A, Redwine DB: Complications of laparoscopic surgery: how to avoid them and how to repair them, *J Minim Invasive Gynecol* 13:352, 2006.

Tian YF, Lin YS, Lu CL, Chia CC, Huang KF, Shih TY, Shen KH, Chung MT, Tsai YC, Chao CH, WuShirk MP: Major complications of operative gynecologic laparoscopy in Southern Taiwan: a follow-up study, *J Minim Invasive Gynecol* 14:284-292, 2007.

Anesthetic Complications

Gerges FJ, Kanazi GE, Jabbour-Khoury SI: Anesthesia for laparoscopy: a review, *J Clin Anesth* 18:67-78, 2006.

Goldberg JM, Maurer WG: A randomized comparison of gasless laparoscopy and CO2 pneumoperitoneum, *Obstet Gynecol* 90:416-420, 1997.

Joshi GP: Complications of laparoscopy, *Anesthesiol Clin North Am* 19:89-105, 2001.

Sprung J, Whalley DG, Falcone T, Wilks W, Nvaratil JE, Bourke DL: The effects of tidal volume and respiratory rate on oxygenation and respiratory mechanics during laparoscopy in morbidly obese patients, *Anesth Analg* 97:268-274, 2003.

Neurologic Injury

Barnett JC, Hurd WW, Rogers RM Jr, Williams NL, Shapiro SA: Laparoscopic positioning and nerve injuries, *J Minim Invasive Gynecol* 14:664-672, 2007.

Coppieters MW, Can de Velde M, Stappaerts KH: Positioning in anesthesiology: toward a better understanding of stretch-induced perioperative neuropathies, *Anesthesiology* 97:75-81, 2002.

Irvin W, Andersen W, Taylor P, Rice L: Minimizing the risk of neurologic injury in gynecologic surgery. *Obstet Gynecol* 103:374, 2004.

Romanowski L, Reich H, McGlynn F, Adelson MD, Taylor PJ: Brachial plexus neuropathies after advanced laparoscopic surgery, *Fertil Steril* 60:729-732, 1993.

Warner MA, Martin JT, Schroeder DR, Offord KP, Chute CG: Lower extremity neuropathy associated with surgery carried out on patients in lithotomy position, *Anesthesiology* 81:6-12, 1994.

Warner MA, Warner DO, Harper CM, Schroeder DR, Maxson PM: Lower extremity neuropathies associated with lithotomy positions, *Anesthesiology* 93:938, 2000.

Whiteside JL, Barber MD, Walters MD, Falcone T: Anatomy of ilioinguinal and iliohypogastric nerves in relation to trocar placement and low transverse incisions, *Am J Obstet Gynecol* 189:1574-1578, 2003.

Winfree CJ, Kline DG: Intraoperative positioning nerve injuries, *Surg Neurol* 63:5-18, 2005.

Vascular Injury

Champault G, Cazacu F, Taffinder N: Serious trocar accidents in laparoscopic surgery: a French survey of 103,852 operations, *Surg Laparosc Endosc* 6:367-370, 1996.

Bowel Injury

Bishoff JT, Allaf ME, Kirkels W, et al: Laparoscopic bowel injury: incidence and clinical presentation, *J Urol* 161:887-890, 1999.

Duepree HJ, Senagore AJ, Delaney CP, Marcello PW, Brady KM, Falcone T: Laparoscopic resection of deep pelvic endometriosis with rectosigmoid involvement, *J Am Coll Surg* 195:754-758, 2002.

Nezhat C, de Fazio A, Nicholson T, Nezhat C: Intraoperative sigmoidoscopy in gynecologic surgery, *J Minim Invasive Gynecol* 12:391-395, 2005.

Nezhat CH, Seidman D, Nezhat F, Nezhat CR: The role of intraoperative proctosigmoidoscopy in laparoscopic pelvic surgery, *J Am Assoc Gynecol Laparosc* 11:47-49, 2004.

Urinary Tract Injury

Grainger DA, Soderstrom RM, Schiff SF, et al: Ureteral injuries at laparoscopy: insights into diagnosis, management, and prevention, *Obstet Gynecol* 75.839, 1990.

Jelovsek JE, Chen CCG, Roberts SL, Paraiso MFR, Falcone T: Incidence of lower urinary tract injury and the value of routine intraoperative cystoscopy at the time of total laparoscopic hysterectomy, *JSLS* 11:422-427, 2007.

Nezhat CH, Nezhat F, Seidman D, Nezhat C: Laparoscopic ureteroureterostomy: a prospective follow-up of 9 patients, *Prim Care Update Ob Gyns* 5:200, 1998.

Ostrzenski A, Radolinski B, Ostrzenska K: A review of laparoscopic ureteral injury in pelvic surgery, *Obstet Gynecol Surv* 58:794-799, 2003.

Tamussino KF, Lang PFJ, Breinl E: Ureteral complications with operative gynecologic laparoscopy, *J Urol* 160;2313-2314, 1998.

Tulikangas PK, Gill IS, Falcone T: Laparoscopic repair of ureteral injuries, *J Am Assoc Gynecol Laparosc* 8:259-262, 2001.

Walter AJ, Magtibay PM, Morse AN, et al: Perioperative changes in serum creatinine after gynecologic surgery, *Am J Obstet Gynecol* 186:1315, 2002.

Index